Laboratory Techniques with Reagents and Solutions

The Author

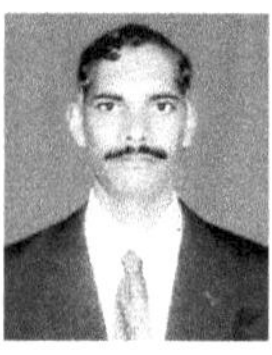

Dr U D Chavan obtained his M.Sc. (Ag) Biochemistry degree from Mahatma Phule Krishi Vidyapeeth, Rahuri in 1987. He received his Ph.D. degree in Food Science from Memorial University of Newfoundland

St. John's Canada in 1999. He has done International training on "Global Nutrition 2002" at Uppsala University Uppsala, Sweden in 2002. He also attended follow-up International workshop on "Global Nutrition 2002" at Hanoi, Vietnam in 2002. Dr. Chavan visited Denmark, Finland, Ireland, France, Switzerland, Poland, Spain, Vietnam, Thailand, England, and U.S.A. under "Global Nutrition 2002" Programme. Dr. Chavan worked as Senior Research Assistant in the Department of Biochemistry and Food Science and Technology at Mahatma Phule Krishi Vidyapeeth Rahuri from 1988 to 2000. During his Ph.D., he worked as Technician/Research Associate at Atlantic Cool Climate Crop Research Center and Agriculture and Agri-Food Canada. He received D.Sc. degree in 2006 from USA. He has guided 22 students for M.Sc. (Agri.) in Biochemistry and Food Science and Technology. From 2000 to 2004 he worked as an Assistant Professor of Biochemistry at Mahatma Phule Krishi Vidyapeeth Rahuri. Now, he is working as a Professor in the Department of Food Science and Technology, Senior Cereal Food Technologist in Sorghum Improvement Project and Foreign Student Advisor at Mahatma Phule Krishi Vidyapeeth, Rahuri, Dist, Ahmednagar, Maharashtra, India.

Laboratory Techniques with Reagents and Solutions

U D Chavan
Professor
Department of Food Science and Technology
Mahatma Phule Krishi Vidyapeeth, Rahuri

2018
Daya Publishing House®
A Division of
Astral International Pvt. Ltd.
New Delhi – 110 002

ISBN 9789388173056 (Int. Edition)

Published by : **Daya Publishing House®**
A Division of
Astral International Pvt. Ltd.
– ISO 9001:2015 Certified Company –
4736/23, Ansari Road, Darya Ganj
New Delhi-110 002
Ph. 011-43549197, 23278134
E-mail: info@astralint.com
Website: www.astralint.com

Digitally Printed at : **Replika Press Pvt. Ltd.**

Preface

There was a great demand from students and research workers for having reagents and solutions book. From last few decades have been a tremendous expansion of knowledge in the field of Science and Technology particularly new research findings. Therefore, a book on **"Laboratory Techniques with Reagents and Solutions"** for Practical and Research Laboratory Purpose is prepared. An important part of working in any laboratory is the proper use and calibration of instruments and equipment, as well as more detailed information about the step-by-step procedures for the specific instruments that you use.

This book contains most suitable procedure of laboratory techniques. It describes the basic laboratory rules, equipment and instrumentation, basic concepts, types of stock standard solutions, equivalent concentration, normality, normal solution, molar solution, molal solution, percent solution, parts per million (ppm), various types of buffer solutions, pH, spectrophotometry, atomic absorption spectrophotometry, chromatography viz. paper chromatography, thin layer chromatography (TLC), gas chromatography (GC), liquid chromatography (LC), gas-liquid chromatography (GLC), high performance liquid chromatography (HPLC), polymerase chain reaction (PCR), scanning electron microscope (SEM), radiation, enzyme assays and radioactivity and related calculations. These equipment and instruments are commonly used in practical laboratory. Important references have been also cited for detailed reading. It is hoped that the book is quite useful for students, teachers, researchers, biochemists, chemist, food chemist and person engaged in various laboratories. Constructive suggestions of students, teachers and researchers are invited for further improvement of this book.

U. D. Chavan

Contents

CHAPTER 1

Introduction

GENERAL PRINCIPLES

In all laboratories all first aids material should be kept ready. All hazards chemicals should be kept in lock and key storage. All students working the laboratory should give guidelines for safety and first aids while any injury during working in the laboratory. Before preparation of all types of solutions students as well as staff should read the content and other information given on the packet or bottles. While preparation of solutions first make the necessary calculations and check with laboratory attendance/teacher/senior staff and then do the necessary solutions. Follow the guidelines given in the practical manual and protocols and take necessary safety precautions while working in the research laboratory. While working in the chemical laboratory wear safety glasses, aprons and hand goose whenever necessary. See the following instructions and act accordingly.

1. BASIC LABORATORY RULES

Safety first, so we have always to get a look at laboratory main rules:

General Rules

1. Do not work with hazardous substances without a second person being present.
2. Do not eat, drink or smoke in the laboratory under any circumstances.
3. Always Keep your working area clean and tidy and free of clutter.
4. Always Keep benches tidy and gangways clear.
5. Always support gas cylinders, and always close cylinder valves after use.
6. Always label containers in plain English with the common known name of the substance and the appropriate hazard warning sign.
7. Always secure the tops of reagent bottles immediately after use.
8. Always work with fume cupboard when dealing with organic solvent or acid or volatile substance.
9. Always clear up spillages immediately.
10. Do not leave equipment using water, gas or electricity on overnight.

Personal Protection Rules

1. Always wear a lab coat and appropriate eye protection, *e.g.* safety spectacles, goggles or face shield.
2. Always use the appropriate gloves whenever handling chemicals or hazardous substances.
3. Always check their integrity before use, ensuring they will give you protection against the substance being used.
4. Always wear proper footwear, do not wear open toed footwear.

Hygiene Rules

1. Do not pipette by mouth.
2. Always wash hands after using any substances hazardous to health, on leaving the laboratory and before visiting the toilet.
3. Do not touch surfaces with your contaminated gloves if they may be touched by others (phones, door handles *etc.*,).

Emergencies Rules

1. Always know where your nearest fire extinguisher and first aid kit are.
2. Always know your emergency escape route and assembly point.

Storage and Disposal Rules

1. Always keep broken glassware and sharps separate from other waste.
2. Always dispose of in the appropriate containers.
3. Always return stock bottles/jars/dewar's etc of highly flammable liquids or acids to their correct store cupboard after work has finished.
4. Do not have more than 500 ml of a flammable solvent in use at any one time on the bench.

2. BASIC EQUIPMENT AND INSTRUMENTATION

There measurements in lab are made using appropriate equipment or instruments. The array of equipment and instrumentation used in analytical chemistry is impressive, ranging from the simple and inexpensive, to the complex and costly. The instrumentation used to measure mass and much of the equipment used to measure volume is important to all analytical techniques and are therefore discussed in this section.

Instrumentation for Measuring Mass

An object's mass is measured using a balance. The most common type of balance is an electronic balance in which the balance pan is placed over an electromagnet. The sample to be weighed is placed on the sample pan, displacing the pan downward by a force equal to the product of the sample's mass and the acceleration due to gravity. The balance detects this downward movement and generates a counterbalancing force using an electromagnet. The current needed to produce this force is proportional to the object's mass. A typical electronic balance has a capacity of 100–200 g and can measure mass to the nearest ± 0.01 to ± 1 mg. Another type of balance is the single-pan, unequal arm balance. In this mechanical balance the balance pan and a set of removable standard weights on one side of a beam are balanced against a fixed counterweight on the beam's other side. The beam itself is balanced on a fulcrum consisting of a sharp knife edge. Adding a sample to the balance pan tilts the beam away from its balance point. Selected standard weights are then removed until the beam is brought back into balance. The combined mass of the removed weights equals the sample's mass. The capacities and measurement limits of these balances are comparable to an electronic balance.

The mass of a sample is determined by difference. If the material being weighed is not moisture-sensitive, a clean and dry container is placed on the balance. The mass of this container is called the tare. Most balances allow the tare to be automatically adjusted to read a mass of zero. The sample is then transferred to the container, the new mass is measured and the sample's mass determined by subtracting the tare. Samples that absorb moisture from the air are weighed differently. The sample is placed in a covered weighing bottle and their combined mass is determined. A portion of the sample is removed, and the weighing bottle and remaining sample are reweighed. The difference between the two masses gives the mass of the transferred sample.

Several important precautions help to minimize errors in measuring an object's mass. Balances should be placed on heavy surfaces to minimize the effect of vibrations in the surrounding environment and should be maintained in a level position. Analytical balances are sensitive enough that they can measure the mass of a fingerprint. For this reason, materials placed on a balance should normally be handled using tongs or laboratory tissues. Volatile liquid samples should be weighed in a covered container to avoid the loss of sample by evaporation. Air currents can significantly affect a sample's mass. To avoid air currents, the balance's glass doors should be closed, or the balance's wind shield should be in place. A sample that is cooler or warmer than the surrounding air will create convective air currents that adversely affect the measurement of its mass. Finally, samples dried in an oven should be stored in desiccators to prevent them from reabsorbing moisture from the atmosphere.

Equipment for Measuring Volume

Analytical chemists use a variety of glassware to measure volume. The type of glassware used depends on how exact the volume needs to be. Beakers, dropping pipettes, and graduated cylinders are used to measure volumes approximately, typically with errors of several percept. Pipettes and volumetric flasks provide a more accurate means for measuring volume. When filled to its calibration mark, a volumetric flask is designed to contain a specified volume of solution at a stated temperature, usually 20 °C. The actual volume contained by the volumetric flask is usually within 0.03–0.2% of the stated value. Volumetric flasks containing less than 100 mL generally measure volumes to the hundredth of a milliliter, whereas larger volumetric flasks measure volumes to the tenth of a milliliter. For example, a 10-mL volumetric flask contains 10.00 mL, but a 250-mL volumetric flask holds 250.0 mL (this is important when keeping track of significant figures).

Because a volumetric flask contains a solution, it is useful in preparing solutions with exact concentrations. The reagent is transferred to the volumetric flask, and enough solvent is added to dissolve the reagent. After the reagent is dissolved, additional solvent is added in several portions, mixing the solution after each addition. The final adjustment of volume to the flask's calibration mark is made using a dropping pipette. To complete the mixing process, the volumetric flask should be inverted at least ten times.

A pipette is used to deliver a specified volume of solution. Several different styles of pipettes are available. Transfer pipettes provide the most accurate means for delivering a known volume of solution; their volume error is similar to that from an equivalent volumetric flask. A 250-mL transfer pipette, for instance, will deliver 250.0 mL. To fill a transfer pipette, suction from a rubber bulb is used to pull the liquid up past the calibration mark (never use your mouth to suck a solution into a pipette). After replacing the bulb with your finger, the liquid's level is adjusted to the calibration mark, and the outside of the pipette is wiped dry. The pipette's contents are allowed to drain into the receiving container with the tip of the pipette touching the container walls. A small portion of the liquid remains in the pipette's tip and should not be blown out. Measuring pipettes are used to deliver variable volumes, but with less accuracy than transfer pipettes. With some measuring pipettes, delivery of the calibrated volume requires that any solution remaining in the tip be blown out. Digital pipettes and syringes can be used to deliver volumes as small as a microliter.

Three important precautions are needed when working with pipettes and volumetric flasks. First, the volume delivered by a pipette or contained by a volumetric flask assumes that the glassware is clean. Dirt and grease on the inner glass surface prevents liquids from draining evenly, leaving droplets of the liquid on the container's walls. For a pipette this means that the delivered volume is less than the calibrated volume, whereas drops of liquid above the calibration mark mean that a volumetric flask contains more than its calibrated volume. Commercially available cleaning solutions can be used to clean pipettes and volumetric flasks.

Second, when filling a pipette or volumetric flask, set the liquid's level exactly at the calibration mark. The liquid's top surface is curved into a meniscus, the bottom of which should be exactly even with the glassware's calibration mark. The meniscus should be adjusted with the calibration mark at eye level to avoid parallax errors. If your eye level is above the calibration mark the pipette or volumetric flask will be overfilled. The pipette or volumetric flask will be under filled if your eye level is below the calibration mark.

Finally, before using a pipette or volumetric flask you should rinse it with several small portions of the solution whose volume is being measured. This ensures that any residual liquid remaining in the pipette or volumetric flask is removed.

WORKING SAFELY

Hazard

A hazard is defined as the potential of a substance to cause harm. Hazards are a property of a substance and cannot be reduced (see 'Hazard Warning Signs' for the common hazards).

Risk

Risk is how likely that a substance will be harmful under the conditions it is used. Risks can be reduced by using smaller amounts of chemicals and taking precautions such as containment in fume hoods.

Risk Assessment

An effective risk assessment will take into account the hazards involved, who will be at risk, the steps needed to minimise risks and the safe means of disposal of the substances used.

Basic Laboratory Rules

Here are a few simple rules that form the basis of good, safe lab practice. There might be particular procedures however that requires special rules. For this reason it is vital to read any scripts thoroughly and to seek the advice of demonstrators / lab - supervisors.

Always do this things	**Never do this things**
Wear Safety Glasses	Work Alone or Unsupervised
Wear a Buttoned Up Lab Coat	Eat or Drink in the Laboratory
Tie Back Long Hair	Touch, Sniff or Taste Chemicals
Wear Gloves if Necessary	Wear Open Toed Shoes or Sandals in the Laboratory
Be Aware of the Risks and Hazards Involved in Any Experiment	Pipette Liquids By Mouth
Use a Fume Cupboard if Necessary	Dispose of Hazardous Materials Down the Drain
Minimise Risks By Working Tidily	Return Unused Chemicals to Their Containers
Clear Up Spillages Immediately	
Clear Up at the End of a Practical	

FOR SAFELY HANDLING CHEMICALS

Harmful and Toxic Chemicals

The difference between a harmful chemical and a toxic one is a matter of degree; chemicals which are particularly harmful being classified as toxic. Harmful and toxic chemicals must always be handled in a fume cupboard with the glass front pulled down as far as is practicable to ensure that a good air-flow. It is also essential to wear protective gloves and take particular note of any special instructions about disposal and what to do in case of spillage.

Examples of harmful and toxic materials are aniline, bromine, chloroform, methanol and cyanide salts.

Flammable Chemicals

Many solvents and reagents used in the laboratory are highly flammable and so there should never be naked flames in places where they are being used. The heating of flammable materials should be carried out using water baths, heating mantles or hot plates.

Examples of highly flammable solvents are diethyl ether, petroleum ether, toluene, acetone (propanone) and ethyl acetate (ethylethanoate).

Corrosive Chemicals

The most commonly encountered corrosive materials are acids and alkalis although many other types of chemical fall into this category. It is essential to wear appropriate protective gloves when handling corrosive material and if there is contact with the skin it should be washed off immediately with plenty of water. It may also be necessary to seek medical attention.

Examples of corrosive materials are the mineral acids (hydrochloric, nitric, sulphuric and phoshoric acids), strong alkalis such as sodium hydroxide and potassium hydroxide.

Oxidising Agents

Oxidising agents are dangerous because they can cause fires if they make contact with any combustable material, particularly if they are disposed of carelessly.

Examples of oxidising agents are potassium dichromate (VI), potassium manganate (VII), concentrated nitric acid as well as hydrogen peroxide.

Explosive Reagents

Many substances are explosion hazards because of their extreme reactivity with water. Other compounds are explosive because they are unstable, particularly if heated or when dry. When handling such chemicals it is essential to use only small amounts and protect yourself with a face mask and a safety screen.

Examples of explosion hazards are the alkali metals sodium and potassium.

Irritants

Chemicals which can irritate the eyes and or the skin should always be handled in fume cupboards.

Examples of irritants are acid chlorides, thionyl chloride as well as certain chloro compounds.

HANDLING GLASSWARE SAFELY

Careless use of glassware in the laboratory can cause many minor accidents all of which can be avoided by observing a few simple rules. If mishaps do occur always place broken glassware in the glass bins.

Hazard Warning Signs

Hazard

Always make yourself aware of the hazards associated with the chemicals involved in a practical before you even start. Here are the most common hazard symbols that all chemical containers must display. If you ever come across a chemical you do not know the hazard of you must assume that is very hazardous until you find otherwise.

Personal Protection

Proper protective clothing must be worn at all times in the chemistry laboratory to prevent contact of harmful material with the body.

WORKING SAFELY

The chemistry laboratory is full of potential hazards and dangers and it is your responsibility to work safely for your own wellbeing as well as that of others. This section covers basic rules and procedures that should be followed to reduce any risks to a minimum.

3. LAB TECHNIQUES

Good practical technique is essential for a successful and safe outcome of any experiment. This section sets out to illustrate how to assemble the apparatus, use animations to illustrate the science behind the techniques as well as provide instructional videos for the most common techniques likely to be encountered in a chemistry laboratory.

Assemble Apparatus

There are many different ways to assemble apparatus and it is important that you carefully follow the guidelines that might be in the practical script. This section illustrates the basic principles and good practice involved in putting together equipment.

CHROMATOGRAPHY

Chromatography is a versatile technique used to separate compounds in a mixture. It relies on differences in interaction of molecules with a solvent system (the mobile phase) and a solid or gel known as the stationary phase. There are two main types of chromatography carried out in the lab; Thin Layer Chromatography (TLC) and Column Chromatography.

Thin Layer Chromatography

The technique of Thin Layer Chromatography (TLC) is normally used as an analytical method to follow the progress of a reaction, to analyse mixtures or to establish conditions for a preparative separation of compounds using column chromatography. The stationary phase (often silica) is coated on plastic or aluminium plates. The mixture is spotted on the plate and solvent is allowed to run up the plate and separate the compounds.

Column Chromatography

The separation of mixtures produced in reactions is often carried out by supporting the stationary phase in a column and allowing the solvent to move the mixtures through whilst collecting fractions of the emerging solvent. This can be carried out by allowing the solvent to flow under gravity or under a moderate pressure to increase the solvent flow rate ('Flash Chromatography'). The fractions are usually analysed by TLC in order to identify which contain the components of the mixture.

COOLING

There are many instances where you will need cooling as part of the procedure, for example in recrystallization, carrying out reactions at low temperatures, controlling exothermic reactions as well as in vapour traps.

DEAN-STARK APPARATUS

There are many equilibrium reactions that yield water as a co-product where removal of the water as it is produced is necessary to drive the reaction to completion and this is done using a Dean - Stark apparatus. The reaction is carried out under reflux in a solvent which is less dense than water, both immiscible with it and forms an azeotrope. The apparatus allows the water to be separated from the condensed azeotrope preventing it from returning to the reaction mixture.

DISTILLATION

Distillation separates liquids on the basis of them having different boiling points. Simple Distillation is a technique used to purify a liquid.

Vacuum Distillation is a distillation carried out at reduced pressure to lower boiling points. Fractional Distillation is used to separate compounds with boiling points that are close. The extraction of a crude mixture containing water-insoluble material (such as natural products) can be achieved by the co-distillation with steam. A technique to remove a volatile product from a reaction mixture to prevent further reaction taking place.

Drying Liquids

There are many instances when it is necessary to remove traces of water from a solution or liquid. One common example is the drying of an organic layer after a solvent extraction. The technique involves adding a suitable solid drying agent to the liquid followed by its removal by gravity filtration.

Filtration

Filtration is commonly carried out to separate a solid from a liquid. If the solid is to be discarded (such as in the removal of insoluble impurities) it is done by gravity filtration. If the solid is to be collected it is done under a reduced pressure using a Buchner Funnel and Buchner Flask.

This is the simplest kind of filtration when the solution to be filtered is poured through a filter paper in a filter funnel. The filtration of hot solutions through a heated funnel and fluted filter paper is often carried out as part of a recrystallization. Gravity filtration is generally carried out to remove impurities rather than to isolate solids.

When a solid needs to be isolated from a solution it is normally done at a reduced pressure using a Buchner flask and Buchner funnel.

Heating

There are many instances when heat is needed in a laboratory practical, it is needed to reflux reaction mixtures, to distil liquids as well as help to dissolve solids in recrystallizations. The use of the appropriate method of heating is most important.

IR SPECTROSCOPY

Infra-Red (IR) spectroscopy is a technique which reveals the bonds present in a compound and therefore can be used to identify functional groups. A sample of reaction product can be analysed to confirm its composition by comparison to a pure sample, or to judge the extent of reaction by comparison with the starting material.

Measuring Melting Points

The measurement of melting points is a relatively straightforward procedure that is carried out to determine the purity of a compound or to assist with its identification. A pure compound will melt over a relatively narrow temperature range, impurities both lowering temperature and widening the range over which it melts. The apparatus used to measure melting points can be simple oil baths to 'hot-stage' apparatus where the melting process is observed with the aid of a microscope. In each case the range of temperatures a compound melts is recorded and compared with known data.

Recrystallization

Recrystallization is a means of purifying solids. If carried out correctly the final product will be both of a high yield as well as pure.

Reflux

The term 'reflux' describes an arrangement when a reaction is carried out in a boiling solvent with the vapour being condensed and returned to the reaction vessel. Refluxing is carried out when reactions need to be heated to give a reasonable yield of product in a reasonable time.

The reactants are dissolved in a suitable solvent in a flask fitted with a condenser. Heat is supplied via a heating mantle or an oil bath fitted with a stirrer.

Rotary Evaporation

A reactant is added to the refluxing reaction mixture in a controlled way via an addition funnel. This can be done to prevent exothermic reactions getting out of control.

A rotary evaporator is used to remove large amounts of solvent from solutions at a reduced pressure. This is often done to isolate a product from a chromatographic separation or a solvent extraction.

Solvent Extraction

This technique uses two solvents which are immiscible, for example an organic solvent such as dichloromethane can be used to extract an organic compound from an aqueous solution leaving water soluble impurities behind. A variation of this is acid - base extraction where acidic or basic compounds are extracted out of organic solutions using basic or acidic aqueous solutions.

Soxhlet Extraction

When a compound of low solubility needs to be extracted from a solid mixture a Soxhlet exatraction can be carried out. The technique places a specialised piece of glassware in-between a flask and a condenser. The refluxing solvent repeatedly washes the solid extracting the desired compound into the flask.

Volumetric Analysis

The technique of volumetric analysis uses the reaction between solutions of known concentration with a solution of unknown concentration. The most common reactions are between acids and bases although many other reactions can be used as the basis of a volumetric method.

A standard solution is a solution of accurately known concentration prepared from a primary standard (a compound which is stable, of high purity, highly soluble in water and of a high molar mass to allow for accurate weighing) that is weighed accurately and made up to a fixed volume.

The addition of one reagent (the titrant) from a burette to another reagent until and end-point is reached is known as a titration. These have to be done with great care and precision to establish reliable and accurate results.

Some reactions used in volumetric analysis are self-indicating because the reaction uses strongly coloured reactants (for example manganite (VII) titrations). In the case of acid - base titrations an indicator is needed to visualise the end-point. The correct choice of indicator is essential to get a distinct end-point. The indicator must undergo a complete colour change within the pH change at the equivalence point.

Weighing

Weighing is done to ensure the correct amount of a reactant is added to a reaction, for the preparation of standard solutions or the weighing of a product to calculate a yield. There is also a branch of analytical chemistry called 'Gravimetric Analysis' where precipitates are accurately weighed as a means to determine concentrations.

4. LAB APPRATUS

This section shows the standard pieces of equipment found in most university chemistry laboratories.

Addition Funnels

Addition funnels (or dropping funnels) are used to add reagents to reactions. Self-equalising dropping funnels are used stoppered to add reagents that might be air sensitive, or for the addition of reagents under reduced pressure.

Balances

The most commonly encountered balance is a general purpose top-pan balance which will be able to weigh to the nearest 0.01g. For more accurate work an analytical balance must be used. This balance has many similarities with the simple top-ban balance but it can weigh to the nearest 0.0001g. The doors of the balance must be closed before taking a reading to prevent any disturbances in the air effecting the measurement.

Column Chromatography

Column chromatography is a technique used for the separation of mixtures. Chromatography columns are designed to be filled with a 'stationary phase' (usually silica gel) and the mixture to be separated is passed through the column with a solvent system. A simple column has to be plugged with a small amount of glass wool to retain the stationary phase, whereas this is unnecessary in a column fitted with a sintered glass support.

Condensers

Water cooled condensers are the ones encountered most commonly. The double surfaced condenser and the coiled condenser are the most efficient and are often used for reflux of solvents with low boiling points. For solvents with boiling points in excess of 150 °C an air condenser should be used. The dry ice condenser is designed for use with dry ice/acetone mixtures or even liquid nitrogen as the coolant.

Dean-Stark Apparatus

The Dean-Stark apparatus is designed to collect water produced in synthetic reactions carried out under reflux. The reactions are normally done in solvents (for example toluene) that remove water formed in a reaction as an azeotrope. The condensed mixture of toluene and water collects in the burette and the denser water separates and falls to the bottom. The tap allows the water to be removed.

Desiccators

Desiccators are used to dry solids and keep them dry by containing them in a sealed vessel containing a drying agent. A vacuum desiccator has a tap, usually on the lid which allows the desiccator to be evacuated to speed up the drying process.

Distillation Receivers

Receiver adapters are used to allow collection of distillates emerging from a condenser. The simple receiver adapter can be used to direct the distillate into a conical flask. The jointed adapter would be used with a round bottomed flask, the vented side arm preventing a closed system which would otherwise form an explosion hazard. Adapter is designed for vacuum distillations. The 'pig' adapter allows collection of three different fractions without interrupting the distillation. The receiving flask can be swapped by rotating the 'pig' about its joint.

Filtration

For straightforward filtrations where only the filtrate is required (e.g. removing unwanted solids or decolourising charcoal) a filter funnel and fluted filter paper is used. In situations where the solid is required, a Buchner flask is fitted with a

Buchner funnel using a Buchner collar to form a good seal when under suction. Flat filter paper of the appropriate diameter is used in the Buchner funnel.

Flasks

Round bottomed flasks are generally used for reactions carried out under reflux. Twin necked flasks and three necked flasks allow the fitting of other jointed glassware such as dropping funnels and stirrers. Pear shaped flasks are the best choice for distillations, their shape allowing more of the product to be distilled. The twin necked flask can be used to add a reagent whilst the product is being removed by distillation.

Fraction Column

There are several types of fractionating column but the most common is the Vigreux column which has indentations designed to force condensing liquid into the rising vapour. This is necessary to achieve the equilibrium needed for efficient fractionation. The Vigreux column is often incorporated into a still head. Alternative columns are packed with glass beads or open columns.

Lab Jack

A 'Lab Jack' is an adjustable platform that can be used to raise or lower apparatus by turning the knob at the front. It is particularly useful for the raising and lowering of heat sources (*e.g.* heating mantles) in distillations.

Manometers

A manometer is designed to measure the pressure during a reduced pressure (vacuum) distillation. The Anschutz manometer gives a continuous reading of the pressure throughout the distillation, most often in combination with water pumps. The Vacustat manometer gives a very accurate 'snap shot' reading of the vacuum at a particular point and is usually restricted for use with rotary oil pumps.

Melting Point Apparatus

The simplest method of measuring a melting point is by use of an oil bath. A round bottomed flask is partly filled with a mineral oil and the capillary tube containing the sample is attached to a thermometer with a rubber band. The oil is carefully heated with a micro burner. The heated block apparatus can be found in many shapes and sizes but the principle is the same; the sample is heated placed in an electrically heated block and the observations are made through a magnified port. The 'hot-stage' apparatus allows the observer to look at the sample through a microscope while its temperature is increased.

Pipettes

Graduated pipettes are designed for adding approximate volumes of solutions or reagents. Some pipettes are graduated so that the 0 reading is at the top. These can be filled up to the 0 mark and the appropriate volume added. Others have the full volume at the top. These can be used by drawing the correct volume into the pipette and then allowing it to discharge its contents. Volumetric (bulb) pipettes are designed for accurate work and the volume will be printed or etched onto the pipette body. Pasteur pipettes are used for the transfer or addition of small amounts of liquids. These have no volume markings.

Rotary Evaporators

Rotary (film) evaporators are used to remove large volumes of solvent from solutions by rotating the solution under vacuum in combination with a water bath (optional).

Separating Funnels

Separating funnels are used to separate immiscible solvents such as water from organic solvents and are most commonly used in solvent extraction. Their tapered shapes allows for efficient separation of the two layers. There are two types of funnel, those fitted with a ground glass tap and those with a PTFE (Rota flow) screw type tap.

Soxhlet Apparatus

A Soxhlet extractor is a piece of apparatus designed to extract substances with a low solubility in the extracting solvent. It does this by allowing condensed solvent to wash through a paper thimble placed in the extractor which is designed to return the washings to the boiling flask by siphon action.

Still Heads

Still heads are designed to connect a flask to a condenser in distillations. The simplest allows a thermometer to be attached to follow the temperature of the distillate. The Claisen still head has an additional socket to allow a dropping funnel or mechanical stirrer to be fitted. The splash head is used to prevent the 'raw' distilling liquid from carrying over into the vapour. This type of still head is often used in steam distillations.

Stopper and Adapters

1. Ground glass stopper.
2. Screw capped adapter, used for thermometers or air bleeds in vacuum distillations.

3. Gas inlet adapter, used to allow delivery of a gas (e.g. a protective layer of nitrogen) to a reaction.
4. Step down adapter, used to connect ground glass joints of different diameters.
5. Step up adapter, used to connect ground glass joints of different diameters.
6. Guard tube, when filled with a drying agent, such as calcium chloride, it can be used to protect reactions from moisture.

Volumetric Apparatus

1. Volumetric flask, used to prepare accurately diluted solutions.
2. Analytical pipette, used to deliver an accurate volume (aliquot) of solution.
3. Pipette filler.
4. Burette (black graduations), used for titrations where the solution is clear or of a pale colour.
5. Burette (white graduations), used for titrations with dark, highly coloured solutions.

Common Conversions

Converting from one unit to a different one can cause all kinds of problems if it is not done correctly. Here is some of the most common conversion that is often necessary.

Mass Conversions

$$\text{microgram } (\mu g) \underset{\times 1000}{\overset{\div 1000}{\rightleftarrows}} \text{milligram (mg)} \underset{\times 1000}{\overset{\div 1000}{\rightleftarrows}} \text{gram (g)} \underset{\times 1000}{\overset{\div 1000}{\rightleftarrows}} \text{kilogram (kg)}$$

Volume Conversions

$$cm^3 \underset{\times 1000}{\overset{\div 1000}{\rightleftarrows}} dm^3 \underset{\times 1000}{\overset{\div 1000}{\rightleftarrows}} m^3$$

Temperature Conversions

$$^{o}C \underset{-273}{\overset{+273}{\rightleftarrows}} K$$

Physical Constants

The use of physical constants will be inevitable in practical write - ups where calculations are required. Here are some of the more common ones.

Item	Symbol	Value
Avogadro Constant	L, N_A	6.022×10^{23} mol^{-21}
Molar Gas Constant	R	8.314 J K^{-1} mol^{-1}
Faraday Constant	F	9.649×10^4 C mol^{-1}
Molar Volume of an Ideal Gas at 100kPa and 273K	V_M	22.7 dm^3
Atomic Mass Unit	a.m.u.	1.661×10^{-27} kg

Terminology Generally used in the Laboratory

Terminology	Meaning / words explanations
Accuracy	The 'closeness' of a measurement to the true value.
Acetic Acid	The trivial name for ethanoic acid.
Acetone	The trivial name for propanone.
Acid Wash	A technique where a dilute solution of acid is used to extract basic compounds out of an organic solution using a separating funnel.
Aliquot	A portion of solution, usually measured with a volumetric pipette.
Analyte	A substance that is determined in a quantitative procedure such as volumetric analysis.
Anti - Bumping Granule	Small pieces of a ceramic material that are added to solutions to prevent the solution 'bumping'.
Aqueous Wash	A technique where water is used to extract ionic impurities out of an organic solution using a separating funnel.
Aspirator	Also known as a filter pump, a device that produces a vacuum (reduced pressure) using a flow of tap water. This can be used in Buchner filtrations, vacuum distillations or with rotary evaporators.
Azeotrope	A mixture of two or more liquids that cannot be separated by simple distillation. An application of this is the addition of a second solvent to a solution to produce a lower boiling zoetrope of the two solvents which is easier to remove by evaporation.
B sizes	Sizes of ground glass joints which are usually printed on the joints of 'Quickfit' apparatus.
Boiling Stick	A thin stick of wood added to solutions to prevent 'bumping' (see also).
Buchner Flask	A thickened glass conical flask with a side arm for connection to a water pump. Used for reduced pressure filtration in conjunction with a Buchner funnel (see below).

Terminology	Meaning / words explanations
Buchner Funnel	A ceramic funnel used in conjunction with flat filter papers for collecting solids under reduced pressure.
Bumping	A term used to describe the sudden uncontrollable boiling of a solution which shoots hot liquid out of a container. This is prevented by using anti-bumping granules, a magnetic stirrer or a boiling stick.
Calibration (Thermometers)	To ensure accurate temperature readings (for example when measuring melting points) thermometers are often calibrated by measurement of melting points of pure compounds. A graph of measured melting points against actual ones. Can then be used to correct the thermometer.
Capillary (Tubes)	Thin walled tubes of a small diameter. These can be sealed at one end for use in melting point determinations or they can be 'drawn out' to make micropipettes for spotting TLC plates.
Chromophore	A group which will absorb radiation in the visible or UV spectrum. Compounds containing chromophores can be visualised on developed TLC plates under UV light providing the plate has been pre-treated with a suitable fluorescing agent.
Clear	A liquid that is free of any solids or suspended material. A clear solution may be coloured.
Colourless	Any material that has no colour (as opposed to white).
Decant	Pouring a liquid away from a solid residue.
Decolourising	The removal of coloured impurities from a solution by heating with a small amount of decolourising charcoal followed by filtration.
Desiccant	Another word for drying agent.
Develop	The rise of a solvent up a TLC plate.
Distillate	The liquid that is collected from a distillation.
Drop wise	Addition of a solution or liquid at a very slow (drop-by-drop) rate to ensure accuracy (as in titrations) or to prevent unctrollable reactions.
Drying Agent	A solid material (for example an anhydrous salt) that is used to remove moisture from solvents or in desiccators or guard tubes.
Drying Over	Removal of moisture from organic solvents by adding anhydrous salts (such as sodium sulphate) followed their removal by filtration.
Effervescence	Bubbling by the liberation of a gas (for example when acid is added to a carbonate solution).

Contd...

Terminology	Meaning / words explanations
End Point	The point in which a titration results in a colour change and where the titre is recorded.
Equivalence Point	When the correct (stoichiometric) amount has been added in a titration. This is not the same as the end point but if the titration is carried out properly and a suitable indicator is used the end point will be an accurate reflection of the equivalence point.
Eluate	The solvent that emerges from the column in a chromatographic separation.
Eluent	The solvent used in a chromatographic separation.
Elute	Literally means 'to wash' and it is the term used to describe the passage of solvent through the stationary phase in chromatography.
Erlenmeyer Flask	An alternative name for a conical flask.
Ether	The trivial name for diethyl ether.
Ethyl Acetate	The trivial name for ethyl ethanoate.
Extract (verb)	The action of removing a compound from a solution by shaking with an immiscible solvent.
Extract (noun)	The separated immiscible liquid that has been used to extract a compound from a solution.
Extrapolation	The process of constructing new data points beyond measured points, for example by extending a line of best fit beyond the plotted points.
Filtrate	The filtered liquid that has passed through a filter.
Finely Divided	Any solid material that is of a small particle size and therefore a large surface area.
Flash Chromatography	A form of column chromatography that uses a smaller size of absorbent material for the stationary phase and is therefore capable of separating compounds with closer Retention Factors (see also) than gravity chromatography. Flash chromatography is carried out with pressurised solvent to increase the flow rate.
Flea	An alternative name for a magnetic follower.
Fluted (Filter Paper)	Filter paper that has been folded in a way to allow the filtrate to pass through quickly.
Follower (Magnetic)	A plastic (often Teflon) coated magnet that is used to stir liquids on stirrer hot plates.
Forerun	The lower boiling material in a distillation.

Terminology	Meaning / words explanations
Gas Liquid Chromatography (GLC)	A form of analytical chromatography where compounds are carried in a stream of gas through a column which contains a non-volatile liquid either on the walls of the column or on the surface of a finely divided solid.
Gravimetric (Analysis)	A form of analysis where a reagent is used to form a precipitate which is in turn weighed accurately.
Gravity Chromatography	A form of chromatography where the solvent is allowed to drain through the solid phase under gravity.
Gravity Filtration	The simplest form of filtration where the filtrate is allowed to run through a filter under the influence of gravity.
High Performance Liquid Chromatography (HPLC)	A form of analytical or preparative chromatography where the mobile phase is forced through a chromatography column under high pressure.
Hirsch Funnel	A ceramic funnel with a perforated plate onto which flat filter paper is placed for the purpose of a reduced pressure filtration. A Hirsch funnel is similar to a Buchner funnel but smaller.
Hygroscopic	Readily absorbs moisture from the air.
	A form of analytical or preparative chromatography where the mobile phase is forced through a chromatography column under high pressure.
Immiscible (liquids)	Liquids that will not dissolve in each other
Interpolation	The construction of data points in-between those that have been measured.
Joint Clips	Plastic clips that are used to secure jointed glassware ('Quick fit') together.
Keck Clip	A trade name for joint clips.
Manometer	A device used to measure pressure in reduced pressure distillations.
Micro (Bunsen) Burner	A small burner which is used to heat test tubes and boiling tubes.
Micropipette	Used to spot TLC plates.
Mobile Phase	The solvent that is used in a chromatographic separation (see also Eluent).
Molality	A concentration term expressed as mole per kilogram of solution.
Molarity	A concentration term expressed as mole per cubic decimeter.
Mull	A paste of a finely ground solid sample in Nujol (a paraffin oil) used as a sample in Infra-Red spectroscopy.

Contd...

Terminology	Meaning / words explanations
Nujol	A paraffin oil used to disperse solid samples prior to Infra-Red spectroscopy (see also Mull).
Nucleation	The process by which crystal growth from a solution takes place. This can be aided by scratching the inside of the flask with a spatula or by adding a rough surface such as a single anti-bumping granule.
'Oil Out '	When oil, instead of a crystalline solid is produced in a recrystallization process.
Partition	The equilibrium that takes place when a compound dissolves in a pair of immiscible liquids.
Partition Coefficient	The ratio of concentrations of a compound when it is partitioned between two immiscible liquids.
'Pig'	A type of receiver adapter used in distillations which allows several flasks to be attached.
Precision	The closeness of repeated measurements (not to be confused with accuracy).
Primary Standard	A compound that is use to make up standard solutions (such as in volumetric analysis) which is; 1. Obtainable in a highly pure form. 2. Of a high molar mass to help the accuracy of weighing. 3. Should not be hygroscopic (see also). 4. Readily soluble in in an appropriate solvent. 5. Should react rapidly with the substance it is analysing in stoichiometric (see also) amounts.
Qualitative	The determination of the presence of a specific species.
Quantitative	The determination of the amount of specific species.
'Quick fit'	The trade name given to interchangeable jointed glassware.
Reflux	The heating of a reaction (in a suitable solvent) in a flask fitted with a condenser so that evaporated solvent is returned to the flask.
Residue	The proportion of material that remains in the boiling flask after a distillation is completed.
Retention Factor (R_f)	A measurement of how far a compound has moved up a thin layer chromatography plate. It is calculated by dividing the distance the compound has moved by the distance the solvent has moved and so has a value between 0 and 1.
'Rotoflow' Tap	Often fitted to separating and addition funnels and is made up of a plastic tap which screws into a glass thread. The advantage of this kind of tap is the added control of addition rate.

Terminology	Meaning / words explanations
Sealing Film	A polymeric film used to temporarily seal aqueous solutions.
Silica Gel	1. A desiccant (drying agent) used in desiccators which is often treated with cobalt chloride which will turn from blue to pink as the desiccant becomes exhausted. 2. The stationary phase in chromatographic separations
Silicone Grease	A grease that is used to as a thin film on glass joints to prevent them from seizing and to seal them in reduced pressure distillations. It may also be used to seal the lids of desiccators.
Sintered Glass	A type of glass that is made by heating powdered glass below its melting point so that the particles stick to each other. The result is a material which will allow liquids to pass through it but it will retain solid material. Sintered glass can be used to make filters as well as the support for the stationary phase in chromatography columns.
Standard (Solution)	A solution of precisely known concentration used in volumetric analysis.
Standardisation	Using volumetric analysis to determine the exact concentration of a standard solution.
Stoichiometry	The number of moles involved in a reaction in accordance with the balanced equation.
Stationary Phase	The solid phase in a chromatographic separation.
Tare	To zero a balance once an empty weighing vessel is placed on it.
Titrant	The solution of unknown concentration in the conical flask in a titration.
Titrant	The solution of known concentration in the burette in a titration.
Toluene	The trivial name for methyl benzene.
Turbidity	The cloudiness or haziness of a liquid or solution
Volatile	Evaporating easily under normal conditions (for example solvents with low boiling points).
Washing	1. The removal of impurities from a solution by extracting with an immiscible solvent. 2. The washing away of soluble impurities from a solid filtered in a Buchner funnel using cold solvent. 3. The complete transfer of a solid or solution by repeated washing out with solvent (for example in the preparation of a standard solution).
Washings	The material produced from a washing procedure.
'Work Up'	The final stages of a reaction where the product is isolated and purified.

Contd...

ABBREVIATIONS

There are many abbreviations you will meet in laboratory situations. The more common ones you will pick up pretty quickly, others less so. Here is a list of the most common and more useful ones.

Abbreviation	Meaning
AAS	Atomic absorption spectroscopy
ACS	American Chemical Society
AMS	Accelerated mass spectrometry
AMS	Accelerator mass spectrometer
API	Active pharmaceutical ingredients
A_r	Relative Atomic Mass
b.pt.	Boiling Point
Bq	Becquerel
CCC	Counter current chromatography
CCD	Charge coupled device
CEC	Capillary electromatography
CEMS	Capillary electrophoresis
Ci	Curie
CID	Collision induced dissociation
CME	Coronal mass ejections
CODATA	Committee on Data for Science and Technology
COSHH	Control of Substances Hazardous to Health
COSY	Correlation spectroscopy
CS AAS	Continuum source atomic absorption spectroscopy
CSIRO	Commonwealth Scientific and Industrial Research Organization
CWA	Chemical warfare agents
DART	Direct analysis in real time
DCM	Dichloromethane
DIOS	Desorption ionization on silicon
DNA	Deoxyribonucleic acid
DSC	Differential scanning calorimeter
EBA	Expanded bed adsorption

Abbreviation	Meaning
ECD	Electron capture dissociation
EDD	Electron detachment dissociation
EDL	Electrodeless discharge lamps
EDTA	Ethylene diamine tetraacetic Acid
EIA	Enzyme immuno assay
ELF	Extremely low frequency
ELISA	Enzyme linked immuno sorbent assay
EM	Electromagnetic
EMIA	Enzyme mobilized immuno assay
EMSA	Electrophoretic mobility shift assay
En	Ethylenediamine
ESI	Electrospray ionization
ET	Electro thermal
ETD	Electron transfer dissociation
F	Faraday Constant
FAB	Fast atom bombardment
FD	Field desorption
FFA	Face field analyser
FIA	Fourier immuno assay
FIM	Field ion microscopy
FPLC	Fast protein liquid chromatography
FT-IR	Fourier Transform Infrared (Spectroscopy)
FTMS	Fourier transform mass spectrometry
GC	Gas Chromatography
GC-MS	Gas chromatography Mass spectroscopy
GDU	Gelatine digesting units
GFAA	Graphite furnace atomic absorption
GLC	Gas liquid chromatography
GPC	Gel permeation chromatography
GRB	Gamma ray bursts
GY	Gray

Contd...

Abbreviation	Meaning
HASAW	Health and Safety at Work
HCL	Hollow cathode lamp
HPLC	High Performance Liquid Chromatography
HR	High-resolution
IAC	International Avogadro Coordination
ICR	Ion cyclotron resonance
IMAC	Immobilized metal affinity chromatography
IMMS	Ion mobility mass spectrometry
IMS	Ion mobility spectrometry
IR	Infra-Red
IRMPD	Infrared multiphoton dissociation
IRMS	Isotope ratio mass spectrometry
IUPAC	International Union of Pure and Applied Chemistry
K_a	Acid Dissociation Constant
K_s	Solubilty Product
K_w	Ionic Product of Water
LDPE	Low density polyethylene
LS AAS	Line source atomic absorption spectroscopy
M	Molarity
m	Molality
m.pt.	Melting Point
MALDI	Matrix assisted laser desorption ionization
MCU	Milk clotting units
Mr	Relative Molecular Mass
MS	Mass spectroscopy
MSD	Mass selective detector
N	Normality
NIR	Near-Infrared reflectance spectroscopy
NMR	Nuclear Magnetic Resonance
NOESY	Nuclear over Hauser effect spectroscopy
NPLC	Normal phase liquid chromatography
PAGE	Polyacrylamide gel electrophoresis

Abbreviation	Meaning
PCR	Polymer chain reaction
PMF	Peptide mass fingerprinting
PTFE	Polytetrafluoroethylene (e.g Teflon)
PTR	Proton transfer reaction
PTV	Programmable temperature vaporizer
R	Universal Gas Constant
R_f	Retention Factor
RIA	Radioactive immuno assay
RNA	Ribonucleic acid
RPC	Reversed phase chromatography
RSC	Roal Society of Chemistry
SDS	Sodium dodecyl sulphate
SEC	Size exclusion chromatography
SEM	Scanning electron microscopy
SFC	Supercritical fluid chromatography
SI	System Internationale d'Unites
SID	Surface induced dissociation
SIFT	Selected ion flow tube
SIMS	Secondary ion mass spectroscopy
SIMS	Secondary ion mass spectrometry
SLD	Soft laser desorption
SPME	Solid phase micro extraction
SRM	Selected reaction monitoring
STEM	Scanning transmission electron microscope
STP	Standard Temperature and Pressure
STPF	Stabilized temperature platform furnace
Sv	Sievert
TCA	Trichloroacetic Acid
TEM	Transmission electron microscope
TIMS	Thermal ionization mass spectrometry
TLC	Thin Layer Chromatography

Contd...

Abbreviation	Meaning
TMS	Tetramethylsilane
TOCSY	Total correlation spectroscopy
TOF	Time of flight
UPS	Ultraviolet photoelectron spectroscopy
UV	Ultraviolet
VLF	Very low frequency
XPS	X – ray photoelectron spectroscopy
XPS	X-ray photoelectron spectroscopy

Various Analytical Techniques are Generally Used in the Laboratory.

- Colourimetry
- Spectrophotometry
- Spectroscopy
- Chromatography
    - Adsorption chromatography
    - Paper chromatography
        - Ascending
        - Descending
        - Circular Thin layer chromatography
        - Partition chromatography
        - Ion-exchange chromatograph
        - Gel filtration chromatography
- Centrifugation
    - Solid wall centrifugation
    - Perforated wall centrifugation

  Density gradient ultracentrifugation
    - Stabilized moving boundary centrifugation
    - Zone centrifugation
    - Isopycnic gradient centrifugation
- Electrophoresis

  1. Paper electrophoresis 2. Disc gel electrophoresis 3. PAGE
  4. SDS-PAGE 5. SDS-Disc gel electrophoresis
  6. Moving boundary electrophoresis 7. Zone electrophoresis

Isotachophorcsis

Isoelectric focusing

Electroosmosis

Micellar electrokinetic capillary chromatography

Immuno electrophoresis

a. FIA b. RIA c. EIA

- ELISA
- EMIA

- Flame photometry • Atomic absorption technique
- Inductively coupled plasma technique
- Fluorimetry • Infrared spectroscophy
- Radio immunoassay
- Fourier transform infrared spectroscophy
- Scanning electron micrography (SEM)
- Differential scanning calorimeters (DSC)
- X-ray diffraction technique
- Brabender viscoamylography
- High performance liquid chromatography (HPLC)
- Gas chromatography (GC)
- Mass spectroscophy (MS)
- Gas chromatography-Mass spectroscophy (GC-MS)
- Polymer chain reaction technique (PCR)
- Nuclear magnetic resonance (NMR)
- Near-Infrared reflectance spectroscophy (NIR)
- Dialysis, Salting in and Salting out techniques

LABORATORY FIRST AID

Information on First Aid

This information outlines the first aid treatment of the type of injury which is most likely to be sustained in a chemical laboratory. Such injuries are caused not only by chemical substances; they often consist of cuts from broken glass tubes or apparatus, burns from hot pipes or steam, abrasions caused by contact with carboys or packing cases etc. The treatments suggested must be considered as first aid: they are not substitutes for attention by a doctor or trained nurse.

Any injury, however small, must receive prompt treatment. Delay may result in a minor injury becoming a major one due to infection in the cause of a slight wound or scratch or due to shock in the case of a slightly burned or gassed casualty. The first aid measures suggested are necessarily brief; they must be applied with common sense. For example, if medical attention is required a doctor or an ambulance must be summoned at once. In the cause of shock the casualty must be made to lie down and rest; he/she should be kept warm by covering him/her with a light blanket (hot water bottles should not be applied). Should a casualty stop breathing artificial respiration must be started without delay, before any other treatment is resorted to and must be continued until breathing is resumed. Wash your hands thoroughly before treating a casualty suffering from a cut or wound, a burn or any eye injury. In all cases of skin, eye or mouth contact with an injurious chemical substance, thorough irrigation or rinsing with water should be the first treatment.

Treatment of Cuts and Scratches

Wounds, cuts or scratches, however small, should receive immediate attention. The wound should be covered as soon as possible with a sterilized wound dressing. If the skin around the wound is dirty or is contaminated with a water-soluble chemical substance, careful washing with clean water should be carried out. If the wound area is contaminated with a water-insoluble chemical, careful swabbing with cotton wool and surgical spirit should be carried out, followed by the application of a dressing in the normal manner. Except in the case of small cuts or scratches, it is advisable to obtain medical attention as stitching of the wound may be necessary. In any case should an injury become inflamed or painful, medical attention must be obtained.

Treatment of Burns

Heat burns or scalds: A serious heat burn or scaled should have a dry sterilized dressing applied (not an adhesive wound dressing) and medical attention should be obtained immediately. An extensive burn should be covered loosely with a clean towel. Clothing which is sticking to a burn should not be removed, nor should blisters be pricked.

Chemical Burns

Chemical burns should be flushed gently with plenty of cold water and all contaminated clothing should be removed.

Suggested Minimum Requirements and Additional Provisions

Subject to the legal requirements: It is suggested as guide, that the following items be kept in a clearly labeled first aid box or cupboard. The quantities indicated are recommended for establishments employing up to fifty persons.

1. A sufficient number (not less than twelve) of small sterilized un-medicated dressings for injured fingers.

2. A sufficient number (not less than six) of medium sized sterilized un-medicated dressings for injured hands or feet.
3. A sufficient number (not less than six) of large sterilized un-medicated dressings for other injured parts.
4. A sufficient number (not less than twenty four) of adhesive wound dressings of an approved type and of associated sizes.
5. A sufficient number (not less than four) of triangular bandages of un-medicated calico, the longest side of which should measures not less than 130 cm and each of the other side's not less than 92 cm.
6. A sufficient supply of adhesive plaster.
7. A sufficient supply of absorbent sterilized cotton wool in half-ounce packets.
8. A sufficient supply of approved eye ointment in a container of an approved type and size.
9. A sufficient number (not less than four) of sterilized eye-pads in separate sealed packets.
10. A rubber bandage or pressure bandage.
11. Safety pins.

It is suggested that in addition to the above provisions, which cater primarily for cuts and heat burns, each laboratory first aid box should contain the following:

- Eye irrigation bottle ½ liter capacity.
- Tablespoon
- Bottle of common salt
- Bottle of Magnesium sulphate (Epsom salts)
- Bottle of milk of Magnesia (dose: two tablespoonfuls)
- Bottle of vinegar of 1% Acetic acid.

*The following remedies and antidotes for specific chemicals should be included in the first aid box if these chemicals are being handled in the laboratory concerned:

- **Bromine, Formic acid and Hydrofluoric acid:** (splashed on skin). A 350 mL bottle containing dilute ammonium solution (1 volume 0.88 sp. gm. ammonia added to 15 volumes of water).
- **Cyanides:** (Antidote to be taken when cyanides have been swallowed).

The following solutions must be made up and kept ready for immediate use:

A: One hundred fifty eight grams (158 g) of ferrous sulphate crystals ($FeSO_4.7H_2O$) and 3 g citric acid crystals dissolved in a liter of distilled water (the solution must be regularly inspected and replaced if any deterioration occurs).

B: Sixty grams (60 g) of anhydrous sodium carbonate (Na_2CO_3) dissolved in a liter of distilled water. 50 mL of solution A is placed in a 175 mL wide neck bottle closed by a polythene covered cork and labeled clearly "Cyanide antidote A". 50 mL of solution B is similarly bottled and labeled "Cyanide antidote B". Both bottles should bear the legend mix the whole contents of bottles "A" and "B" and swallow the mixture.

- **Hydrogen cyanide and nitriles:** Inhaled by gassing casualties with Amyl nitrite capsules 3 minims.
- **Iodine:** (after skin contact or ingestion). Sodium thiosulphate crystals in bottles for fresh preparation of 1% solution in water.
- **Phosphorus:** (skin burns). 350 mL bottle containing a 3% solution of copper sulphate in water.
- **Emetics:** The response of different people to the various first aid methods used to induce vomiting is by no means uniform. A simple method is that of ticking the back of the throat with two fingers or a spoon. A useful and quickly available emetic is salt water (one tablespoonful of common salt in each cupful of tepid water) repeated until vomiting occurs.

*It is emphasized that vomiting should never be induced in cases of unconsciousness or the ingestion of corrosive poisons such as strong acids or alkalis or phenolic substances.

* The information contained in this chapter for laboratory first aid is for immediate reference for giving first aid by authorized qualified first aiders. MSDS of the respective chemicals involved must be sent along with the causality to the Doctor.

Mouth-to-Mouth Artificial Respiration

For a great majority of casualties, when breathing has stopped the mouth-to-mouth method of artificial respiration is probably the most effective. It is simple to apply, even by operators with the minimum of training. Where injuries to the mouth or face are apparent or where cyanide poisoning is known or suspected, the well-known Holger-Nielson back pressure arm-lift method should be adopted; in all other cases where breathing has stopped the mouth-to-mouth method should be immediately applied.

1. Positioning the Head

a. The casualty is quickly turned on his back.
b. The casualty's head is tilted back to open the air passages. If a cushion folded coat or blanket can be placed under the shoulders without delay, this should be done immediately.

2. Inflation

The casualty's nose kept closed by pinching. The operator takes a deep breath, applies his mouth to the casualty's mouth and inflates the lungs by blowing air into the mouth.

3. Exhalation

When the casualty's chest rises, the operator removes his mouth and turns his head to one side to allow air escape from the casualty's lungs. The inflation exhalation cycle (steps 2 and 3) is repeated continuously at a rate not exceeding 10-12 breaths per minute, until there are signs or returning natural respiration. The operator adjusts his breathing to coincide with the casualty's returning respiration.

NOTE:

1. When it is apparent that a casualty has stopped breathing, medical attention must be obtained as soon as possible, but this must not delay starting artificial respiration.
2. If the stomach contents are regurgitated the casualty's head should be turned to one side and his mouth cleaned out.
3. When natural breathing is restored the casualty should be kept warm (but not overheated) with blankets.

Table 1: Affected area and first aid measures

Affected area	Symbol	First aid measures
Eye	–	Irrigate the eyes thoroughly with water. Obtain medical attention: 1. In severe cases 2. When splashing or direct contact has occurred. In the case of hydrofluoric acid the eyes must be irrigated with cold water for at least 15 minutes and 0.03% (1 in 30 000) BKC solution to be used for prolonged irrigation for 1 to 3 hr.
Lungs	A	Remove from exposure, rest and keep warm.
	B	Remove from exposure, rest and keep warm in severe cases, or if exposure has been great. Obtain medical attention.
	C	Remove from exposure, rest and keep warm. Obtain medical attention.
	D	Remove from exposure first and keep warm. If breathing, break a capsule of Amyl nitrite and give to casualty by inhalation for 15-30 seconds. Repeat every 2-3 minutes. Apply artificial respiration if breathing has stopped. In any case obtain medical attention at once.

Contd...

Affected area	Symbol	First aid measures
	E	Remove from exposure, rest and keep warm. In severe cases obtain medical attention and apply artificial respiration if breathing gas stopped.
Skin	F	Drench the skin with plenty of water. Remove contaminated clothing and wash before re-use in severe cases obtain medical attention.
	G	Drench the skin with water and wash with soap and water. Remove contaminated clothing and wash re-use.
	Ga	Clothing to be thoroughly aired instead of washed.
	H	Drench the skin with water and then bath with a dilute solution of Sodium thiosulphate in water. Obtain medical attention.
	I	Drench the skin with water. Blisters or burns must receive medical attention. Do not prick the blusters, remove contaminated clothing and wash before re-use.
	J	Drench the skin with water and wash thoroughly with soap and water. Blister or burns must receive medical attention. Remove contaminated clothing and wash before re-use.
	K	Drench the skin with water after removing any adhering metal or penetrating particles. Except when contact has been slight. Obtain medical attention.
	L	Irrigate the skin immediately and continuously with cold water until medical attention is obtained. Pay particular attention to the skin under the finger-nails. If medical attention is delayed. Apply a dilute Solution of ammonia in water. Remove contaminated clothing and wash before re-use in case of hydrofluoric acid apply paste of Calcium gluconate on affected part.
	M	If skin contact is believed to have been prolonged, medical observation will be required.
	N	Drench the skin with plenty of water and then swab with a 3% solution of copper sulphate in water (this will convert phosphorus to a black copper salt which can be readily seen and re-moved). Obtain medical attention.

Affected area	Symbol	First aid measures
Mouth	O	Wash out the mouth thoroughly with water and given an emetic. Obtain medical attention.
	P	Wash out the mouth thoroughly with water and given plenty of water to drink, followed by milk of magnesia. Obtain medical attention.
	Q	Wash out the mouth thoroughly with water and given plenty of water, followed by vinegar or 1% acetic acid to drink. Obtain medical attention.
	R	Wash out the mouth thoroughly with water and given two tablespoonfuls of Magnesium sulphate (Epsom salts) in water and then an emetic rest and keep warm. Obtain medical attention.
	S	Wash out the mouth thoroughly with water and given plenty of water to drink, following by two tablespoons of Magnesium sulphate (Epsom salts) in water. Obtain medical attention.
	T	Wash out the mouth thoroughly with water and give large quantities of water to drink. Obtain medical attention.
	U	Give cyanide antidote. If breathing break capsule of amyl nitrite and give inhale for 15-30 seconds, repeat every 2-3 minutes. Apply artificial respiration if breathing has stopped. In any case obtain medical attention.
	V	Wash out the mouth with water. Obtain medical attention.
	W	Wash out the mouth thoroughly with a 1% Solution of Sodium thiosulphate in water and give some solution to drink. Followed by an emetic, medical attention.
	X	If swallowed obtain medical attention.
	Y	Wash out the mouth thoroughly with water and give a large quantity of milk to drink. Obtain medical attention.

Table 2: Suggested treatment for burns caused by skin contact with certain chemical compounds.

Ether	Affected area			
Ethyl bromide	**Eye**	**Lungs**	**Skin**	**Mouth**
Ethyl chloro-acetate		A	–	O
Ethyl chloro formate		A	F	P
Ethylene chlorhydrin		A	F	P
Ethylene chloride		B	Ga	O
Ethylene dibromide		B	F	P
Ethylene dichloride		E	F	O

Contd...

Ether	Affected area		
Ethylene diamine	B	F	O
Ethylene glycol	A	G	O
Ethylene oxide	B	G	O
Ferric chloride anhydrous	A	F	P
Fluorides	B	F	Q
Fluoro boric acid and salts	B	F	Q
Flurosilic acid and salts	B	F	O
Formaldehyde solution	B	–	O
Formalin	B	G	O
Formic acid	–	G	O
Fuming sulphuric acid	B	G	O
Hydrazine hydrate	–	–	R
Hydriodic acid	B	Ga	O
Hydrogen iodide	–	G	O
Hydrobromic acid	A	G	P
Hydrogen bromide	A	G	O
Hydrochloric acid	A	G	O
Hydrogen chloride	C	K	O
Hydrocyanic acid	B	F	P
Hydrogen cyanide	B	H	T
Hydrofluoric acid	–	I	P
Hydrogen fluoride	B	G	O
Hydrogen peroxide	B	J	T
Hydrogen sulphide	B	–	O
Hydroxyl-ammonium salts	E	–	O
Carbon monoxide	E	–	–
Carbon tetrachloride	E	Ga	O
Caustic potash	–	F	Q
Caustic soda	–	F	Q
Chlorine	B	F	–
Chloro-acetic acid	–	J	P
Chloro-aniline	A	G	O
1-chloro-2, 4-dinitro benzene	B	G	O
1-chloro-2, 3-epoxy propane	B	G	O

Ether	Affected area		
2-chloro-ethanol	C	G	O
Chloroform	E	–	O
Chloro-nitro-aniline	–	G	O
Chloro-phenols	A	G	S
Chloro-sulphonic acid	B	I	P
Chromates and dichromates	A	F	O
Chromic acid	A	F	P
Chromium trioxide	A	F	P
Coal gas	E	–	–
Copper compounds	A	–	O
Cresols	A	G	S
Cyanide	D	F	U
Diamino-ethane	A	F	O
1,2-dibromo-ethane	A	G	O
1,2-dichloro-ethane	E	–	O
1,2-dichloro-ethylene	A	–	O
Dichloro-methane	B	–	O
Diethyl ether	B	–	O
Dimethylamine and solutions	B	F	T
N-N-dimethyl-aniline	B	G	O
Dimethyl sulphate	C	F	P
Dinitro-*o*-cresol	B	G	O
Dinitro-phenols	B	G	O
Dioxin (dioxane)	B	–	O
Epichlorhydrin	B	G	O
Ethane-diol	–	–	O
Ether	B	–	O
Ethyl bromide	B	G	O
Ethyl chloro-acetate	B	G	O
Ethyl chloro formate	B	G	O
Ethylene chlorhydrin	C	G	O
Ethylene chloride	E	–	O
Ethylene dibromide	A	G	O
Ethylene dichloride	E	–	O

Contd...

Ether	**Affected area**		
Ethylene diamine	A	F	O
Ethylene glycol	–	–	O
Ethylene oxide	E	Ga	V
Ferric chloride anhydrous	A	F	P
Fluorides	B	G	O
Fluoro boric acid and salts	A	F	T
Flurosilic acid and salts	A	F	T
Formaldehyde solution	B	F	Y
Formalin	B	F	Y
Formic acid	A	F	P
Fuming sulphuric acid	B	F	P
Hydrazine hydrate	–	F	T
Hydriodic acid	A	F	P
Hydrogen iodide	A	F	P
Hydrobromic acid	A	F	P
Hydrogen bromide	A	F	P
Hydrochloric acid	A	F	P
Hydrogen chloride	A	F	P
Hydrocyanic acid	D	F	U
Hydrogen cyanide	D	F	U
Hydrofluoric acid	B	L	P
Hydrogen fluoride	B	L	P
Hydrogen peroxide	–	F	T
Hydrogen sulphide	E	–	–
Hydroxyl-ammonium salts	–	F	T
Hydroxylamine salts	–	F	T
Iodic acid	A	F	P
Iodine	A	H	W
Iodine pentoxide	A	F	P
Iodo-methane	B	F	O
Lead salts	–	–	R
Mercury	B	M	X
Mercury compounds	C	G/M	Y
Methanolic compounds	B	Ga	O

Ether	Affected area		
Methyl alcohol	B	Ga	O
Methylamine and solutions	B	F	T
N-methyl-alanine	B	G	O
Methyl bromide	B	J	T
Methyl cyanide	B	Ga	O
Methylene chloride	B	–	O
Methyl iodide	B	F	O
Methyl sulphate	C	F	P
Naphthylamine and salts	–	G	O
Nickel salts	A	G	O
Nitric acid	B	F	P
Nitro-anilines	A	G	O
Nitro-benzene	B	G	O
Nitrogen dioxide	B	–	–
Nitro-phenols	A	F	S
p-nitro-phenyl-hydrazine	A	G	O
Nitro-toluenes	B	G	O
Nitrous fumes	B	–	–
Oleum	B	F	P
Orthophosphoric acid	–	F	P
Oxalates	–	G	O
Oxalic acid	C	F	P
Pentachloro ethane	B	G	O
Pentachloro-phenol	B	G	S
Perchloric acid	–	F	P
Perchloro-ethylene	A	G	O
Phenol	A	J	S
Phenol-disulphonic acid	–	F	P
Phenylene-diamines	–	G	O
Phenyl-hydrazine	B	G	O
Phosgene	C	Ga	O
Phosphoric acid	–	F	P
Phosphoric oxide	B	F	P
Phosphorus (yellow)	B	N	O

Contd...

Ether	**Affected area**		
Phosphorus oxychloride	B	F	P
Phosphorus pentachloride	B	F	P
Phosphorus pentoxide	B	F	P
Phosphorus trichloride	B	F	P
Phosphoryl chloride	B	F	P
Picric acid	–	G	Y
Potassium metal	–	K	V
Potassium dichromate	A	F	O
Potassium bisulphate	–	F	P
Potassium cyanide	D	F	U
Potassium hydrogen sulphate	–	F	P
Potassium hydroxide	–	F	Q
Prussic acid	D	F	U
Pyridine	A	F	O
Resorcinol	–	G	S
Selenium and compounds	A	G	O
Silicon tetrachloride	A	F	P
Silver nitrate	–	F	O
Soda asbestos	A	G	Q
Sodium metal or amalgam	–	K	V
Sodium chromate	A	F	O
Sodium bisulphate	–	F	P
Sodium cyanide	D	F	U
Sodium dichromate	A	F	O
Sodium ethoxide	–	F	Q
Sodium fluoride	B	G	O
Sodium hydrogen sulphate	–	F	P
Sodium hydroxide	–	F	Q
Sodium hypochlorite solution	–	F	T
Sodium methoxide	–	F	Q
Sodium oxalate	–	G	O
Sodium sulphide	–	F	O
Stannic chloride anhydrous	A	G	P
Sulphonic acid	–	F	P

Ether	Affected area		
Sulphur chloride	B	I	P
Sulphur dichloride	B	I	P
Sulphur dioxide	B	–	–
Sulphuretted hydrogen	E	–	–
Sulphuric acid	–	I	P
Sulphuryl chloride	B	I	P
Tellurium and compounds	A	G	O
Tetrachloro-ethane	B	–	O
Tetrachloro-ethylene	A	G	O
Thallium and salts	B	G	O
Thionyl chloride	B	I	P
Titanic chloride	B	G	P
Titanium tetrachloride	B	G	P
Toluene	A	Ga	O
Toluidines	A	G	O
Trichloro-acetic acid	–	I	P
Trichloro-ethylene	A	–	O
Trimethylamine and solutions	B	F	T
Uranium compounds	B	–	O
Vanadium compounds	B	–	O
Xylenes	A	Ga	O
Xylenols	A	G	S

CHAPTER 2

Some Basic Concepts

1. SCIENTIFIC NOTATION

Scientific notation is simply a method for expressing, and working with, very large or very small numbers. It is a short hand method for writing numbers, and an easy method for calculations. Numbers in scientific notation are made up of three parts: the coefficient, the base and the exponent. Scientific notation expression:

$$N \times 10^n$$

Where $(1 < N < 10)$

Example:

Number 2,890,000,000 becomes 2.89×10^9 in scientific notation

Number 0.0000672 expressed as 6.72×10^{-5}

2. SIGNIFICANT FIGURES

Definition: The digits that are considered correct and the first doubtful digit are called significant figures.

Every experiment (except in some counting situations) involves a degree of uncertainty. Thus, suppose that several people measure the length of a sheet of paper, using a ruler that is divided into tenths of a centimeter, and get the following results: 27.92 cm, 27.96 cm, 27.90 cm, 2.10 cm. Notice that everyone agrees as to the first three digits (except the last person who is measuring from the wrong end of a 30 cm long ruler). Clearly the fourth digit, which has been estimated by everyone, is a doubtful figure (in fact even the third figure may be doubtful if the ruler is too short or too long due to manufacturing defect or environmental factors).

The number of significant figures in a measurement depends upon the precision of the instrument and, to some extent, upon the skill of the measure. An effort should always be made to obtain as many figures as an instrument will allow. Conversely, only significant figures should be recorded in taking data – i.e., a measurement should not be written in such a way as to imply a greater precision than is actually inherent in the measuring device and/or measuring technique.

For example, if we weigh a sample on a balance and record its mass as 1.2637 g, we assume that all digits, except the last, are known exactly. We assume that the last digit has an uncertainty of at least ± 1, giving an absolute uncertainty of at least ± 0.0001 g or a relative uncertainty of at least.

$$\frac{+0.0001\ g}{1.2637\ g} \times 100 = \pm 0.0079\%$$

Significant figures are a reflection of a measurement's uncertainty. The number of significant figures is equal to the number of digits in the measurement; with the exception that a zero (0) used to fix the location of a decimal point is not considered significant. This definition can be ambiguous. For example, how many significant figures are in the number 100? If measured to the nearest hundred, then there is one significant figure. If measured to the nearest ten, however, then two significant figures are included. To avoid ambiguity we use scientific notation. Thus, 1×10^2 has one significant figure, whereas 1.0×10^2 has two significant figures.

For measurements using logarithms, such as pH, the number of significant figures is equal to the number of digits to the right of the decimal, including all zeros. Digits to the left of the decimal are not included as significant figures since they only indicate the power of 10. A pH of 2.45, therefore, contains two significant figures.

Exact numbers, such as the stoichiometric coefficients in a chemical formula or reaction, and unit conversion factors, have an infinite number of significant figures. A mole of $CaCl_2$, for example, contains exactly two moles of chloride and one mole of calcium. In the equality 1000 mL = 1 L. Both numbers have an infinite number of significant figures. Recording a measurement to the correct number of significant figures is important because it tells others about how precisely you made your measurement. For example, suppose you weigh an object on a balance capable of measuring mass to the nearest ±0.1 mg, but record its mass as 1.762 g instead of 1.7620 g. By failing to record the trailing zero, which is a significant figure, you suggest to others that the mass was determined using a balance capable of weighing to only the nearest ±1 mg. Similarly, a buret with scale markings every 0.1 mL can be read to the nearest ±0.01 mL. The digit in the hundredth's place is the least significant figure since we must estimate its value. Reporting a volume of 12.241 mL implies that your buret's scale is more precise than it actually is, with divisions every 0.01 mL.

Significant figures are also important because they guide us in reporting the result of an analysis. When using a measurement in a calculation, the result of that calculation can never be more certain than that measurement's uncertainty. Simply put, the result of an analysis can never be more certain than the least certain measurement included in the analysis.

Finding the number of significant figures in a measurement is usually easy but can be troublesome if zeros are present. Look at the following four quantities:

4.803 cm Four significant figures: 4, 8, 0, 3

0.006 61 g Three significant figures: 6, 6, 1

55.220 K Five significant figures: 5, 5, 2, 2, 0

34,200 m Anywhere from three (3, 4, 2) to five (3, 4, 2, 0, 0) significant figures.

The fourth rule shows why it's helpful to write numbers in scientific notation rather than ordinary notation. Doing so makes it possible to indicate the number of significant figures. Thus, writing the number 34,200 as 3.42×10^4 indicates three significant figures, but writing it as 3.4200×10^4 indicates five significant figures.

One further point about significant figures: Certain numbers, such as those obtained when counting objects, are exact and have an effectively infinite number of significant figures. For example, a week has exactly 7 days, not 6.9 or 7.0 or 7.1, and a foot has exactly 12 in., not 11.9 or 12.0 or 12.1. In addition, the power of 10 used in scientific notation is an exact number. That is, the number is exact, but the number has one significant figure.

The Following Rules Cover the Different Situations that can Arisc:

1. Zeros in the middle of a number are like any other digit; they are always significant. Thus, 4.803 cm has four significant figures.
2. Zeros at the beginning of a number are not significant; they act only to locate the decimal point. Thus, 0.00661 g has three significant figures. (Note that 0.00661 g can be rewritten as 6.61×10^{-3} or as 6.61 mg.)
3. Zeros at the end of a number and after the decimal point are always significant. The assumption is that these zeros would not be shown unless they were significant. Thus, 55.220 K has five significant figures. (If the value were known to only four significant figures, we would write 55.22 K.)
4. Zeros at the end of a number and before the decimal point may or may not be significant. We can't tell whether they are part of the measurement or whether they only locate the decimal point. Thus, 34,200 m may have three, four, or five significant figures. Often, however, a little common sense is helpful. A temperature reading of 20°C probably has two significant figures rather than one, since one significant figure would imply a temperature anywhere from 10–30°C and would be of little use. Similarly, a volume given as 300 mL probably has three significant figures. On the other hand, a figure of 93,000,000 mi for the distance between the earth and the sun probably has only two or three significant figures.

Example:

How many significant figures in each of the following numbers:

(a) 6.07×10^{-15}

(b) 0.003840

(c) 463.8052

Solution:

(a) Three significant figures 6, 0, 7

(b) Four significant figures 3, 8, 4, 0

(c) Seven significant figures 4, 6, 3, 8, 0, 5, 2

3. RECORDING OF RESULTS

When a value contains too many significant figures, it must be rounded off. Rounding method involves underestimating the value when rounding the five digits 0, 1, 2, 3, and 4, and overestimating the value when rounding the five digits 5, 6, 7, 8, and 9. With this approach, if the value of the digit to the right of the last significant figure is smaller than 5, drop this digit and leave the remaining number unchanged. Thus, 2.794 become 2.79. If the value of the digit to the right of the last significant digit is 5 or larger, drop this digit and add 1 to the preceding digit. Thus, 2.795 become 2.80.

In chemistry there are several rules or bases to round final result of calculations:

1. Rounding to correct number of significant figures which are mostly applicable for laboratory reported final results
2. Rounding result to specific number of decimal places, 1, 2, 3, 4 or more depend upon the precision or calculation purpose we would like to reach.

Unless specified otherwise all this book examples we will follow second rule of rounding final results, because this book prepared to help analyst to find the exact weight and most analytical balances are prepared to weigh up to four decimal places (0.0000 ± 0.0001).

4. PREPARING SOLUTIONS

Solutions of known concentration can be prepared in a number of different ways depending on the nature of the analyte and/or the concentration required:

1. Weighing out a solid material of known purity, dissolving it in a suitable solvent and diluting to the required volume
2. Weighing out a liquid of known purity, dissolving it in a suitable solvent and diluting to the required volume
3. Diluting a solution previously prepared in the laboratory
4. Diluting a solution from a chemical supplier.

Remember to record all masses and volumes used in the preparation of solutions in a laboratory workbook, and to show how you calculated the concentration of the solution. The procedure for preparing a solution by dilution of a more concentrated solution (either prepared in the laboratory or from a chemical supplier).

5. LABELING AND STORING SOLUTIONS

Once you have prepared the solution you need to think about how you will store it and how it will be identified in the future. Remember the following key points:

A. Solutions should not be stored in volumetric flasks – transfer them to a suitable container for storage;

B. Ensure that solutions are stored correctly. Some solutions will need to be stored in a refrigerator while others may be light-sensitive and need to be stored in amber bottles;

C. All solutions should be clearly labeled with the following information:
   1. The name and concentration of the solution;
   2. Date of preparation;
   3. Name of analyst;
   4. Review or expiry date;
   5. Hazard information (if appropriate);

D. The label must be securely attached to the container and be written in water insoluble ink.

In some cases, particularly where volatile solvents are used, it is useful to check for any changes in the mass of the solution during storage. After the solution has been prepared, it is transferred to a suitable container and the mass of the sealed container and the solution is recorded. Prior to an aliquot of the solution being used, the container is re-weighed. The mass should not be significantly different from that recorded prior to the solution being stored. After the required volume of the solution has been transferred from the storage container, the solution is reweighed before being returned to storage. If a significant change in mass is observed after the solution has been stored then it should not be used.

Checklist for Preparing Solutions of Known Concentration

Table 1: Do this and don't do this for preparing solutions of known concentration.

Do this	Don't do this
Preparing a solution by dissolving a solid material	
Use a material with a suitable purity (grade) and ensure that it has been stored correctly and is within its expiry date.	Use material that appears to have been stored incorrectly or that has passed its expiry date.
Use a clean, dry spatula to transfer the required amount of material.	Return unused material to the original bottle.
Make sure you have correctly calculated the amount of material required.	
Weigh accurately the required amount of material.	
Ensure that all glassware used is clean, dust free and undamaged.	Use dirty glassware or glassware that is damaged and/or has faded graduation marks.
Transfer the material to a beaker and dissolve in a small amount of solvent.	Transfer the material directly to the volumetric flask.
Make sure that material has dissolved completely.	

Contd...

Use a small glass funnel to transfer the solution from the beaker to the volumetric flask.	
Rinse the beaker with solvent and transfer the rinsing to the volumetric flask.	
Make sure that the solution is at ambient temperature before making the solution up to the calibration mark with solvent.	Make the solution up to the calibration mark if its temperature is significantly different from the ambient temperature. (Note that if the ambient temperature is significantly different from the calibration temperature of the glassware used this will increase the uncertainty in the concentration of the solution.)
Make sure the solution is mixed thoroughly before use.	
Preparing solutions by dilution of a stock solution	
Make sure the stock solution is at room temperature.	Use a stock solution straight from the refrigerator.
Plan a dilution scheme to minimize the uncertainty in the concentration of the diluted solution.	Carry out large dilutions in a single step.
Ensure that all glassware used is clean, dust free and undamaged.	Use dirty glassware or glassware that is damaged and/or has faded graduation marks.
Ensure the stock solution is well mixed before use.	
Transfer the stock solution to a beaker or conical flask for pipetting.	Pipette directly from the stock solution bottle/flask.
Make sure the diluted solution is well mixed before use.	Return unused solution to the stock bottle.
All Solutions	
Transfer the solution to a suitable container for storage.	Store solutions in volumetric flasks.
Clearly label containers with: the name and concentration of the solution; date of preparation; name of analyst; review or expiry data; hazard labels (if appropriate).	
Store solutions correctly (e.g. in a refrigerator if necessary).	

6. HANDLING, CALCULATIONS, PREPARATION AND STORAGE OF STANDARDS

Overview

This section contains basic information on the handling, preparation and storage of standards, as well as basic calculations and nomenclature.

Handling

Observing the following recommendations will save considerable time, money, and frustration:

1. Never put solution transfer devices into the standard solution. This precaution avoids possible contamination from the pipette or transfer device.
2. Always pour an aliquot from the standard solution to a suitable container for the purpose of volumetric pipette solution transfer and do not add the aliquot removed back to the original standard solution container. This precaution is intended to avoid contamination of the stock standard solution.
3. Perform volumetric pipette solution transfer at room temperature. Aqueous standard solutions stored at 'lower' temperature will have a higher density. Weight solution transfers avoid this problem provided the density of the standard solution is known or the concentrations units are in wt./wt. rather than wt./volume.
4. Never use glass pipettes or transfer devices with standard solutions containing HF. Free HF attacks glass but it is sometimes considered safe to use glass when the HF is listed as trace and/or as a complex. However, many fluorinated compounds will attack glass just as readily as free HF.
5. Don't trust volumetric pipette standard solution transfer. Weigh the aliquot of the standard taken. This can be easily calculated provided the density of the standard solution is known. There are too many possible pipetting errors to risk a volumetric transfer without checking the accuracy by weighing the aliquot.
6. Uncap your stock standard solutions for the minimum time possible. This is to avoid transpiration concentration of the analytes as well as possible environmental contamination.
7. Replace your stock standard solutions on a regular basis. Regulatory agencies recommend or require at least annual replacement. Why is this precaution taken in view of the fact that the vast majority of inorganic standard solutions are chemically stable for years? This is due to the changing concentration of the standard through container transpiration and the possibility of an operator error through general usage. A mistake may occur the first time you use the stock standard solution or it may never occur with the probability increasing with use and time. In addition, the transpiration concentration effect occurs whether the standard solution is opened / used or not and increases with use and increased vapor space (transpiration rate is proportional to the ratio of the circumference of the bottle opening to vapor space).

CALCULATIONS

The concentration units for chemical standard solutions used for ICP applications are typically expressed in μg/mL (micrograms per milliliter) or ng/mL (nanograms per milliliter). For example, a 1000 μg/mL solution of Ca^{+2} contains 1000 micrograms of Ca^{+2} per each mL of solution and a 1 μg/mL solution of Ca^{+2} contains 1000 ng of Ca^{+2} per milliliter of solution. To convert between metric concentration units the following conversions apply:

Table 2: Mass portion of concentration unit where g = gram

Prefix	Scientific Notation	Decimal equivalents	Example Units
kilo- (k)	$= 10^{3}$	= 1000 g	kilogram (kg)
milli- (m)	$= 10^{-3}$	= 0.001 g	milligram (mg)
micro- (μ)	$= 10^{-6}$	= 0.000001 g	microgram (μg)
nano- (n)	$= 10^{-9}$	= 0.000000001 g	nanogram (ng)
pico- (p)	$= 10^{-12}$	= 0.000000000001 g	picogram (pg)

Table 3: Volume portion of concentration unit where L = liter

Prefix	Scientific Notation	Decimal equivalents	Example Units
milli- (m)	$= 10^{-3}$	= 0.001 L	milliliter (mL)
micro- (μ)	$= 10^{-6}$	= 0.000001 L	microliter (μL)
nano- (n)	$= 10^{-9}$	= 0.000000001 L	nanoliter (nL)
pico- (p)	$= 10^{-12}$	= 0.000000000001 L	picoliter (pL)

The difference between ppm and μg/mL is often confused. A common mistake is to refer to the concentration units in ppm as a short cut (parts per million) when we really mean μg/mL. One ppm is in reality equal to 1 μg/g. In similar fashion ppb (parts per billion) is often equated with ng/mL. One ppb is in reality equal to 1 ng/g. To convert between ppm or ppb to μg/mL or ng/mL the density of the solution must be known. The equation for conversion between wt./wt. and wt./vol. units is:

(μg/g) (density in g/mL) = μg/mL and/or (ng/g) (density in g/mL) = ng/mL

Therefore, if we have a solution that is 1000 μg/mL Ca^{+2} and know or measure the density to be 1.033 g/mL then the ppm Ca^{+2} = (1000 μg/mL) / (1.033 g/mL) = 968 μg/g = 968 ppm.

When making dilutions the following equation is useful:

$(mL_A)(C_A) = (mL_B)(C_B)$

For example, to determine how much of a 1000 μg/mL solution of Ca^{+2} required to prepare 250 mL of a 0.3 μg/mL solution of Ca^{+2} we would use the above equation as follows:

$(mL_A)(1000\ \mu g/mL) = (250\ mL)(0.3\ \mu g/mL)$

$(mL_A) = [(250\ mL)(0.3\ \mu g/mL)]/(1000\ \mu g/mL)$

$(mL_A) = 0.075\ mL = 75\ \mu L$

Preparation

Weight ≠ Volume

Standard chemical solutions can be prepared to weight or volume. The elimination of glass volumetric flasks may be necessary to eliminate certain contamination issues with the use of borosilicate glass or to avoid chemical attack of the glass. It is often assumed that 100 grams of an aqueous solution is close enough to 100 mL to not make a significant difference since the density of water at room temperature is very close to 1.00 (0.998203 at 20.0 °C). Diluting / preparing standard solutions by weight are much easier. Still, the above assumption should not be made. The problem is that trace metals standards are most commonly prepared in water + acid mixtures where the density of the common mineral acids is significantly greater than 1.00. For example, a 5% v/v aqueous solution of nitric acid will have a density of ~1.017 g/mL which translates into a fixed error of ~1.7%. Higher nitric acid levels will result in larger fixed errors. This same type of problem is true for solutions of other acids to a degree that is a function of the density and concentration of the acid in the standard solution as described by the following equation (to be used for estimation only):

$$d_S = [(100\text{-}\%) + (d_A)(\%)] / 100$$

Where:

d_S = density of final solution

% = The v/v % of a given aqueous acid solution

d_A = density of the concentrated acid used

For example, lets estimate the density of a 10% v/v aqueous solution of nitric acid made using 70% concentrated nitric acid with a density of 1.42 g/mL.

$D_S = [(100\text{-}\%) + (d_A)(\%)]/100 = [(100\text{-}10) + (1.42)(10)]/100 = (90 + 14.2)/100 = 1.042$ g/mL

Acid Content

Another area of confusion is the expression of the acid content of the solution. We all agree that it is important to matrix match the standard and sample solutions to avoid a fixed error in the solution uptake rate and/or nebulization efficiency sometimes referred to as a matrix interference. If a solution is labeled as 5% HNO_3 what does this mean? If we take 5 mL of 70% concentrated nitric acid and dilute to a volume of 100 mL then this is 5% HNO_3 (v/v) where the use of 70% concentrated acid is assumed. However, nitric acid can be purchased as 40%, 65%, 70%, and > 90%. Therefore, note the concentration of the concentrated acid used if different from the 'norm' as well as the method of preparation i.e. v/v or wt/wt or wt/v or v/wt. The wt. % concentrations of the common mineral acids, densities, and other information are shown in the following table:

Table 4: Weight, percentage and Concentrations

Acid	Mol wt.	Density (g/mL)	Wt %	Molarity
Hydrochloric acid	36.46	1.19	37.2	12.1
Hydrofluoric acid	20.0	1.18	49.0	28.9
Nitric acid	63.01	1.42	70.4	15.9
Perchloric acid	100.47	1.67	70.5	11.7
Phosphoric acid	97.10	1.70	85.5	14.8
Sulfuric acid	98.08	1.84	96.0	18.0

Acid Content in Molarity

It is important to know what the concentration units of the concentrated acid being used mean. Taking 70% concentrated nitric acid as an example means that 100 grams of this acid contains 70 grams of HNO_3. The concentration is expressed at 70% wt./wt. or 70 wt. % HNO_3. Some analysts prefer to work in matrix acid concentrations units of Molarity (moles/liter). To calculate the Molarity of 70 wt. % nitric acid we calculate how many moles of HNO_3 are present in 1 liter of acid. Let's say that we take a 1 liter volumetric flask and then dilute to the mark with 70.4 wt. % HNO_3. We would then measure the weight of the solution to be 1420 grams. Knowing that the solution is 70.4 wt % would then allow us to calculate the number of grams of HNO_3 which would be (0.704)(1420g) = 999.7 grams HNO_3 per liter. Dividing the grams HNO_3 by the molecular weight of HNO_3 (63.01 g/mole) gives the moles HNO_3 / L or Molarity which is 15.9 M. The above logic explains the following equation used for calculating the Molarity of acids where the concentration of the acid is given in wt %:

$[(\% \times d) / MW] \times 10 = \text{Molarity}$

Where:

% = wt. % of the acid

d = density of acid (specific gravity can be used if density not available) MW = molecular weight of acid

Using the above equation to calculate the Molarity of the 70 wt % nitric acid we have:

$[(70.4 \times 1.42) / 63.01] \times 10 = 15.9\ M$

Dilutions of the concentrated acid to prepare specific volumes of specified Molarity can be make using the $(mL_A)\ (C_A) = (mL_B)\ (C_B)$ equation.

Avoiding Precipitates

In the preparation of mixtures of the elements, it is good to avoid the formation of precipitates. It is common to form precipitates when concentrates of elements that are considered compatible are mixed. Many precipitates are not reversible (i.e., will not go into solution upon dilution). It is therefore best to add all of the acid and most of the water to the volumetric flask or standard solution container (dilutions to weight) before adding the individual element concentrates aliquots. Mixing after each aliquot addition is strongly advised. When diluting to volume it is often found that the solution is above room temperature. Therefore allow the solution to cool to room temperature and adjust to the mark with DI water. It is best to prepare the dilution the day before needed to allow for proper volume adjustment.

Storage

The following are some considerations you may want to make before the storage of chemical standard solutions:

1. Know the chemical stability of your standard. Chemical stability can be altered by changes in starting materials and preparation conditions. It is therefore advisable to perform stability studies on all standard solutions to avoid time consuming and costly delays or mistakes and to strictly adhere to preparation methodology, including order of addition for multi-component standard solutions.
2. Note the temperature during storage and attempt to maintain a storage temperature at or around 20 °C. Some standards are not stable for long periods at room temperature and require refrigeration or even freezing.
3. Perform the stability study in the container material selected for storage. It is not advisable to use volumetric flasks as storage containers due to expense, contamination, and transpiration issues.
4. Determine if the standard is photosensitive and/or store in the dark if there is a concern. This is an issue with some of the precious metals and is a function of matrix. Photosensitivity will increase in the presence of higher energy light (sunlight as opposed to artificial light) and trace or minor amounts of organics especially if there is an extractable proton alpha to an electron withdrawing functional group such as a carbonyl group. The presence of chloride may increase instability to photo reduction. A classic example is Ag^+ in HCl solutions.
5. Store the standard in containers that will not contribute to contamination of the standard. LDPE is an excellent container for most inorganic standards.
6. Weigh the standard solution before storage and then just before the next use. If there is measurable transpiration the weight will decrease with time.

7. DILUTION OF CONCENTRATION SOLUTIONS

Diluting a solution involves adding additional solvent to decrease the solution's concentration.

Key Points for Dilutions:

A. Most commonly, a solution's concentration is expressed in terms of mass percent, mole fraction, molarity, molality, and normality. When calculating dilution factors, it is important that the units of volume and concentration remain consistent.

B. Dilution calculations can be performed using the formula $M_1V_1 = M_2V_2$.

C. A serial dilution is a series of stepwise dilutions, where the dilution factor is held constant at each step.

Terms used While Dilutions:

- Serial dilution: stepwise dilution of a substance in solution.
- Dilution: a solution that has had additional solvent, such as water, added to make it less concentrated.

Dilution refers to the process of adding additional solvent to a solution to decrease its concentration. This process keeps the amount of solute constant, but increases the total amount of solution, thereby decreasing its final concentration. Dilution can also be achieved by mixing a solution of higher concentration with an identical solution of lesser concentration. Diluting solutions is a necessary process in the laboratory, as stock solutions are often purchased and stored in very concentrated forms. For the solutions to be usable in the lab (for a titration, for instance), they must be accurately diluted to a known, lesser concentration.

The volume of solvent needed to prepare the desired concentration of a new, diluted solution can be calculated mathematically. The relationship is as follows:

$$M_1V_1 = M_2V_2$$

M_1 denotes the concentration of the original solution, and V_1 denotes the volume of the original solution; M_2 represents the concentration of the diluted solution, and V_2 represents the final volume of the diluted solution. When calculating dilution factors, it is important that the units for both volume and concentration are the same for both sides of the equation.

Example 1:

175 mL of a 1.6 M aqueous solution of LiCl is diluted with water to a final volume of 1.0 L. What is the final concentration of the diluted solution?

Solution:

$$M_1V_1 = M_2V_2$$
$$(1.6 \text{ M})(175 \text{ mL}) = M_2(1000 \text{ mL})$$
$$M_2 = 0.28 \text{ M}$$

You dilute a solution whenever you add solvent to a solution. Adding solvent results in a solution of lower concentration. You can calculate the concentration of a solution following a dilution by applying this equation:

$$\text{M}_1\text{V}_1 = \text{M}_2\text{V}_2$$

where M is molarity, V is volume, and the subscripts 1 and 2 refer to the initial and final values.

Example 2:

How many milliliters of 5.5 M NaOH are needed to prepare 300 mL of 1.2 M NaOH?

Solution:

$$5.5 \text{ M} \times \text{V}_1 = 1.2 \text{ M} \times 0.3 \text{ L}$$
$$\text{V}_1 = 1.2 \text{ M} \times 0.3 \text{ L} / 5.5 \text{ M}$$
$$\text{V}_1 = 0.065 \text{ L V}_1 = 65 \text{ mL}$$

So, to prepare the 1.2 M NaOH solution, you pour 65 mL of 5.5 M NaOH into your container and add water to get 300 mL final volume.

Serial Dilutions

Serial dilutions involve diluting a stock or standard solution multiple times in a row. Typically, the dilution factor remains constant for each dilution, resulting in an exponential decrease in concentration. For example, a ten-fold serial dilution could result in the following concentrations: 1 M, 0.1 M, 0.01 M, 0.001 M, and so on. As is evidenced in this example, the concentration is reduced by a factor of ten in each step. Serial dilutions are used to accurately create extremely diluted solutions, as well as solutions for experiments that require a concentration curve with an exponential or logarithmic scale. Serial dilutions are widely used in experimental sciences, including biochemistry, pharmacology, microbiology, and physics.

8. HOW TO CALCULATE UNITS OF CONCENTRATION

Once you have identified the solute and solvent in a solution, you are ready to determine its concentration. Concentration may be expressed several different ways, using percent composition by mass, volume percent, mole fraction, molarity, molality, or normality.

1. Percent Composition by Mass (%)

This is the mass of the solute divided by the mass of the solution (mass of solute plus mass of solvent), multiplied by 100.

Example:

Determine the percent composition by mass of a 100 g salt solution which contains 20 g salt.

Solution:

20 g NaCl / 100 g solution x 100 = 20% NaCl solution.

2. Volume Percent (% v/v)

Volume percent or volume/volume percent most often is used when preparing solutions of liquids. Volume percent is defined as:

v/v % = [(volume of solute)/(volume of solution)] × 100%

Note that volume percent is relative to volume of solution, not volume of *solvent*. For example, wine is about 12% v/v ethanol. This means there are 12 ml ethanol for every 100 ml of wine. It is important to realize liquid and gas volumes are not necessarily additive. If you mix 12 ml of ethanol and 100 ml of wine, you will get less than 112 ml of solution.

See as another example. 70% v/v rubbing alcohol may be prepared by taking 700 ml of isopropyl alcohol and adding sufficient water to obtain 1000 ml of solution (which will not be 300 ml).

3. Mole Fraction (X)

This is the number of moles of a compound divided by the total number of moles of all chemical species in the solution. Keep in mind, the sum of all mole fractions in a solution always equals 1.

Example:

What is the mole fractions of the components of the solution formed when 92 g glycerol is mixed with 90 g water? (molecular weight water = 18; molecular weight of glycerol = 92).

Solution:

90 g water = 90 g x 1 mol / 18 g = 5 mol water

92 g glycerol = 92 g x 1 mol / 92 g = 1 mol glycerol

total mol = 5 + 1 = 6 mol

x_{water} = 5 mol / 6 mol = 0.833

$x_{glycerol}$ = 1 mol / 6 mol = 0.167

It's a good idea to check your math by making sure the mole fractions add up to 1:

$x_{water} + x_{glycerol}$ = .833 + 0.167 = 1.000

4. Molarity (M)

Molarity is probably the most commonly used unit of concentration. It is the number of moles of solute per liter of solution (not necessarily the same as the volume of solvent).

Example:

What is the molarity of a solution made when water is added to 11 g $CaCl_2$ to make 100 mL of solution?

Solution:

11 g $CaCl_2$ / (110 g $CaCl_2$ / mol $CaCl_2$) = 0.10 mol $CaCl_2$

100 mL x 1 L / 1000 mL = 0.10 L

molarity = 0.10 mol / 0.10 L

molarity = 1.0 M

5. Molality (m)

Molality is the number of moles of solute per kilogram of solvent. Because the density of water at 25°C is about 1 kilogram per liter, molality is approximately equal to molarity for dilute aqueous solutions at this temperature. This is a useful approximation, but remembers that it is only an approximation and doesn't apply when the solution is at a different temperature, isn't dilute, or uses a solvent other than water.

Example:

What is the molality of a solution of 10 g NaOH in 500 g water?

Solution:

10 g NaOH / (40 g NaOH / 1 mol NaOH) = 0.25 mol NaOH

500 g water x 1 kg / 1000 g = 0.50 kg water

molality = 0.25 mol / 0.50 kg

molality = 0.05 M / kg

molality = 0.50 m

6. Normality (N)

Normality is equal to the *gram equivalent weight* of a solute per liter of solution. A gram equivalent weight or equivalent is a measure of the reactive capacity of a given molecule. Normality is the only concentration unit that is reaction dependent.

Example:

1 M sulfuric acid (H_2SO_4) is 2 N for acid-base reactions because each mole of sulfuric acid provides 2 moles of H^+ ions. On the other hand, 1 M sulfuric acid is 1 N for sulfate precipitation, since 1 mole of sulfuric acid provides 1 mole of sulfate ions.

CHAPTER 3

Types of Stock Standard Solutions

1. STOCK STANDARD SOLUTION

Analysis in any laboratory mainly based on reference materials like Stock standard solution. The accuracy in the preparation of stock standard reflects accuracy of the results. Stock standard solution is defined as a solution with high concentration of stable analyte(s) that can be stored at specific conditions in laboratory for long time and used as a standard reference material for analysis of the target analyte(s) in the daily use. Example of stock standard solutions for like Sodium (Na) solution with a concentration of 1000 mg Na /L (ppm) used as stock solution for Sodium analysis by Inductively Coupled Plasma (ICP), Flame Photometry, Ion Chromatography (IC) etc., that can be stored at 4 ^{0}C for a minimum of 6 months. All stock standards shall be checked before use with another standard that has been prepared separately from different source.

To prepare stock standard solution in lab you should first make sure that you understand the concentration unit principles and some mathematical rules which will help to find exact answer for reporting.

2. IONIC STANDARD SOLUTIONS

Ionic Compounds

Ionic compounds are basically defined as being compounds where two or more ions are held next to each other by electrical attraction. One of the ions has a positive charge (called a "cation") and the other has a negative charge ("anion"). Cations are usually metal atoms and anions are either nonmetals or polyatomic ions (ions with more than one atom).

Ions can be single atoms, as the sodium and chloride in common table salt sodium chloride, or more complex groups such as the carbonate in calcium carbonate. But to be considered an ion, they must carry a positive or negative charge. Thus, in an ionic bond, one 'bonder' must have a positive charge and the other a negative one. By sticking to each other, they resolve, or partially resolve, their separate charge imbalances. Positive to positive and negative to negative ionic bonds do not occur.

Ionic standard solutions are mostly used in analysis of all kind of ions, anions such as chloride (Cl^-), bromide (Br^-), sulfate (SO_4^{2-}) or cations such as sodium (Na^+), magnesium (Mg^{2+}) and potassium (K^+). The analysis procedure is either in wet-chemistry by titration or by using instrument like ion-chromatography or spectrophotometer or else. But regardless of the procedure used in the analysis the accuracy in the analysis depends on the accuracy of standards.

To prepare stock standard solution of ion analyte, first we have to find a salt starting reagent either in liquid or solid state contain such ion then make sure the salt is fully dissociated in water such as sodium chloride (NaCl) and sodium sulfate (Na_2SO_4).

$$NaCl \longrightarrow Na^+ + Cl^-$$

$$Na_2SO_4 \longrightarrow 2Na^+ + SO_4^{2-}$$

Sodium chloride dissociate in water into one sodium cation (Na^+) and one chloride anion (Cl^-) as per equation above. Sodium sulfate dissociate into two sodium cations and one sulfate anion.

After find the starting reagent to prepare standard solution check the chemical formula of the substance and find how many ion(s) are produced from dissociation of single molecule. Example each molecule of NaCl produces one sodium ion (Na^+) but each molecule of Na_2SO_4 produce two sodium ions. Use the conversion factor equation to make calculations.

We consider some examples below will show how to prepare and make calculations for different kinds of ionic standard solutions.

Example 1:

Calculate amount required to prepare 500 mL solution of 1000 ppm (mg/L) Na starting from sodium chloride (NaCl).

Solution:

We will use conversion factor and we will start with conversion we will prepare:

Molecular weight for NaCl = 58.44 g/mol

Atomic weight for Na = 22.99 g/mol

Each 58.44 g of NaCl contain 22.99 g of Na by convert grams to milligrams

Each 58.44 mg of NaCl contain 22.99 mg of Na

$$\frac{1000\,mg\ Na}{L} \times \frac{1g Na}{1{,}000\,mg\ Na} \times \frac{58.44g\ NaCl}{22.99\,g\ Na} \times 0.5L = 1.271g\ NaCl$$

Example 2:

Calculate how to prepare sulfate (SO_4^{2-}) stock standard solution 1000 ppm (mg/L) in 1 Liter starting from magnesium sulfate hexahydrate ($MgSO_4.7H_2O$).

Solution:

First will calculate the molecular weight for starting reagent formula and for sulfate ion

Molecular weight for $MgSO_4.7H_2O$ = 246.48 g/mol

Formula weight for sulfate ion (SO_4^{2-}) = 96.06 g/mol

From starting reagent formula $MgSO_4.7H_2O$ each molecule produce after dissociate in water one sulfate anion (SO_4^{2-}) i.e each 246.48 grams of $MgSO_4.7H_2O$ have 96.06 grams of sulfate anion. Use this relation to write the conversion factor. Start always from the concentration we need to prepare 1000 ppm (mg/L).

$$\frac{1000\ mg\ SO_4^{2-}}{L} \times \frac{1g SO_4^{2-}}{1,000\ mg\ SO_4^{2-}} \times \frac{246.48g\ MgSO_4.7H_2O}{96.06g SO_4^{2-}} \times 1L$$

$$= 2,565.90mg = 2.5659\ g\ MgSO_4.7H_2O$$

To prepare stock solution dissolve 2.5659 grams of $MgSO_4.7H_2O$ in small amount of solvent then complete to total volume 1 Liter.

Example 3:

Nitrate (NO_3^-) anion solution prepared by dissolving 3.0 g of KNO_3 in 250 mL of water. What is the concentration of Nitrate ion, express the concentration in Molarity and ppm.

Solution:

Molecular weight of KNO_3 = 101.10 g/mol

Formula weight of NO_3^- = 62.00 g/mol

Starting from the information we have:

$$\frac{3.0g\ KNO_3}{0.250L} \times \frac{62.00g NO_3^-}{101.10g\ KNO_3} \times \frac{1000\ mg\ NO_3^-}{1.0\ g\ NO_3^-} = 7359.05\ mg/L\ NO_3^-$$

$$\frac{3.0g\ KNO_3}{0.250L} \times \frac{1\ mol\ KNO_3}{101.10g\ KNO_3} \times \frac{1\ mol\ NO_3^-}{1\ mol\ KNO_3} = 0.1187\ mol/L\ (M) NO_3^-$$

Example 4:

A student needs to prepare mixed anion standard solution 1 Liter to be used in Ion Chromatography contains the following:

1. Sulfate (SO_4^{2-}) 10,000 ppm
2. Nitrate (NO_3^-) 1,000 ppm
3. Bromide (Br^-) 1,000 ppm

Student has the following reagent in his lab, Aluminum sulfate hexadecahydrate $Al_2(SO_4)_3.16H_2O$, Sodium bromide NaBr, Calcium nitrate $Ca(NO_3)_2$.

Explain to the student how to prepare stock standard.

Solution:

First we have to find a source for each ion as per the following table:

Ion	Source	Concentration (ppm)	Number of ion in each molecule
Sulfate (SO_4^{2-})	Aluminum sulfate hexadecahydrate $Al_2(SO_4)_3.16H_2O$	10,000	3
Nitrate (NO_3^-)	Calcium nitrate $Ca(NO_3)_2$	1,000	2
Bromide (Br^-)	Sodium bromide NaBr	1,000	1

Above table shows each ion in stock standard and it's starting reagent source and concentration in ppm (mg/L). The last column shows number of ions produced from each molecule of starting reagents after dissociation in water.

To calculate the amount required we assume all starting reagents are pure 100 % w/w. Start calculate from the target concentration:

a. Sulfate (SO_4^{2-})

Molecular weight of $Al_2(SO_4)_3.16H_2O$ = 630.40 g/mol

$$\frac{10,000\ mg\ SO_4^2}{L} \times \frac{1g SO_4^{-2}}{1,000\ mg\ SO_4^{2-}} \times \frac{630.40\ gAl_2(SO_4)_3.16H_2O}{3\times 96.06g\ SO_4^{2-}} \times 1L$$

$$= 21.8752g\ Al_2(SO_4)_3.16H_2O$$

b. Nitrate (NO_3^-)

Molecular weight of $Ca(NO_3)_2$ = 164.09 g/mol

$$\frac{1,000\ mg\ NO_3^-}{L} \times \frac{1g\ NO_3^-}{1,000\ mg\ NO_3} \times \frac{164.09mgCa(NO_3)_2}{2\times 62.00\ mg\ NO_3^-} \times 1L$$

$$= g = 1.3233g\ Ca(NO_3)_2$$

c. Bromide (Br^-)

Molecular weight of NaBr = 102.89 g/mol

$$\frac{1,000\ mg\ Br^-}{L} \times \frac{1g\ Br^-}{1,000\ mg\ Br^-} \times \frac{102.89\ g\ Na3r}{79.90.00\ g\ Br^-} \times 1L$$

$$= 1.2877g\ NaBr$$

To prepare standard we weigh exactly 21.8752 g, 1.3233 g and 1.2877 g from $Al_2(SO_4)_3.16H_2O$, $Ca(NO_3)_2$ and NaBr respectively and transfer all to same 1 liter volumetric flask then add solvent (water) to dissolve all substances then we complete to marked volume with solvent.

Example 5:

A solution prepared by add 5.0 g of KNO_3 and 5.0 g of $Hg(NO_3)_2$ in 1 L volumetric flask and complete with water to volume, what is the concentration of Nitrate anion (NO_3^-) in the final solution? Express concentration in Molarity unit.

Solution:

First we calculate how many grams or how many moles of nitrate ion in the solution from each source reagent, we start always from the information we know:

Molecular weight of KNO_3 = 101.10 g/mol

$$5.0g\ KNO_3 \times \frac{1\ mol\ KNO_3}{101.10\ g\ KNO_3} \times \frac{1\ mol\ NO_3^-}{1\ mol\ KNO_3}$$

$$= 0.04946\ moles = 49.46\ mmoles\ of\ NO_3^-$$

Molecular weight of $Hg(NO_3)_2$ = 324.60 g/mol

$$5.0g\ Hg(NC_3)_2 \times \frac{1\ mol\ Hg(NO_3)_2}{324.60\ gHg(NO_3)_2} \times \frac{2\ mol\ NO_3^-}{1\ mol\ Hg(NO_3)_3}$$

$$= 0.03080\ moles = 0.03080\ moles\ of\ NO_3^-$$

Total number of moles of nitrate ions from both source =

49.46 mmoles + 30.80 mmoles = 80.26 mmoles = 0.08026 moles NO_3^-

$$Molarity = \frac{Moles}{Sclution\ Volume\ (L)} = \frac{0.08026\ moles\ NO_3^-}{1L} = 0.08026\ M\ NO_3^-$$

Example 6:

Sulfide (S^{2-}) ion solution prepared from sodium sulfide Na_2S solid with purity of 30% (w/w). How many grams of sodium sulfide required preparing 500 mL of 2,000 ppm sulfide (S^{2-}) stock standard solution?

Solution:

Purity of starting reagent is important, 30% w/w means for each 100 grams of sodium sulfide powder there are 30 grams of sodium sulfide, we will start calculations from the target concentration 2,000 ppm:

$$\frac{2,000\ mg\ S^{2-}}{L} \times \frac{1gS^{2-}}{1,000\ mg\ S^{2-}} \times \frac{1\ mol\ S^{2-}}{32.07\ g\ S^{2-}} \times \frac{1\ mol\ Na_2S}{1\ mol\ Na_2S} \times \frac{100\ g\ Na_2S\ Powder}{30g\ Na_2S} \times 0500\ L =$$

$$= 8.1125 \text{ g of } Na_2S \text{ powder}$$

To prepare standard weigh exactly 8.1125 g of Na_2S powder dissolved it in water then complete to total volume 500 mL.

Example 7:

A solution prepared by mixing 50 mL from 0.5 M orthophosphate (PO_4^{3-}) and 35 mL from 5,000 ppm (mg/L) PO_4^{3-} solutions then completed to 250 mL total volume. What is the final concentration of phosphate anion PO_4^{3-} in both ppm and molarity.

Solution:

First we calculate number of moles of orthophosphate ion we took from each solution:

- 50 mL of 0.5 M PO_4^{3-} solution (M = mol/L)

$$\frac{0.5\ mol\ PO_4^{3-}}{L} \times 0.050\ L = 0.025\ mol\ PO_4^{3-}$$

- 35 mL of 5,000 ppm PO_4^{3-} solution (ppm = mg/L)

$$\frac{5,000\ mg\ PO_4^{3-}}{L} \times \frac{1\ g\ PO_4^{3-}}{1,000\ mg\ PO_4^{3-}} \times \frac{1 mol PO_4^{3-}}{94.97\ g\ PO_4^{3-}} \times 0.035\ L = 0.00184\ mol\ PO_4^{3-}$$

Total number of moles = 0.025 + 0.00184 = 0.02684 mol PO_4^{3-}

Calculate concentration of final solution in Molarity (M):

$$Molarity = \frac{Moles}{L} = \frac{0.02684\ mols\ PO_4^{3-}}{0.250\ L} = 0.1074\ M\ PO_4^{3-}.$$

Calculate concentration in ppm(mg/L):

$$0.02684\ mol\ PO_4^{3-} \times \frac{94.97\ g\ PO_4^{3-}}{1\ mol\ PO_4^{3-}} \times \frac{1}{0250L} = 10,195.97\ ppm\ (mg/L)\ PO_4^{3-}$$

Final concentration of solution is 0.1074 M or 10,195.97 ppm PO_4^{3-}.

Example 8:

Nitrite anion (NO_2^-) stock solution prepared from Sodium nitrite $NaNO_2$, the concentration of nitrite are expressed in terms of nitrogen element. For example if we said Nitrite-N 1,000 ppm mg N/L means 1 liter of the solution contains one thousand milligrams of nitrogen element sourced from nitrite anion.

Notice: Express nitrite and nitrate anions concentrations by nitrogen element source make it easy for comparison between them; most of national environmental protection agencies for water in many countries around the world are expressing thus kind of ions by nitrogen element.

How many grams of Sodium nitrite $NaNO_2$ powder required to prepare 1 liter of Nitrite-N solution with concentration of 1,000 mg N/L if the purity of $NaNO_2$ powder is 97.1 % w/w.

Solution:

Calculation is depend on nitrogen element in Sodium nitrite, there is only on nitrogen atom produced from each molecule of Sodium nitrite

$$\frac{1,000\ mg\ N}{L} \times \frac{1gN}{1,000\ mg\ N} \times \frac{1molN}{4.00\ gN} \times \frac{1\ mol\ NaNC_4}{1\ mol\ NO_2^-} \times \frac{69.00\ g\ NaNO_2}{1\ mol\ NaNO_2} \times \frac{100\ g\ NaNO_2pwd}{97.1\ g\ NaNO_2} =$$

$$= 5.0758\ g\ of\ NaNO_2\ powder$$

3. ELEMENT STANDARD SOLUTIONS

Element stock standard solutions used in the analysis of elements by analytical instruments like Inductively Coupled Plasma (ICP), Flame Photometer (FP) and Atomic Absorption (AA) which are the most commonly used in analysis of elements. Following are some examples for preparations of elements stock standard solutions.

Example 1:

How many grams required from Iron (III) chloride $FeCl_3.6H_2O$ powder to prepare Iron (Fe) stock standard solution in 1 Liter with concentration of 1,000 ppm Fe if the purity of Iron (III) chloride is 96.5% w/w?

Solution:

Each molecule of Iron (III) chloride contains one mole of iron (Fe) element:

Molecular weight of $FeCl_3.6H_2O$ = 270.30 g/mol

Atomic weight of Fe = 55.85 g/mol

$$\frac{1,000\ mg\ Fe}{L} \times \frac{1g\ Fe}{1,000\ mg\ Fe} \times \frac{1\ mol\ Fe}{55.85\ g\ Fe} \times \frac{1\ mol\ FeCl_3 6H_2O}{1\ mol\ Fe} \times$$

$$\frac{270.30\ g\ FeCl_3.6H_2O}{1\ mol\ FeCl_3.6H_2O} \times \frac{100\ g\ FeCl_3.6H_2Opwd}{96.5\ FeCl_3.6H_2O}$$

$$= 5.0153 \text{ g of } FeCl_3.6H_2O \text{ powder}$$

To prepare stock solution it required to weight 5.0153 g of Iron (III) chloride powder and dissolve it in small amount of water then complete to volume 1 L.

Example 2:

A 500 mL of Mercury (Hg) solution prepared by mixing 2.45 g of mercury chloride ($HgCl_2$) and 4.68 g of mercury sulfate ($HgSO_4$) in one container then dissolve and complete to volume with solvent 2% nitrice acid. What is the final concentration Mercury (Hg) in the final solution? Express concentration in Molarity and % (w/v).

Solution:

Each mole of either mercury chloride or mercury sulfate contain one mole of mercury element (Hg)

Molecular weight of mercury chloride ($HgCl_2$) = 271.50 g/mole

Molecular weight of mercury sulfate ($HgSO_4$) = 296.65 g/mole

Atomic weight of mercury element (Hg) = 200.59 g/mole

Calculate number of total number of moles of mercury element from each source.

Mercury from mercury chloride ($HgCl_2$):

$$2.45\ g\ HgCl_2 \times \frac{1\ mol\ HgCl_2}{271.50\ g\ HgCl_2} \times \frac{1 mol\ Hg}{1\ mol\ HgCl_2} = 0.00902\ mole = 9.02\ mmoles\ Hg$$

Mercury from mercury sulfate ($HgSO_4$):

$$4.68\ g\ HgSO_4 \times \frac{1\ mol\ HgSO_4}{296.65\ g\ HgSO_4} \times \frac{1\ mol\ Hg}{1\ mol\ HgCl_2} = 0.0158\ mole = 15.8\ mmoles\ Hg$$

Total number of millimoles = 9.02 + 15.8 = 24.8 mmoles = 0.0248 moles mercury (Hg) in solution

Concentration of mercury in solution in molarity (M)

$$Molarity = \frac{\#\ of\ moles\ of\ Hg}{Solution\ volume\ (L)} = \frac{0.0248\ mols\ Hg}{0.500\ L} = 0.0496\ M\ Hg$$

To concentration of mercury in solution in % (w/v) first we calculate grams of mercury in the solution:

Weight of mercury(Hg) = molecular weight × number of moles = 200.59 g/mol × 0.0248 moles = 4.97 g Hg

$$\%(w/v) = \frac{g\ of\ solute}{100\ mL\ of\ Solution} = \frac{g\ of\ solute}{mL\ of\ Solution} \times 100\%$$

$$= \frac{4.97 g\ Hg}{500\ mL} \times 100\% = 0.994\%(w/v) Hg$$

Example 3:

A student has got three stock standard solutions of 3 different elements, zinc (Zn) 2000 ppm, cadmium (Cd) 1500 ppm and lead (Pb) 1000 ppm. A student took 10 mL from each solution and transfers it to 200 mL volumetric flask then completed to total volume with solvent. What is the final concentration of each element in the diluted mix solution?

Solution:

In this example simple dilution process was made, to calculate the concentration of each element in the final solution use dilution equation from chapter one:

$Cf \times Vf = Ci \times Vi$

Final concentration of zinc (Zn)

$$C_f = \frac{C_i \times V_i}{V_f} = \frac{2000\ ppm \times 10\ mL}{20\ mL} = 100\ ppm\ Zn$$

Final concentration of cadmium (Cd):

$$C_f - \frac{C_i \times V_i}{V_f} - \frac{1500\ ppm \times 10\ mL}{200\ mL} - 75\ ppm\ Cd$$

Final concentration of cadmium (Pb):

$$C_f = \frac{C_i \times V_i}{V_f} = \frac{1000\ ppm \times 10\ mL}{200\ mL} = 50\ ppm\ Pb\,.$$

Example 4:

Lead chloride ($PbCl_2$) powder has purity of 89% w/w, a chemist need to prepare 1 L of 0.5 M lead (Pb) stock solution. How many grams of $PbCl_2$ required for preparing such stock solution.

Solution:

Each mole of lead chloride contains one mole of lead (Pb) element:

$PbCl_2 \longrightarrow Pb$

Molarity of lead (Pb) = 0.5 M

Total volume (L) = 1 L

Purity of $PbCl_2$ = 89% (w/w) à each 100 grams of $PbCl_2$ powder contains 89 grams of $PbCl_2$

Starting from concentration required as first item in conversion factor equation:

$$\frac{0.5\ mol\ P_b}{L} \times \frac{1\ mole\ PbCl_a}{1\ mole\ Pb} \times \frac{278.1054\ g\ PbCl_2}{1\ mole\ PbCl_2} \times \frac{100\ g\ PbCla\ powder}{89\ g\ PbCl_2}$$

$$= 156.24 \text{ g of } PbCl_2 \text{ powder}$$

It required 156.24 grams of lead chloride powder to prepare stock solution, dissolve it in solvent and complete to total volume 1 Liter.

4. FORMULA STANDARD SOLUTIONS

Formula stock standard solutions means the analyte is the molecular formula of starting reagent. In ion standard solutions calculations are based on the analyte ion formula, also for elements stock solutions the calculations are based on the element atomic weight and number of elements in molecular formula. In this kind of standard the analyte is molecular formula of the starting reagent regardless if is dissociate in solvent or not.

Examples of stock standard solutions:

Stock standard type	Example solution
Ion	1000 ppm Sulfate (SO_4^{2-})
Element	1000 ppm Iron (Fe)
Formula	1000 ppb Naphthalene.

Example 1:

Naphthalene ($C_{10}H_8$) is one of aromatic hydrocarbons measured by GC-MS. If molecular weight of naphthalene is 128.6 g/mol; how many milligrams are required to prepare 100 mL of 2,000 ppb stock standard solution of naphthalene from powder Naphthalene (purity of 91.5 % w/w)?

Solution:

Concentration of naphthalene = 2,000 ppb (μg/L)

Purity of naphthalene = 91.5 % w/w ⟶ each 100 mg of Naphthalene powder contains 91.5 mg of pure naphthalene.

$$\frac{2,000\ \propto g\ Naphthalcn\ c}{L} \times \frac{1\ mg\ Naphthalcn\ c}{1000\ \propto g\ Naphthalene} \times \frac{100\ mg\ Naphthalcn\ c\ powder}{91.5\ mg\ Naphthalene}$$

= 2.1858 mg napthalene powder.

Example 2:

Kerosene Range Organic (KRO) tested in all environmental and petroleum laboratories. The standard of KRO is prepared from commercial Kerosene fuel available from fuel station. How many grams required from kerosene to prepare 250 mL of 5000 ppm of KRO?

Solution:

KRO concentration = 5,000 ppm (mg/L)

Total volume = 250 mL = 0.250 L

$$\frac{5,000\ mg\ KRO}{L} \times \frac{1\ g\ KRO}{1,000\ mg\ KRO} \times 0.250\ L = 1.250\ C\ g\ KRO$$

Example 3

How many grams of methanol (CH_3OH) are contained in 0.100 L of 1.71 M aqueous methanol (i.e., 1.71 mol CH_3OH/L solution?

Solution:

Molecular weight of methanol (CH_3OH) = 32.042 g/mol

$$\frac{1.71\ mole}{L} \times \frac{32.042\ g\ methanol}{1\ mole\ methanol} \times 0.100\ L = 5.4792\ g\ methanol.$$

CHAPTER 4

Equivalent Concentration

INTRODUCTION

This chapter reviews the basic chemical concepts and units used to quantitative reagents. Equations for calculating the amounts and concentrations of reagents are derived immediately after the relevant chemical concept has been explained. A guideline on reagent preparation is then given, and, finally, practical examples addressing various aspects of calculating for reagent preparation, concentrations, and amounts are presented.

ATOMIC MASS UNIT

By international agreement, 1 amu is defined as $^1/_{12}$ the mass of an atom of carbon-12 (^{12}C). When converted to grams, 1 amu = 1.66×10^{-24} g.

MOLE (mol)

Weighing out or counting individual atoms or molecules is impossible because they are extremely small. The unit of measure, the mole, was introduced to enable scientists to weigh out the amount of any chemical substance that contains a given number of atoms, molecules, or other chemical particles. One mole of atoms is the number of atoms in exactly 12 g of ^{12}C, which is 6.02×10^{23}. In a broader sense, 1 mole of any substance contains 6.02×10^{23} units. One mole of a chemical element or compound contains 6.02×10^{23} atoms or molecules, respectively, and its weight in grams is equal to the numerical value of the atomic weight (at. wt) or molecular weight (mol wt).

By definition, mol = wt. (g) ÷ mol wt. (g/mol).

Wt (g) = mol × mol wt. (g/mol)

If the substance is an element, molecular weight is substituted with atomic weight.

ATOMIC WEIGHT (at. wt.)

Atomic weight is the weight (in amu) of one atom of an element. It comprises the weight of the protons and neutrons in the atomic nucleus. The gram-atomic weight of any element is the weight (in grams) of 6.02×10^{23} atoms or 1 mole of that element. The gram-atomic weight is numerically equal to the atomic weight.

MOLECULAR WEIGHT (MOL WT) AND GRAM MOLECULAR WEIGHT (G-MOL WT)

The molecular weight of a compound is the sum of the atomic weight (in amu) of all the atoms that make up one molecule of the compound. The molecular weight (in g) of any compound contains 6.02×10^{23} molecules or 1 mole of the compound. For this reason, the molecular weight, expressed in grams, is termed gram-molecular weight. The gram-molecular weight of a compound is numerically equal to its molecular weight.

Molecular Formula

The atoms that make up one molecule of a compound constitute the chemical or molecular formula of that compound. For example, the formula of a molecule of glucose, which consists of 6 atoms of carbon, 12 atoms of hydrogen and 6 atoms of oxygen, is $C_6H_{12}O_6$. The atoms in this formula are covalently linked and do not dissociate in solution. Therefore, $C_6H_{12}O_6$ exists as a discrete molecule. In contrast discrete molecules of some compounds exist only in concept because the molecules are formed by associated ions. For example the formula of magnesium sulfate is $MgSO_4$. In solution, it dissociates into one magnesium ion (Mg^{2+}) and one sulfate ion (SO_4^{2-}). A discrete molecule of magnesium sulfate or any other dissociable compound, therefore, exists only in concept.

AVOGADRO'S NUMBER

In chemistry and physics, the Avogadro constant (symbols: L, N_A) is the number of constituent particles, usually atoms or molecules, that are contained in the amount of substance given by one mole. Thus it is the proportionality factor that relates the molar mass of a material to its mass. It has the dimension of reciprocal amount of substance. Avogadro's constant has the value 6. 022140857(74) $\times 10^{23}$ mol^{-1} in the International System of Units (SI).

Previous definitions of chemical quantity involved Avogadro's number, a historical term closely related to the Avogadro constant but defined differently: Avogadro's number was initially defined by Jean Baptiste Perrin as the number of atoms in one gram-molecule of atomic hydrogen, meaning (in modern terminology) one gram of (atomic) hydrogen. It was later redefined as the number of atoms in 12 grams of the isotopecarbon-12 (^{12}C) and still later generalized to relate amounts of a substance to their molecular weight. For instance, to a first approximation, 1 gram of hydrogen element (H), which has a mass number of 1 (atomic number 1), has 6.022×10^{23} hydrogen atoms. Similarly, 12 grams of ^{12}C, with the mass number of 12 (atomic number 6), has the same number of carbon atoms, 6.022×10^{23}. Avogadro's number is a dimensionless quantity and has the numerical value of the Avogadro constant given in base units.

The Avogadro constant is fundamental to understanding both the makeup of molecules and their interactions and combinations. For instance, since one atom of oxygen will combine with two atoms of hydrogen to create one molecule of water (H_2O), one can similarly see that one mole of oxygen (6.022×10^{23} of O atoms) will combine with two moles of hydrogen ($2 \times 6.022\times10^{23}$ of H atoms) to make one mole of H_2O.

Mole and *moles* are frequently abbreviated as *mol* in chemical and mathematic notation. Revisions in the base set of SI units necessitated redefinitions of the concepts of chemical quantity and so Avogadro's number, and its definition, was deprecated in favor of the Avogadro constant and its definition. Changes in the SI units are proposed that will precisely fix the value of the constant to exactly $6.02214X\times10^{23}$ when it is expressed in the unit mol^{-1}.

GENERAL ROLE IN SCIENCE

Avogadro's constant is a scaling factor between macroscopic and microscopic (atomic scale) observations of nature. As such, it provides the relation between other physical constants and properties. For example, it establishes a relationship between the gas constant R and the Boltzmann constant k_B,

$$R = k_B N_A = 8.3144621(75)\ \text{J mol}^{-1}\text{K}^{-1}$$

and the Faraday constant F and the elementary charge e,

$$F = N_A e = 96485.3365(21)\ C\ \text{mol}^{-1}$$

The Avogadro constant also enters into the definition of the unified atomic mass unit, u,

$$1\ u = \frac{M_u}{M_A} = 1.660538921(73) \times 10^{-27}\ \text{kg}$$

where M_u is the molar mass constant.

MEASUREMENT

Coulometry

The earliest accurate method to measure the value of the Avogadro constant was based on coulometry. The principle is to measure the Faraday constant, F, which is the electric charge carried by one mole of electrons, and to divide by the elementary charge, e, to obtain the Avogadro constant.

$$N_A = \frac{F}{e}$$

The classic experiment is that of Bower and Davis at NIST, and relies on dissolving silver metal away from the anode of an electrolysis cell, while passing a constant electric current I for a known time t. If m is the mass of silver lost from the anode and A_r the atomic weight of silver, then the Faraday constant is given by:

$$F = \frac{A_r M_u I t}{m}$$

The NIST scientists devised a method to compensate for silver lost from the anode by mechanical causes, and conducted an isotope analysis of the silver used to determine its atomic weight. Their value for the conventional Faraday constant is $F_{90} = 96485.39(13)$ C/mol, which corresponds to a value for the Avogadro constant of 6.0221449 (78)×10^{23} mol^{-1}: both values have a relative standard uncertainty of 1.3×10^{-6}.

Electron Mass Measurement

The Committee on Data for Science and Technology (CODATA) publishes values for physical constants for international use. It determines the Avogadro constant from the ratio of the molar mass of the electron $A_r(e)M_u$ to the rest mass of the electron m_e:

$$N_A = \frac{A_r(e)M_u}{m_e}$$

The relative atomic mass of the electron, $A_r(e)$, is a directly-measured quantity, and the molar mass constant, M_u, is a defined constant in the SI. The electron rest mass, however, is calculated from other measured constants:

$$m_e = \frac{2R\infty h}{c\alpha^2}$$

X-Ray Crystal Density (XRCD) Methods

A modern method to determine the Avogadro constant is the use of X-ray crystallography. Silicon single crystals may be produced today in commercial facilities with extremely high purity and with few lattice defects. This method defines the Avogadro constant as the ratio of themolar volume, V_m, to the atomic volume V_{atom}:

$$N_A = \frac{V_m}{V_{atom}}, \text{ where } V_{tom} = \frac{V_{cell}}{n}$$

and n is the number of atoms per unit cell of volume V_{cell}.

The unit cell of silicon has a cubic packing arrangement of 8 atoms, and the unit cell volume may be measured by determining a single unit cell parameter, the length of one of the sides of the cube, a. In practice, measurements are carried out on a distance known as d_{220}(Si), which is the distance between the planes denoted by the Miller indices {220}, and is equal to $a/\sqrt{8}$. The 2006 CODATA value for d_{220} (Si) is 192.0155762(50) pm, a relative uncertainty of 2.8×10^{-8}, corresponding to a unit cell volume of 1.60193304(13)×10^{-28} m^3.

The isotope proportional composition of the sample used must be measured and taken into account. Silicon occurs in three stable isotopes (^{28}Si, ^{29}Si, ^{30}Si), and the natural variation in their proportions is greater than other uncertainties in the measurements. The atomic weight A_r for the sample crystal can be calculated, as the relative atomic masses of the three nuclides are known with great accuracy. This, together with the measured density ρ of the sample, allows the molar volume V_m to be determined:

$$V_m = \frac{A_r M_u}{\rho}$$

where M_u is the molar mass constant. The 2006 CODATA value for the molar volume of silicon is 12.058 8349(11) cm^3mol^{-1}, with a relative standard uncertainty of 9.1×10^{-8}.

As of the 2006 CODATA recommended values, the relative uncertainty in determinations of the Avogadro constant by the X-ray crystal density method is 1.2×10^{-7}, about two and a half times higher than that of the electron mass method.

International Avogadro Coordination

The International Avogadro Coordination (IAC), often simply called the "Avogadro project", is a collaboration begun in the early 1990s between various national metrology institutes to measure the Avogadro constant by the X-ray crystal density method to a relative uncertainty of 2×10^{-8} or less. The project is part of the efforts to redefine the kilogram in terms of a universal physical constant, rather than the International Prototype Kilogram, and complements the measurements of the Planck constant using watt balances. Under the current definitions of the International System of Units (SI), a measurement of the Avogadro constant is an indirect measurement of the Planck constant:

$$h = \frac{c\alpha^2 A_r(e) M_u}{2R_\infty N_A}$$

The measurements use highly polished spheres of silicon with a mass of one kilogram. Spheres are used to simplify the measurement of the size (and hence the density) and to minimize the effect of the oxide coating that inevitably forms on the surface. The first measurements used spheres of silicon with natural isotopic composition, and had a relative uncertainty of 3.1×10^{-7}. These first results were also inconsistent with values of the Planck constant derived from watt balance measurements, although the source of the discrepancy is now believed to be known. The main residual uncertainty in the early measurements was in the measurement of the isotopic composition of the silicon to calculate the atomic weight so, in 2007, a 4.8-kg single crystal of isotopically enriched silicon (99.94% ^{28}Si) was grown, and two one-kilogram spheres cut from it. Diameter measurements on the spheres are repeatable to within 0.3 nm and the uncertainty in the mass is 3 μg. Full results from these determinations were expected in late 2010. Their paper, published in January 2011, summarized the result of the International Avogadro Coordination and presented a measurement of the Avogadro constant to be 6.02214078 (18) $\times10^{23}$ mol^{-1}.

Formula Weight (FW)

This unit is used in place of molecular weight to designate the weight of the formula of a compound that does not exist as a discrete molecule (section E). It is defined as the sum of the atomic weights of all the elements that comprise the chemical formula of the compound. The formula weight (g) of any compound contains 6.02×10^{23} molecules or 1 mole of the compound.

Equivalent Weight (Equiv Wt)

This is the weight of an acid or a base containing 1 mole of replaceable H^+ or OH^-, respectively, or the weight of a redox compound that contains 1 mole of exchangeable electrons, or the weight of an ionic substance carrying 1 mole of ions. Gram equivalent weight is used when equivalent weight is expressed in grams.

Equivalent weight = mol wt ÷ n, where n = Number of replaceable H^+ or OH^-.

Equivalent weight (also known as gram equivalent) is a term which has been used in several contexts in chemistry. In its most general usage, it is the mass of one equivalent that is the mass of a given substance which will

- Combine or displace directly or indirectly with 1.008 parts by mass of hydrogen or 8 parts by mass of oxygen or 35.5 parts by mass of chlorine; or
- Supply or react with one mole of hydrogen cations H^+ in an acid–base reaction; or
- Supply or react with one mole of electrons *e* - in a redox reaction.

Equivalent weight has the dimensions and units of mass, unlike atomic weight, which is dimensionless. Equivalent weights were originally determined by experiment, but (insofar as they are still used) are now derived from molar masses. Additionally, the equivalent weight of a compound can be calculated by dividing the molecular weight by the number of positive or negative electrical charges that result from the dissolution of the compound.

Equivalent weights were not without problems of their own. For a start, the scale based on hydrogen was not particularly practical, as most elements do not react directly with hydrogen to form simple compounds. However, one gram of hydrogen reacts with 8 grams of oxygen to give water or with 35.5 grams of chlorine to give hydrogen chloride: hence 8 grams of oxygen and 35.5 grams of chlorine can be taken to be *equivalent* to one gram of hydrogen for the measurement of equivalent weights. This system can be extended further through different acids and bases.

Much more serious was the problem of elements which form more than one oxide or series of salts, which have (in today's terminology) different oxidation states. Copper will react with oxygen to form either brick red *cuprous oxide* (copper (I) oxide, with 63.5 g of copper for 8 g of oxygen) or black *cupric oxide* (copper (II) oxide, with 32.7 g of copper for 8 g of oxygen), and so has *two* equivalent weights. Supporters of atomic weights could turn to the Dulong–Petit law (1819), which relates the atomic weight of a solid element to its specific heat capacity, to arrive at a unique and unambiguous set of atomic weights. Most supporters of equivalent weights -- which were the great majority of chemists prior to 1860, simply ignored the inconvenient fact that most elements exhibited multiple equivalent weights. Instead, these chemists had settled on a list of what were universally called "equivalents" (H = 1, O = 8, C = 6, S = 16, Cl = 35.5, Na = 23, Ca = 20, and so on). However, these nineteenth-century "equivalents" were not equivalents in the original or modern sense of the term. Since they represented dimensionless numbers that for any given element were unique and unchanging, they were in fact simply an alternative set of atomic weights, in which the elements of even valence have atomic weights one-half of the modern values. This fact was not recognized until much later.

The final death blow for the use of equivalent weights for the elements was Dmitri Mendeleev's presentation of his periodic table in 1869, in which he related the chemical properties of the elements to the approximate order of their atomic weights. However, equivalent weights continued to be used for many compounds for another hundred years, particularly in analytical chemistry. Equivalent weights of common reagents could be tabulated, simplifying analytical calculations in the days before the widespread availability of electronic calculators: such tables were commonplace in textbooks of analytical chemistry.

Use in General Chemistry

The use of equivalent weights in general chemistry has largely been superseded by the use of [molar masses]. Equivalent weights may be calculated from molar masses if the chemistry of the substance is well known:

- sulfuric acid has a molar mass of 98.078(5) g mol^{-1}, and supplies two moles of hydrogen ions per mole of sulfuric acid, so its equivalent weight is 98.078(5) g mol^{-1}/2 eq mol^{-1} = 49.039(3) g eq^{-1}.
- potassium permanganate has a molar mass of 158.034(1) g mol^{-1}, and reacts with five moles of electrons per mole of potassium permanganate, so its equivalent weight is 158.034 (1) g mol^{-1}/5 eq mol^{-1} = 31.6068(3) g eq^{-1}.

Historically, the equivalent weights of the elements were often determined by studying their reactions with oxygen. For example, 50 g of zinc will react with oxygen to produce 62.24 g of zinc oxide, implying that the zinc has reacted with 12.24 g of oxygen (from the Law of conservation of mass): the equivalent weight of zinc is the mass which will react with eight grams of oxygen, hence 50 g × 8 g/12.24 g = 32.7 g.

Use in Volumetric Analysis

When choosing primary standards in analytical chemistry, compounds with higher equivalent weights are generally more desirable because weighing errors are reduced. An example is the volumetric standardization of a solution of sodium hydroxide which has been prepared to approximately 0.1 mol dm^{-3}. It is necessary to calculate the mass of a solid acid which will react with about 20 cm^3 of this solution (for a titration using a 25 cm^3 burette): suitable solid acids include oxalic acid dihydrate, potassium hydrogen phthalate and potassium hydrogen iodate. The equivalent weights of the three acids 63.04 g, 204.23 g and 389.92 g respectively, and the masses required for the standardization are 126.1 mg, 408.5 mg and 779.8 mg respectively. Given that the measurement uncertainty in the mass measured on a standard analytical balance is ±0.1 mg, the relative uncertainty in the mass of oxalic acid dihydrate would be about one part in a thousand, similar to the measurement uncertainty in the volume measurement in the titration.

However the measurement uncertainty in the mass of potassium hydrogen iodate would be five times lower, because its equivalent weight is five times higher: such an uncertainty in the measured mass is negligible in comparison to the uncertainty in the volume measured during the titration.

For sake of example, it shall be assumed that 22.45±0.03 cm^3 of the sodium hydroxide solution reacts with 781.4±0.1 mg of potassium hydrogen iodate. As the equivalent weight of potassium hydrogen iodate is 389.92 g, the measured mass is 2.004 milliequivalents. The concentration of the sodium hydroxide solution is therefore 2.004 meq/0.02245 l = 89.3 meq/l. In analytical chemistry, a solution of any substance which contains one equivalent per liter is known as a normal solution (abbreviated **N**), so the example sodium hydroxide solution would be 0.0893 N. The relative uncertainty (u_r) in the measured concentration can be estimated by assuming a Gaussian distribution of the measurement uncertainties:

$$u_r^2 = \left(\frac{u(V)}{V}\right)^2 + \left(\frac{u(m)}{m}\right)^2 = \left(\frac{0.03}{22.45}\right)^2 + \left(\frac{0.1}{781.4}\right)^2$$

$$= (0.001136)^2 + (0.000128)^2$$

$$\Rightarrow \qquad \underline{u}_r = 0.00134 \Rightarrow \underline{u}(c) = u_r C = 0.01 \text{ me/1}$$

This sodium hydroxide solution can be used to measure the equivalent weight of an unknown acid. For example, if it takes 13.20±0.03 cm^3 of the sodium hydroxide solution to neutralize 61.3±0.1 mg of an unknown acid, the equivalent weight of the acid is:

$$\text{equivalent weight} = \frac{m_{acid}}{c(NaOH)\,V_{eq}} = 52.0 \pm 0.1 \text{ g}$$

Because each mole of acid can only release an integer number of moles of hydrogen ions, the molar mass of the unknown acid must be an integer multiple of 52.0±0.1 g.

Use in Gravimetric Analysis

The term "equivalent weight" had a distinct sense in gravimetric analysis: it was the mass of precipitate which corresponds to one gram of analyte (the species of interest). The different definitions came from the practice of quoting gravimetric results as mass fractions of the analyte, often expressed as a percentage. A related term was the equivalence factor, one gram divided by equivalent weight, which was the numerical factor by which the mass of precipitate had to be multiplied to obtain the mass of analyte.

For example, in the gravimetric determination of nickel, the molar mass of the precipitate bis (dimethylglyoximate) nickel [Ni(dmgH)$_2$] is 288.915(7) g mol^{-1}, while the molar mass of nickel is 58.6934(2) g mol^{-1}: hence 288.915(7)/58.6934(2) = 4.9224(1) grams of [Ni(dmgH)$_2$] precipitate is equivalent to one gram of nickel and the equivalence factor is 0.203151(5). For example, 215.3±0.1 mg of [Ni(dmgH)$_2$] precipitate is equivalent to (215.3±0.1 mg) × 0.203151(5) = 43.74±0.2 mg of nickel: if the original sample size was 5.346±0.001 g, the nickel content in the original sample would be 0.8182±0.0004%.

Gravimetric analysis is one of the most precise of the common methods of chemical analysis, but it is time-consuming and labour-intensive. It has been largely superseded by other techniques such as atomic absorption spectroscopy, in which the mass of analyte is read off from a calibration curve.

Use in Polymer Chemistry

In polymer chemistry, the equivalent weight of a reactive polymer is the mass of polymer which has one equivalent of reactivity (often, the mass of polymer which corresponds to one mole of reactive side-chain groups). It is widely used to indicate the reactivity of polyol, isocyanate, or epoxy thermoset resins which would undergo cross linking reactions through those functional groups. It is particularly important for ion-exchange polymers (also called ion-exchange resins): one equivalent of an ion-exchange polymer will exchange one mole of singly charged ions, but only half a mole of doubly charged ions. Nevertheless, given the decline in use of the term "equivalent weight" in the rest of chemistry, it has become more usual to express the reactivity of a polymer as the inverse of the equivalent weight, which is in units of mmol/g or meq/g.

EQUIVALENT WEIGHT (EQUIV. WT.)

This is the weight of an acid or a base containing 1 mole of replaceable H^+ or OH^-, respectively, or the weight of a redox compound that contains 1 mole of exchangeable electrons, or the weight of an ionic substance carrying 1 mole of ions. Gram equivalent weight is used when equivalent weight is expressed in grams.

$$\text{Equiv. wt.} = \frac{\text{mol. wt.}}{n}$$

where n is the number of equivalents per mole (or the number of replaceable H+ or OH^-, exchangeable electrons or charge, per molecule or ion of the substance). When $n = 1$, then equiv. wt. = mol. wt.

Equivalent (equiv)

This is an operational term that defines the gram-equivalent weight of an acid, a base, an electron transferring substance, or an ion. One equivalent of a compound contains 1 g-equiv wt of the compound. The number of equivalents in a given weight of a substance is calculated using following equations and the weight containing a given number of equivalents is also calculated using below equation.

$$\text{equiv} = \frac{\text{wt(g)}}{\text{equiv wt (g)}}$$

$$\text{wt (g)} = \text{equiv} \times \text{equiv wt}$$

$$\text{mol wt} = \frac{\text{wt}}{\text{mol}} = \text{equiv wt} \times \text{n}$$

or

$$\frac{\text{wt}}{\text{equiv wt}} = \text{n} \times \text{mol}$$

$$\text{equiv} = \text{n} \times \text{mol}$$

Dalton (D)

This unit is used to report the molecular or atomic mass of substances; 1 Dalton is equal to 1 amu, or $^{1}/_{12}$ the mass of one atom of ^{12}C. Although the number of Daltons for a molecule is equivalent to the molecular weight, the Dalton is generally reversed for reporting the masses of macromolecular substances such as proteins.

1. NORMALITY OR NORMAL SOLUTION

In chemistry, the equivalent concentration or normality of a solution is defined as the molar concentration c_i divided by an equivalence factor f_{eq}:

$$\text{Normality} = \frac{C_i}{f_{eq}}$$

Unit Symbol N

The unit symbol "N" is used to denote "Eq/L" (Equivalent per liter) which is normality. Although losing favor, medical reporting of serum concentrations in "mEq/L" (=0.001 N) still occurs.

Usage

There are three common areas where normality is used as a measure of reactive species in solution:

In acid-base chemistry, normality is used to express the concentration of hydronium ions (H_3O^+) or hydroxide ions (OH^-) in a solution. Here, $1/f_{eq}$ is an integer value. Each solute can produce one or more equivalents of reactive species when dissolved.

In redox reactions, the equivalence factor describes the number of electrons that an oxidizing or reducing agent can accept or donate. Here, $1/f_{eq}$ can have a fractional (non-integer) value.

In precipitation reactions, the equivalence factor measures the number of ions which will precipitate in a given reaction. Here, $1/f_{eq}$ is an integer value.

Normal concentration of an ionic solution is intrinsically connected to the conductivity (electrolytic) through the equivalent conductivity.

Examples

Normality can be used for acid-base titrations. For example, sulfuric acid (H_2SO_4) is a diprotic acid. Since only 0.5 mol of H_2SO_4 are needed to neutralize 1 mol of OH^-, the equivalence factor is:

$$f_{eq}(H_2SO_4) = 0.5$$

If the concentration of a sulphuric acid solution is $c(H_2SO_4) = 1$ mol/L, then its normality is 2 N. It can also be called a "2 normal" solution.

Similarly, for a solution with $c(H_3PO_4) = 1$ mol/L, the normality is 3 N because phosphoric acid contains 3 acidic H atoms.

Criticism

Normality is an ambiguous measure of the concentration of a solution. It needs a definition of the equivalence factor, which depends on the definition of equivalents. The same solution can possess different normalities for different reactions. The definition of the equivalence factor varies depending on the type of chemical reaction that is discussed: It may refer to equations, bases, redox species, precipitating ions, or isotopes. For example, a solution of $MgCl_2$ that is 2 N with respect to a Cl^- ion, is only 1 N with respect to an Mg^{2+} ion. Since f_{eq} may not be unequivocal, IUPAC and NIST discourage the use of normality.

Solution:

1. a homogeneous mixture of one or more substances (solutes) dispersed molecularly in a sufficient quantity of dissolving medium (solvent).
2. in pharmacology, a liquid preparation of one or more soluble chemical substances, which are usually dissolved in water. For names of specific solutions, see under the name.
3. the process of dissolving or disrupting.
4. a loosening or separation.

Preparation of solutions: Formula for preparing solutions from a pure drug:

For example, to prepare 2000 mL of a 2 per cent solution from boric acid crystals, the proportion would be

Formula for preparing solutions from stock solutions:

For example, to prepare 1000 mL of a 2 per cent solution from a 4 per cent stock solution, the proportion would be aqueous solution one in which water is used as the solvent.

BCG solution an aqueous suspension of BACILLE CALMETTE- GUÉRIN for instillation into the bladder to activate the IMMUNE SYSTEM in treatment of superficial bladder cancers. It reduces the risk of a subsequent bladder cancer developing, although the exact mechanism of action isunknown.

Buffer solution one that resists appreciable change in its hydrogen ion concentration (pH) when acid or alkali is added to it.

Colloid solution (colloidal solution) imprecise term for colloid.

Hyperbaric solution one having a greater specific gravity than a standard of reference.

Hypertonic solution one having an osmotic pressure greater than that of a standard of reference.

Hypobaric solution one having a specific gravity less than that of a standard of reference.

Hypotonic solution one having an osmotic pressure less than that of a standard of reference.

Isobaric solution a solution having the same specific gravity as a standard of reference.

Isotonic solution one having an osmotic pressure the same as that of a standard of reference.

Molar solution a solution in which each liter contains 1 mole of the dissolved substance; designated 1 M. The concentration of othersolutions may be expressed in relation to that of molar solutions as tenth-molar (0.1 M), etc.

Normal solution a solution in which each liter contains 1 equivalent weight of the dissolved substance; designated 1 N.

Ophthalmic solution a sterile solution, free from foreign particles, for instillation into the eye.

Saturated solution one in which the solvent has taken up all of the dissolved substance that it can hold in solution.

Sclerosing solution one containing an irritant substance (sclerosing agent) that will cause obliteration of a space, as in Sclerotherapy.

Standard solution one that contains in each liter a definitely stated amount of reagent; usually expressed in terms of normality (equivalent weights of solute per liter of solution) or molarity (moles of solute per liter of solution).

Supersaturated solution an unstable solution containing more of the solute than it can permanently hold.

Volumetric solution one that contains a specific quantity of solvent per stated unit of volume.

Solution

1. a liquid preparation of one or more soluble chemical substances usually dissolved in water.
2. the process of dissolving or disrupting.

Aqueous solution: One in which water is used as the solvent.

Buffer solution: One that resists appreciable change in its hydrogen ion concentration (pH) when acid or alkali is added to it.

Colloid solution, colloidal solution: A preparation consisting of minute particles of matter suspended in a solvent.

Hyperbaric solution: One having a greater specific gravity than a standard of reference.

Hypertonic solution: One having an osmotic pressure greater than that of a standard of reference.

Hypobaric solution: One having a specific gravity less than that of a standard of reference.

Hypotonic solution: One having an osmotic pressure less than that of a standard of reference.

Iodine solution:A transparent, reddish brown liquid, each 100 ml of which contains 1.8 to 2.2 g of iodine and 2.1 to 2.6 g of sodium iodide; a localanti-infective.

Iodine solution (strong): Lugol's solution.

Isobaric solution: A solution having the same specific gravity as a standard of reference.

Isotonic solution: One having an osmotic pressure the same as that of a standard of reference.

Molar solution: A solution eachliter of which contains 1 mole of the dissolved csubstance; designated 1 M. The concentration of other solutions maybe expressed in relation to that of molar solutions as tenth-molar (0.1 M), etc.

Normal solution: A solution each liter of which contains 1 chemical equivalent of the dissolved substance; designated 1 N.

Ophthalmic solution: A sterile solution, free from foreign particles, for instillation into the eye.

Physiological saline solution, physiological salt solution, physiological sodium chloride solution: An aqueousolution of sodium chloride and other components, having an osmotic pressure identical to that of blood serum.

Priming solution: The fluid used to fill tubing and the reservoir of a cardiac bypass unit before use.

Saline solution: A solution of sodium chloride, or common salt, in purified water.

Saturated solution: A solution in which the solvent has taken up all of the dissolved substance that it can hold in solution.

Sclerosing solution: One containing an irritant substance that will cause obliteration of a space, such as the lumen of a varicose vein or the cavity of ahernial sac.

Standard solution: One containing a fixed amount of solute.

Supersaturated solution: One containing a greater quantity of the solute than the solvent can hold in solution under ordinary conditions.

Volumetric solution: One that contains a specific quantity of solvent per stated unit of volume.

2. MOLAR CONCENTRATION (MOLARITIES)

Molar concentration, also called molarity, amount concentration or substance concentration, is a measure of the concentration of a solute in a solution, or of any chemical species in terms of amount of substance in a given volume. A commonly used unit for molar concentration used in chemistry is mol/L. A solution of concentration 1 mol/L is also denoted as *1 molar* (1 M).

Definition

Molar concentration or molarity is most commonly expressed in units of moles of solute per liter of solution. For use in broader applications, it is defined as amount of solute per unit volume of solution, or per unit volume available to the species, represented by lowercase *c*:

$$c = \frac{n}{V} = \frac{N}{N_A V} = \frac{C}{N_A}$$

Here, *n* is the amount of the solute in moles, *N* is the number of molecules present in the volume *V* (in liters), the ratio *N*/*V* is the number concentration *C*, and N_A is the Avogadro constant, approximately 6.022×10^{23} mol^{-1}. Or more simply: 1 molar = 1 M = 1 mole/liter.

In thermodynamics the use of molar concentration is often not convenient, because the volume of most solutions slightly depends on temperature due to thermal expansion. This problem is usually resolved by introducing temperature correction factors, or by using a temperature-independent measure of concentration such as molality.

The reciprocal quantity represents the dilution (volume) which can appear in Ostwald's law of dilution.

Units

In the International System of Units (SI) the base unit for molar concentration is mol/m^3. However, this is impractical for most laboratory purposes and most chemical literature traditionally uses mol/dm^3, or mol dm^{-3}, which is the same as mol/L. These traditional units are often denoted by a capital letter M (pronounced *molar*), sometimes preceded by anSI prefix to denote sub-multiples, for example:

mol/m^3 = 10^{-3} mol/dm^3 = 10^{-3} mol/L = 10^{-3} M = 1 mmol/L = 1 mM.

The words "millimolar" and "micromolar" refer to mM and μM (10^{-3} mol/L and 10^{-6} mol/L), respectively.

Name	Abbreviation	Concentration	Concentration (SI unit)
millimolar	mM	10^{-3} mol/dm^3	10^{0} mol/m^3
micromolar	μM	10^{-6} mol/dm^3	10^{-3} mol/m^3
nanomolar	nM	10^{-9} mol/dm^3	10^{-6} mol/m^3
picomolar	pM	10^{-12} mol/dm^3	10^{-9} mol/m^3
femtomolar	fM	10^{-15} mol/dm^3	10^{-12} mol/m^3
attomolar	aM	10^{-18} mol/dm^3	10^{-15} mol/m^3
zeptomolar	zM	10^{-21} mol/dm^3	10^{-18} mol/m^3
yoctomolar	yM	10^{-24} mol/dm^3 (1 particle per 1.6 L)	10^{-21} mol/m^3

Related Quantities

Number concentration

The conversion to number concentration C_i is given by:

$$C_i = c_i \cdot N_A$$

where N_A is the Avogadro constant, approximately 6.022×10^{23} mol^{-1}.

Mass concentration

The conversion to mass concentration ρ_i is given by:

$$\rho_i = c_i \cdot M_i$$

where M_i is the molar mass of constituent i.

Mole fraction

The conversion to mole fraction x_i is given by:

$$x_i = c_i \cdot \frac{M}{\rho} = c_i \cdot \frac{\Sigma x_i M_i}{\rho}$$

$$x_i = c_i \cdot \frac{\Sigma x_j M_j}{\rho - c_i M_i}$$

Where M the average molar mass of the solution is, ρ is the density of the solution and j is the index of other solutes.

A simpler relation can be obtained by considering the total molar concentration namely the sum of molar concentrations of all the components of the mixture.

$$x_i = \frac{c_i}{c} = \frac{c_i}{\Sigma c_i}$$

Mass fraction

The conversion to mass fraction w_i is given by:

$$w_i = c_i \cdot \frac{M_i}{\rho}$$

Molality

The conversion to molality (for binary mixtures) is:

$$b_2 = \frac{c_2}{\rho - \Sigma c_i \cdot M_i}$$

where the solute is assigned the subscript 2.

For solutions with more than one solute, the conversion is:

$$b_i = \frac{c_i}{\rho - \Sigma c_i \cdot M_i}$$

Properties

Sum of molar concentrations – normalizing relations

The sum of molar concentrations gives the total molar concentration, namely the density of the mixture divided by the molar mass of the mixture or by another name the reciprocal of the molar volume of the mixture. In an ionic solution, ionic strength is proportional to the sum of molar concentration of salts.

Sum of products molar concentrations-partial molar volumes

The sum of products between these quantities equals one.

$$\sum_i c_i \cdot \overline{V}_i = 1$$

Dependence on Volume

Molar concentration depends on the variation of the volume of the solution due mainly to thermal expansion. On small intervals of temperature the dependence is:

$$c_i = \frac{c_i, T_0}{(1 + \alpha \cdot \Delta T)}$$

where $c_{i,} T_0$ is the molar concentration at a reference temperature, α is the thermal expansion coefficient of the mixture.

Spatial Variation and Diffusion

Molar and mass concentrations have different values in space where diffusion happens.

Molarity is moles per liter of solution.

$$M = \frac{\text{moles}}{\text{liter}}$$

We use Normality when discussing solutions especially acids and bases.

$$\underset{\text{acid}}{HCl} + \underset{\text{base}}{Na(OH)} \longrightarrow \underset{\text{salt}}{NaCl} + \underset{\text{water}}{HOH}$$

If I had 100 milliliters of a 1 M HCl acid, how many moles of H^+ would I have?

If I had 100 milliliters of a 1 M Na(OH), how many moles of $(OH)^-$ would I have?

Let's look at $H_2(SO_4)$

$$H_2(SO_4) \longrightarrow 2\ H^+ + 1\ (SO_4)^=$$

Each molecule of $H_2(SO_4)$ would give 2 H^+ and 1 $(SO_4)^=$

If I had 100 mL of a 1 M $H_2(SO_4)$

I would have 0.10 moles of $H_2(SO_4)$

I would have 0.10 moles of $(SO_4)^=$

I would have 0.20 moles of H^+ Why? 1 mole of $H_2(SO_4)$ has 2 moles of H^+

1 liter of a 1 M Na(OH) would have 1 mole of $(OH)^-$

l liter of a 1 M $H_2(SO_4)$ would have 2 moles of H^+

If I mixed 1 L of 1 M Na(OH) with 1 L of 1 M $H_2(SO_4)$ I would have an acid solution. Why?

I have 2 times as much H^+'s as I have $(OH)^-$'s.

1 liter of 1 M NaOH has 1 mole of Na and 1 mole of $(OH)^-$

1 liter of 1 M $H_2(SO_4)$ has 1 mole of (SO_4) and 2 moles of H^+

When using acids and bases we use Normality (N) instead of Molarity (M).

1 M HCl = 1 N HCl

1 M $H_2(SO_4)$ = 2 N $H_2(SO_4)$

1 M $H_3(PO_4)$ = __ N $H_3(PO_4)$

$H_2(SO_4) + 2\ Na(OH) \longrightarrow Na_2(SO_4) + 2\ HOH$

If I had 100 milliliters of a 1 M $H_2(SO_4)$, how many moles of H^+ would I have?

a 1 M $H_2(SO_4)$ solution is a 2 N $H_2(SO_4)$

for every mole of sulfuric acid, you would get 2 moles of H^+

1 M $Ca(OH)_2$ = _____ N $Ca(OH)_2$

For every mole of calcium hydroxide, would get 2 moles of hydroxide ions.

HCl has only 1 hydrogen

H_2SO_4 has 2 hydrogens

a 1 M HCl is a 1 N HCl

a 1 M H_2SO_4 is 2 N H_2SO_4

Examples

What is the normality of 3 M $H_2(SO_4)$?

$$1\ M\ H_2(SO_4) = 2\ N\ H_2(SO_4)$$
$$3\ M\ H_2(SO_4) = \times\ N\ H_2(SO_4)$$
$$1 = 2 \text{ criss cross multiply}$$
$$3 \times x = 6$$

What is the molarity of 6 N $H_3(PO_4)$?

$$1\ M\ H_3(PO_4) = 3\ N\ H_3(PO_4)$$
$$x = 6\ N\ H_3(PO_4)$$
$$1 = 3 \times 6x = 2.$$

Examples

Example 1: Consider 11.6 g of NaCl dissolved in 100 g of water. The final mass concentration ρ (NaCl) will be:

$$\rho(NaCl) = 11.6\ g / (11.6\ g + 100\ g) = 0.104\ g/g = 10.4\ \%$$

The density of such a solution is 1.07 g/mL, thus its volume will be:

$$V = (11.6\ g + 100\ g) / (1.07\ g/mL) = 104.3\ mL$$

The molar concentration of NaCl in the solution is therefore:

$$c(NaCl) = (11.6\ g / 58\ g/mol) / 104.3\ mL$$
$$= 0.00192\ mol/mL = 1.92\ mol/L$$

Here, 58 g/mol is the molar mass of NaCl.

Example 2: Another typical task in chemistry is the preparation of 100 mL (= 0.1 L) of a 2 mol/L solution of NaCl in water. The mass of salt needed is:

$$m(NaCl) = 2\ mol/L \times 0.1\ L \times 58\ g/mol = 11.6\ g$$

To create the solution, 11.6 g NaCl are placed in a volumetric flask, dissolved in some water, and then followed by the addition of more water until the total volume reaches 100 mL.

Example 3: The density of water is approximately 1000 g/L and its molar mass is 18.02 g/mol (or 1/18.02=0.055 mol/g). Therefore, the molar concentration of water is:

$$c(H_2O) = 1000 \text{ g/L} / (18.02 \text{ g/mol}) = 55.5 \text{ mol/L}$$

Likewise, the concentration of solid hydrogen (molar mass = 2.02 g/mol) is:

$$c(H_2) = 88 \text{ g/L} / (2.02 \text{ g/mol}) = 43.7 \text{ mol/L}$$

The concentration of pure osmium tetroxide (molar mass = 254.23 g/mol) is:

$$c(OsO_4) = 5.1 \text{ kg/L} / (254.23 \text{ g/mol}) = 20.1 \text{ mol/L}.$$

Example 4: A typical protein in bacteria, such as *E. coli*, may have about 60 copies, and the volume of a bacterium is about 10^{-15} L. Thus, the number concentration C is:

$$C = 60 / (10^{-15} \text{ L}) = 6\times10^{16} \text{ L}^{-1}$$

The molar concentration is:

$$c = C/N_A = 6\times10^{16} \text{ L}^{-1} / (6\times10^{23} \text{ mol}^{-1}) = 10^{-7} \text{ mol/L} = 100 \text{ nmol/L}.$$

Formal Concentration

If the concentration refers to original chemical formula in solution, the molar concentration is sometimes called formal concentration. For example, if a sodium carbonate solution has a formal concentration of $c(Na_2CO_3)$ = 1 mol/L, the molar concentrations are $c(Na^+)$ = 2 mol/L and $c(CO_3^{2-})$ = 1 mol/L because the salt dissociates into these ions.

The equations will be uses are:

M = moles of solute / liters of solution and MV = grams / molar mass <--- The volume here must be in liters.

Typically, the solution is for the molarity (M). However, sometimes it is not, so be aware of that. A teacher might teach problems where the molarity is calculated but ask for the volume on a test question.

Note: Make sure you pay close attention to multiply and divide. For example, look at answer #8. Note that the 58.443 is in the denominator on the right side and you generate the final answer by doing 0.200 times 0.100 times 58.443.

Problem 1: Sea water contains roughly 28.0 g of NaCl per liter. What is the molarity of sodium chloride in sea water?

Solution:

$$MV = \text{grams} / \text{molar mass}$$

$$(x)\,(1.00\text{ L}) = 28.0\text{ g} / 58.443\text{ g mol}^{-1}$$

$$x = 0.4790993\text{ M to three significant figures, } 0.479\text{ M.}$$

Problem 2: What is the molarity of 245.0 g of H_2SO_4 dissolved in 1.000 L of solution?

Solution:

$$MV = \text{grams} / \text{molar mass}$$

$$(x)\,(1.000\text{ L}) = 245.0\text{ g} / 98.0768\text{ g mol}^{-1}$$

$$x = 2.49804235\text{ M}$$

to four sig figs, 2.498 M

If the volume had been specified as 1.00 L (as it often is in problems like this), the answer would have been 2.50 M, NOT 2.5 M. You want three sig figs in the answer and 2.5 is only two SF.

Problem 3: What is the molarity of 5.30 g of Na_2CO_3 dissolved in 400.0 mL solution?

Solution:

$$MV = \text{grams} / \text{molar mass}$$

$$(x)\,(0.4000\text{ L}) = 5.30\text{ g} / 105.988\text{ g mol}^{-1}\ 0.12501415\text{ M}$$

$$x = 0.125\text{ M (to three sig figs).}$$

Problem 4: What is the molarity of 5.00 g of NaOH in 750.0 mL of solution?

Solution:

$$MV = \text{grams} / \text{molar mass}$$

$$(x)\,(0.7500\text{ L}) = 5.00\text{ g} / 39.9969\text{ g mol}^{-1}$$

$$(x)\,(0.7500\text{ L}) = 0.1250097\text{ mol} \text{ <--- threw in an extra step}$$

$$x = 0.1666796\text{ M}$$

$$x = 0.167\text{ M (to three SF).}$$

Problem 5: How many moles of Na_2CO_3 are there in 10.0 L of 2.00 M solution?

Solution:

$$M = \text{moles of solute} / \text{liters of solution}$$

$$2.00\text{ M} = x / 10.0\text{ L}$$

$$x = 20.0\text{ mol}$$

Suppose the molarity was listed as 2.0 M (two sig figs). How to display the answer? Like this: 20. mol.

Problem 6: .How many moles of Na_2CO_3 are in 10.0 mL of a 2.0 M solution?

Solution:

M = moles of solute / liters of solution

2.0 M = x / 0.0100 L <--- note the conversion of mL to L

x = 0.020 mol

Problem 7: How many moles of NaCl are contained in 100.0 mL of a 0.200 M solution?

Solution:

0.200 M = x / 0.1000 L

x = 0.0200 mol.

Problem 8: What weight (in grams) of NaCl would be contained in problem #7?

Solution:

(0.200 mol L^{-1}) (0.100 L) = x / 58.443 g mol^{-1} <--- this is the full set up

x = 1.17 g (to three SF)

You could have done this as well:

58.443 g/mol times 0.0200 mol <--- this is based on knowing the answer from problem #7.

Problem 9: What weight (in grams) of H_2SO_4 would be needed to make 750.0 mL of 2.00 M solution?

Solution:

(2.00 mol L^{-1}) (0.7500 L) = x / 98.0768 g mol^{-1}

x = (2.00 mol L^{-1}) (0.7500 L) (98.0768 g mol^{-1})

x = 147.1152 g to three sig figs, 147 g.

Problem 10: What volume (in mL) of 18.0 M H_2SO_4 is needed to contain 2.45 g H_2SO_4?

Solution:

(18.0 mol L^{-1}) (x) = 2.45 g / 98.0768 g mol^{-1}

(18.0 mol L^{-1}) (x) = 0.0249804235 mol

x = 0.0013878 L

The above is the answer in liters. Multiplying the answer by 1000 provides the required mL value:

0.0013878 L times (1000 mL / L) = 1.39 mL (given to three sig figs).

Problem 11: Phosphoric acid is usually obtained as an 87.0% phosphoric acid solution. If it is 13.0 M, what is the density of this solution? What is its molality?

Solution for density:

1) Determine the moles of H_3PO_4 in 100.0 grams of 87.0% solution:

   87.0 g of the 100.0 g is H_3PO_4

   moles H_3PO_4 = 87.0 g / 97.9937 g/mol = 0.8878 mol

2) Calculate the volume of 13.0 M solution which contains 0.8878 mol of H_3PO_4:

   13.0 mol/L = 0.8878 mol / x

   x = 0.0683 L = 68.3 mL

3) Determine the density of the solution:

   100.0 g / 68.3 mL = 1.464 g/mL = 1.46 g/mL (to three sig fig)

Solution for molality:

1) Let us assume 100.0 grams of solution. Therefore:

   87.0 g is H_3PO_4 13.0 g is H_2O

2) Calculate the molality:

   moles H_3PO_4 = 87.0 g / 97.9937 g/mol = 0.8878 mol kg of water = 0.0130 kg

   molality = 0.8878 mol / 0.0130 kg = 68.3 molal.

Problem 12: Concentrated hydrochloric acid is usually available at a concentration of 37.7% by mass. What is its molar concentration? (The density of the solution is 1.19 g/mL.)

Solution Path 1:

1) Determine moles of HCl in 100.0 g of 37.7% solution:

   37.7 g of this solution is HCl

   37.7 g / 36.4609 g/mol = 1.03398435 mol

2) Determine volume of 100.0 g of solution:

   density = mass / volume

   1.19 g/mL = 100.0 g / x

   x = 84.0336 mL

3) Determine molarity:

   1.03398435 mol / 0.0840336 L = 12.3 M.

Solution Path 2:

1) Assume 1.00 L of solution. Use density to get mass:

   1.19 g/mL = x / 1000 mL

   x = 1190 g

2) (a) Use percent mass to get mass of HCl, then (b) convert to moles:

   1190 g times 0.377 = 448.63 g

   448.63 g / 36.4609 g/mol = 12.3 mol

3) Determine molarity:

   12.3 mol / 1.00 L = 12.3 M.

Problem 13: I have a bottle of NH_3. Its strength is 32.0% and its density is 0.89 g/mL. How do I figure out the molarity?

Solution:

1) Assume 100.0 g of solution is present. Calculate moles of ammonia present:

   32.0 grams of NH_3 are present.

   32.0 g / 17.0307 g/mol = 1.879 mol

2) Determine volume of 100.0 g of solution:

   100.0 g / 0.87 g/mL = 112.36 mL

3) Calculate molarity:

   1.879 mol / 0.11236 L = 16.7 M.

Problem 14: An aqueous solution of hydrofluoric acid is 30.0% HF, by mass, and has a density of 1.101 g cm^{-3}. What are the molality and molarity of HF in this solution?

Solution for molality:

1) Let us assume 100.0 grams of solution. Therefore:

   30.0 g is HF

   70.0 g is H_2O

2) Calculate the molality:

   moles HF = 30.0 g / 20.0059 g/mol = 1.49956 mol kg of water = 0.0700 kg

   molality = 1.49956 mol / 0.0700 kg = 21.4 molal.

Solution for molarity:

1) Determine moles of HF in 100.0 g of 30.0% solution:

   30.0 g of this solution is HF

   30.0 g / 20.0059 g/mol = 1.49956 mol

2) Determine volume of 100.0 g of solution:

   density = mass / volume

   1.101 g/mL = 100.0 g / x

   x = 90.8265 mL

3) Determine molarity:

   1.49956 mol / 0.0908265 L = 16.5 M.

Problem 15: Concentrated nitric acid is a solution that is 70.4% HNO_3 by mass. The density of this acid is 1.42 g/mL. What is the molarity and the molality of the acid?

Solution for molarity:

1) Determine moles of HNO_3 in 100.0 g of 70.4% solution:

   70.4 g of this solution is HNO_3

   70.4 g / 63.0119 g/mol = 1.11725 mol

2) Determine volume of 100.0 g of solution:

   density = mass / volume

   1.42 g/mL = 100.0 g / x

   x = 70.422535 mL

3) Determine molarity:

   1.11725 mol / 0.070422535 L = 15.86 M = 15.9 M (to three sf)

Solution for molality:

1) Let us assume 100.0 grams of solution. Therefore:

   70.4 g is HNO_3

   29.6 g is H_2O

2) Calculate the molality:

   moles HNO_3 = 70.4 g / 63.0119 g/mol = 1.11725

   mol kg of water = 0.0296 kg

   molality = 1.11725 mol / 0.0296 kg = 37.7 molal

Special bonus part to Problem 15: In the above solution, what is the mole fraction of HNO_3?

Solution:

1) Let us assume 100.0 grams of solution. Therefore:

   70.4 g is HNO_3 29.6 g is H_2O

2) Determine the moles of each substance:

   HNO_3 = 1.11725 mol H_2O = 29.6 g / 18.0152 g/mol = 1.643057 mol

3) Determine the mole fraction of HNO_3:

   1.11725 mol / (1.11725 mol + 1.643057 mol) = 0.405.

Problem 16: The density of toluene (C_7H_8) is 0.867 g/mL, and the density of thiophene (C_4H_4S) is 1.065 g/mL. A solution is made by dissolving 9.660 g of thiophene in 260.0 mL of toluene.

a) Calculate the molality of thiophene in the solution.

b) Assuming that the volumes of the solute and solvent are additive, determine the molarity of thiophene in the solution.

Solution to part a:

1) Determine the moles of thiophene:
   9.660 g / 84.142 g/mol = 0.1148 mol
2) Determine mass of toluene in 260.0 mL.
   260.0 mL × 0.867 g/mL = 225.42 g
3) Calculate the molality:
   0.1148 mol / 0.22542 kg = 0.509 molal

Solution to part b:

1) Determine volume of thiophene:
   9.660 g ÷ 1.065 g/mL = 9.07 mL
2) Determine total volume:
   260.0 mL + 9.07 mL = 269.07 mL
3) Calculate molarity:
   0.1148 mol / 0.26907 L = 0.427 M.

Problem 17: An aqueous acetic acid solution is simultaneously 6.0835 molar and 8.9660 molal. Compute the density of this solution.

Solution:

1) Use molality to get moles:
   8.9660 molal = × moles / 1.00 kg solvent
   x = 8.9660 moles
2) Compute the mass of the above solution:
   1000 g solvent + (8.9660 moles × 60.05 g/mol) = 1538.41 g
3) Use molarity to get the volume of solution containing 8.9660 moles
   6.0835 mol/L = 8.9660 moles / x
   x = 1.47382 L
4) Compute the density:
   1538.41 g / 1473.82 mL = 1.0438 g/mL.

Problem 18: What is the density (in g/mL) of a 3.60 M aqueous sulfuric acid solution that is 29.0% H_2SO_4 by mass?

Solution:

1) Assume 100.0 g of solution is present.
2) Detemine the volume of solution that weighs 100.0 g:
   29.0 g of the 100.0 g is H_2SO_4.
   use MV = grams / molar mass to determine the volume.
   (3.60 mol/L) (x) = 29.0 g / 98.1 g/mol
   x = 0.0821 L

3) Determine the density:

   100.0 g / 82.1 mL = 1.22 g/mL.

Problem 19: The density of an aqueous solution of nitric acid is 1.430 g/mL. If this solution contained 36.00% nitric acid by mass, how many mL of the solution would be needed to supply 150.20 grams of nitric acid?

Solution path 1:

1) 1.000 mL of solution weight 1.430 g, of which 36.00% is HNO_3
2) 1.430 × 0.3600 tells you the grams of HNO_3 in each mL of solution.
3) 150.20 g divided by the grams of HNO_3 per one mL of solution.

Solution path 2:

1) Determine how many mL of the solution you need:

   150.20 g nitric acid × (1 g solution/0.3600 g nitric acid) = 417.2 g solution.

2) Determine the volume of solution that weighs 417.2 g:

   417.2 g solution × (1 mL/1.430 g solution)

Problem 20: A bottle of commercial sulfuric acid (density 1.787 g/cc) is labeled as 86% by weight. What is the molarity of acid?

Solution:

1) Determine moles of H_2SO_4 in 100.0 g of 86% solution:

   86 g of this solution is H_2SO_4

   86 g / 98.08 g/mol = 0.876835237 mol

2) Determine volume of 100.0 g of solution:

   density = mass / volume

   1.787 g/mL = 100.0 g / x

   x = 55.96 mL

3) Determine molarity:

   0.876835237 mol / 0.05596 L = 15.67 M = 15.7 M (to three sf)

Note: Try this problem with 96.0% and a density of 1.84 g/mL. The answer is 18.0 M.

Problem 21: Calculate the molarity and mole fraction of acetone in a 2.28-molal solution of acetone (CH_3COCH_3) in ethanol (C_2H_5OH). (Density of acetone = 0.788 g/cm^3; density of ethanol = 0.789 g/cm^3.) Assume that the volumes of acetone and ethanol add.

Solution for molarity:

Remember, 2.28-molal means 2.28 moles of acetone in 1.00 kilogram of ethanol.

1) Determine volumes of acetone and ethanol, then total volume:

   acetone

2.28 mol × 58.0794 g/mol = 132.421 g

132.421 g divided by 0.788 g/cm^3 = 168.047 cm^3

ethanol

1000 g divided by 0.789 g/cm^3 = 1267.427 cm^3

total volume

168.047 + 1267.427 = 1435.474 cm^3

2) Determine molarity:

2.28 mol / 1.435 L = 1.59 M

Solution for mole fraction:

1) Determine moles of ethanol:

1000 g / 46.0684 g/mol = 21.71 mol

2) Determine mole fraction of acetone:

2.28 / (2.28 + 21.71) = 0.0950.

Problem 22.: Calculate the normality of a 4.0 molal sulfuric acid solution with a density of 1.2 g/mL.

Reminders:

N = #equivalents / L solution

#equivalents = molecular weight / n (n = number of H^+ or OH^- released per dissociation.)

molal = moles solute / kg solvent

Solution:

1) Determine grams of H_2SO_4 present:

4.0 molal = 4.0 moles H_2SO_4 / 1000 g solution

4.0 mol times 98.09 g/mol = 392.32 g

2) Determine equivalent weight for H_2SO_4:

98.09 g/mol / 2 dissociable hydrogen/mol = 49.05 g/equivalent

3) Determine # equivalents in 392.32 g:

392.32 g times (1 equivalent / 49.05 g) = 8.0 equivalents

4) Determine volume of solution:

392.32 g + 1000 g = 1392.32 g (total mass of solution)

1392.32 g / 1.2 g/mL = 1160.27 mL

5) Determine normality:

N = 8.0 equivalents / 1.16027 L = 6.9 N.

Problem 23: An car antifreeze mixture is made by mixing equal volumes of ethylene glycol (d = 1.114 g/mL, molar mass 62.07 g/mol) and water (d = 1.000 g/mL) at 20.0 °C. The density of the solution is 1.070 g/mL.

Express the concentration of ethylene glycol as:

(a) volume percent
(b) mass percent
(c) molarity
(d) molality
(e) mole fraction

Solution to (a):

Since the volumes are equal, the volume percent of ethylene glycol is 50%

Solution to (b):

1) Determine the masses of equal volumes (we'll use 50.0 mL) of the two substances: ethylene glycol: (50.0 mL) (1.114 g/mL) = 55.7 g water: (50.0 mL) (1.000 g/mL) = 50.0 g
2) Determine percent due to ethylene glycol:

   55.7 g / 105.7 g = 52.7%.

Solution to (c):

1) Determine moles of ethylene glycol:

   55.7 g / 62.07 g/mol = 0.89737 mol
2) Determine volume of solution:

   105.7 g / 1.070 g/mL = 98.785 mL
3) Determine molarity:

   0.89737 mol / 0.098785 L = 9.08 M.

Solution to (d):

0.89737 mol / 0.050 kg = 17.9 m

Note the large difference between the molarity and the molality.

Solution to (e):

1) Determine moles of water:

   50.0 g / 18.0 g/mol = 2.77778
2) Determine mole fraction for ethylene glycol:

   0.89737 mol / 3.67515 mol = 0.244.

Problem 24: What is the percent of CsCl by mass in a 0.0711 M CsCl solution that has a density of 1.09 g/mL?

Solution:

1) Determine mass of dissolved CsCl:

   Let us assume 100.0 mL of solution.

   MV = grams / molar mass

   (0.0711 mol/L) (0.100 L) = x / 168.363 g/mol

   x = 1.197 g.

2) Determine mass of solution:

   1.09 g/mL times 100.0 mL = 109 g

   Determine mass percent of CsCl in solution:

   1.197 g / 109 g = 1.098%

   to three sig figs: 1.10%.

Problem 25: A 8.77 M solution of an acid, HX, has a density of 0.853 g/mL.The acid, HX, has a molar mass of 31.00 g/mol. Determine the molal concentration of this solution, X_{HX} (mole fraction of HX), and % w/w (percent by mass). The solvent in this solution is water, H_2O.

Comment: Can an 8.77 M solution of an acid have a density of 0.853 g/mL? Who cares? We'll just solve the problem.

Solution:

There is a trick to solving this type of problem: let us assume 1.00 L (or 1000 mL) of the solution is present. (Another place where a similar trick is employed is in determining empirical formulas, where you assume 100 g of the substance is present.)

1) Some preliminary calculations:

   moles acid: 1.00 L × (8.77 moles / L) = 8.77 moles HX (used in molality and mole fraction)

   mass acid: 8.77 moles × 31.00 g / mole = 272 g HX (percent by mass)

   mass of solution: 1000 mL × 0.853 g / mL = 853 g solution (percent by mass)

   mass of solvent: 853 g minus 272 g = 581 g = 0.581 kg (molality)

   moles solvent: 581 g divided by 18.015 g) = 32.25 (mole fraction)

2) Calculations to answer the questions:

   molality = 8.77 moles / 0.581 kg = 15.1m

   mole fraction = 8.77 / (8.77 + 32.25) = 0.214

   % w/w = (272 g / 853 g) × 100 = 31.9%

Problem 26: A solution of hydrogen peroxide, H_2O_2, is 30.0% by mass and has a density of 1.11 g/cm^3. Calculate the (a) molality, (b) molarity, and (c) mole fraction

Solution:

1) Mass of 1 liter of solution:

   1.11 g/cm^3 times (1000 cm^3 / L) = 1110 g/L

2) Mass of the two components of the solution:

   mass of H_2O_2 ---> 30.0% of 1110 g = 333 g mass of H_2O ---> 70.0% of 1110 g = 777 g

3) Moles of hydrogen peroxide:

   333 g / 34.0138 g/mol = 9.79 mol

4) Molality:

   9.79 mol / 0.777 kg = 12.6 m

5) Molarity

   9.79 mol / 1.00 L = 9.79 M

6) Mole fraction

   mole of H_2O_2 = 9.79 mole of H_2O = 43.13

   total moles ---> 9.79 + 43.13 = 52.92

   mole fraction ---> 9.79 / 52.92 = 0.185

Problem 27: Household hydrogen peroxide is an aqueous solution containing 3.0% hydrogen peroxide by mass. What is the molarity of this solution? (Assume a density of 1.01 g/mL.)

Solution:

1) Let us have 1000 g of solution on hand. For the volume of solution:

   1000 g divided by 1.01 g/mL = 990.1 mL

2) Since H_2O_2 is 3% by mass, we know that there are 30 g of H_2O_2 present in the 1000 g of solution.

   MV = mass / molar mass

   (x) (0.9901 L) = 30 g / 34.0138 g/mol

   x = 0.890814 M

   Two sig figs seems reasonable, so 0.89 M.

Problem 28: A 6.90 M KOH solution in water has 30% by weight KOH. Calculate the density of the KOH solution.

Solution:

Let us assume we have 1.00 liter of solution present. This means we have 6.90 mol of KOH. Let us determine the mass of KOH:

6.90 mol times 56.1049 g/mol = 387.124 g

387.124 g represents 30% of the total weight of the solution. (The water makes up the other 70%.) To get the mass of the solution, do this:

387.124 g is to 0.3 as × is to 1

x = 1290 g

density of the solution ---> 1290 g / 1000 mL = 1.29 g/mL.

Problem 29: An aqueous NaCl solution is made using 138 g of NaCl diluted to a total solution volume of 1.30 L.

(A) Calculate the molarity of the solution.

(B) Calculate the molality of the solution.(Assume a density of 1.08 g/mL for the solution.)

(C) Calculate the mass percent of the solution. (Assume a density of 1.08 g/mL for the solution.)

Solution:

Part A:

MV = mass / molar mass

(x) (1.30 L) = 138 g / 58.443 g/mol

x = 1.82 M

Part B:

molality is moles solute per kg of solvent. I will use 2.3613 mol (keeping a few guard digits).

Let us assume 1000 mL of the solution is present. This tells us that 2.3613 mol of the solute is present (that's the 138 g of NaCl).

1.08 g/mL times 1000 mL = 1080 g <--- this is the total mass of the 1000 mL solution

1080 g minus 138 g = 942 g <--- the mass of water in the 1000 mL of solution

942 g = 0.942 kg

2.3613 mol / 0.942 kg = 2.51 m

Part C:

138 g of solute was dissolved in 1080 total grams of solution

(138 / 1080) times 100 = 12.8% <--- NaCl

100% minus 12.8% = 87.2% <--- H_2O

Another type of question is this area is to ask you to determine the mole fraction for each substance. For that you will need to know the moles of water:

942 g / 18.015 g/mol = 52.29 mol

The mole fraction of NaCl is this:

2.3613 mol / (2.3613 mol + 52.29 mol) = 0.0432

The mole fraction of the water is this:

1 - 0.0432 = 0.9568.

Problem 30: A solution is prepared by dissolving 28.0 g of glucose ($C_6H_{12}O_6$) in 350 g of water. The final volume of the solution is 384 mL . For this solution, calculate each of the following:

1) molarity; 2) molality; 3) percent by mass; 4) mole fraction; 5) mole percent

Solution:

1) Molarity is the number of moles divided by volume of solvent in liters.

   28.0 g / 180 g/mol = 0.156 mol

   0.156 mol / 0.384 L = 0.405 M

2) Molality is the number of moles divided by mass of solvent in kilograms.

   0.156 mol / 0.350 kg = 0.444 m

3) Percent by mass, as the name implies, is the mass of solute divided by total mass times 100%.

   28.0 g / (350 g + 28 g) times 100 = 7.41% $C_6H_{12}O_6$ by mass.

4) Mole fraction is the number of moles of solute divided by total moles.

   350 g / 18.015 g/mol = 19.428 mol of water

   0.156 mol / (19.428 + 0.156) = 0.0080 mol fraction $C_6H_{12}O_6$

   The mole fraction of water is:

   1 - 0.0080 = 0.992.

5) Mole percent is mole fraction times 100%.

   0.0080 × 100 = 0.80 % $C_6H_{12}O_6$ by moles.

Problem 31: How many grams of glucose is necessary to dissolve in 3 litres of water to obtain 40% solution?

Solution:

Let × g of glucose dissolve in 3 liters of water to form a 40% solution.

glucose weight = x

water weight = 3 liters = 3000 g (take water density as 1.00 g/mL)

so total solution weight = × + 3000 g

glucose percent ---> × / (x + 3000) = 0.40 <--- that's the 40%

$$x = 0.4\ (x + 3000)$$

$$x = 0.4x + 1200$$

$$x - 0.4x = 1200$$

$$0.6\ x = 1200$$

$$x = 2000\text{ g.}$$

Problem 32: The vinegar sold in the grocery stores is described as 5% (v/v) acetic acid. What is the molarity of this solution (density of 100% acetic acid is 1.05 g/mL)?

Solution:

1) 5% (v/v) means 5% of the volume is acetic acid. So 1.00 L of vinegar contains 50 mL acetic acid:

   (0.05)(1000 mL) = 50 mL

2) The mass of this acetic acid is:

   (1.05 g/mL)(50 mL) = 52.5 g

3) For the molarity, use MV = mass / molar mass

   (x) (1.00 L) = 52.5 g / 60.0516 g/mol

   x = 0.874 M (to three sig figs)

Problem 33: By titration, the molarity of acetic acid in vinegar was determined to be 0.870 M. Convert this to %(v/v). (The density of acetic acid is 1.05 g/mL)

Solution:

1) Assume 1.00 L of the solution to be present. Use MV = mass/molar mass to determine mass of acetic acid present:

   (0.870 mol/L) (1.00 L) = × / 60.0516 g/mol

   x = 52.245 g

2) Determine what volume of pure acetic acid this is:

   52.245 g divided by 1.05 g/mL = 49.757 mL

3) Determine %(v/v):

   (49.757 mL / 1000 mL) * 100 = 4.9757

   Rounded off, this is 4.98%(v/v), usually given as 5%(v/v).

Problem 34: In an aqueous solution of sulfuric acid, the acid concentration is 2.40 mole percent and the density of the solution is 1.079 g/mL. Calculate (1) the molal concentration of the acid, (2) the weight percentage of the acid, and (3) the molarity of the solution

Solution:

2.40 mole percent of acid means 97.60 mole percent water.

Let's assume 100 moles of the solution is present. This means 2.40 mole of the solution is H_2SO_4 and 97.60 mole is water.

(1) For molality, we need to know kg of water ---> 97.60 mol times 18.015 g/mol = 1758.264 g = 1.758264 kg

   molality ---> 2.40 mol / 1.758264 kg = 1.365 m (1.36 m to three sig figs)

(2) For the weight percent, we need the mass of H_2SO_4 ---> 2.40 mol times 98.0768 g/mol = 235.38432 g

   weight percent ---> 235.38432 g / (235.38432 + 1758.264 g) = 0.118067 = 11.8% (three sig figs)

(3) For molarity, we need to know the volume of the solution ---> 1993.64832 g divided by 1.079 g/mL = 1847.68 mL = 1.84768 L

Note: 1993.64832 g is the total mass of the solution.

molarity ---> 2.40 mol / 1.84768 L = 1.2989 M (1.30 M to three sig figs)

By the way, mole percent is mole fraction written as a percent. The mole fractions in the above problem are 0.0240 and 0.9760.

Problem 35: Calculate the molality, molarity, and mole fraction of $FeCl_3$ in a 26.3% (w/w) solution (density = 1.28 g/mL).

Solution:

Molarity:

Assume 100. g of solution present.

26.3 g of $FeCl_3$ is present.

100. g divided by 1.28 g/mL = 78.125 mL

Use MV = mass / molar mass

(x) (0.078125 L) = 26.3 g / 162.204 g/mol

x = 2.08 M (to three sig figs)

Molality

100. g - 26.3 g = 73.7 g <--- the water in the 100 g of solution

molality ---> (26.3 g / 162.204 g/mol) / 0.0737 kg = 2.20 m (to three sig figs)

Mole fraction of $FeCl_3$:

moles $FeCl_3$ ---> 26.3 g / 162.204 g/mol = 0.1621415 mol

moles water ---> 73.7 g / 18.015 g/mol = 4.091035 mol

mole fraction ---> [0.1621415 mol / (0.1621415 mol + 4.091035 mol)] = 0.0381 (to three sig figs)

3. Molal Solution

Molality, also called molal concentration, is a measure of the concentration of a solute in a solution in terms of amount of substance in a specified amount of mass of the solvent. This contrasts with the definition of molarity which is based on a specified volume of solution.

A commonly used unit for molality used in chemistry is mol/kg. A solution of concentration 1 mol/kg is also sometimes denoted as *1 molal*.

Definition - What does Molal Solution mean?

1. A molal solution is a solution that contains 1 molecular weight of solute in a kilogram of solvent. It is the strength or concentration of a solution, especially the amount of dissolved substance in a given volume of solvent. It is a concentration of a solution expressed in moles or molality (m).

Because volume is not part of the molality equation, molality is independent of temperature. Using molalities rather than molarities for lab experiments keeps the results within a closer range.

In the field of electrochemistry and metal corrosion, molality and molarity are applied as concentration units.

2. The molality (b), of a solution is defined as the amount of substance (in mol) of solute, n_{solute}, divided by the mass (in kg) of the solvent, $m_{solvent}$:

$$b = \frac{n_{solute}}{m_{solvent}}$$

Origin

The term *molality* is formed in analogy to *molarity* which is the molar concentration of a solution. The earliest of the intensive property molality and of its adjectival unit, the now-deprecated *molal*, appears to have been published by G. N. Lewis and M. Randall in the 1923 publication of *Thermodynamics and the Free Energies of Chemical Substances.*[2]Though the two terms are subject to being confused with one another, the molality and molarity of a weak aqueous solution are nearly the same, as one kilogram of water (solvent) occupies the volume of 1 liter at room temperature and a small amount of solute has little effect on the volume.

Unit

The SI unit for molality is mol/kg.

A solution with a molality of 3 mol/kg is often described as "3 molal" or "3 m". However, following the SI system of units, the National Institute of Standards and Technology, the United States authority on measurement, considers the term "molal" and the unit symbol "m" to be obsolete, and suggests mol/kg or a related unit of the SI.[3] This recommendation has not been universally implemented in academia yet.

Usage Considerations

Advantages

Compared to molar concentration or mass concentration, the preparation of a solution of a given molality requires only a good scale: both solvent and solute need to be weighed, as opposed to measured volumetrically, which would be subject to variations in density due to the ambient conditions of temperature and pressure; this is an advantage because, in *chemical* compositions, the mass, or the amount, of a pure known substance is more relevant than its volume: a *contained* measured amount of substance may change in volume with ambient conditions, but its amount and mass are unvarying, and chemical reactions occur in proportions of mass, not volume. The mass-based nature of molality implies that it can be readily converted into a mass ratio (or mass fraction, "*w*," ratio),

$$b\,M_{solute} = \frac{m_{solute}}{m_{solvent}} = \frac{W_{solute}}{W_{solvent}},$$

where the symbol *M* stands for molar mass, or into a mole ratio (or mole fraction, "*x*," ratio)

$$b\,M_{solvent} = \frac{n_{solute}}{n_{solvent}} = \frac{x_{solute}}{x_{solvent}}$$

The advantage of molality over other mass-based fractions is the fact that the molality of one solute in a single-solvent solution is independent of the presence or absence of other solutes.

Problem Areas

Unlike all the other compositional properties listed in "Relation" section (below), molality *depends* on the choice of the substance to be called "solvent" in an arbitrary mixture. If there is only one pure liquid substance in a mixture, the choice is clear, but not all solutions are this clear-cut: in an alcohol-water solution, either one could be called the solvent; in an alloy, or solid solution, there is no clear choice or all constituents may be treated alike. In such situations, mass or mole fraction is the preferred compositional specification.

Relation to Other Compositional Properties

In what follows, the solvent may be given the same treatment as the other constituents of the solution, such that the molality of the solvent of an n-solute solution, say b_0, is found to be nothing more than the reciprocal of its molar mass, M_0:

$$b_0 = \frac{n_0}{n_0 M_0} = M_0^{-1}$$

Mass Fraction

The conversions to and from the mass fraction, w, of the solute in a single-solute solution are

$$w = (1 + b\,M)^{-1},\ b = \frac{w}{(1-w)M},$$

where b is the molality and M is the molar mass of the solute.

More generally, for an n-solute/one-solvent solution, letting b_i and w_i be, respectively, the molality and mass fraction of the i-th solute,

$$w_i = w_0 b_i M_i,\ b_i = \frac{w_i}{w_0 M_i},$$

where M_i is the molar mass of the i-th solute, and w_0 is the mass fraction of the solvent, which is expressible both as a function of the molalities as well as a function of the other mass fractions,

$$w_0 = \left(1 + \sum_{j=1}^{n} b_j M_j\right) = 1 - \sum_{j=1}^{n} w_j.$$

Mole Fraction

The conversions to and from the mole fraction, x, of the solute in a single-solute solution are

$$x = (1 + (M_0 b)^{-1},\ b = \frac{x}{M_0(1-x)}$$

where M_0 is the molar mass of the solvent.

More generally, for an n-solute/one-solvent solution, letting x_i be the mole fraction of the i-th solute,

$$x_i = x_0 M_0 b_i,\ b_i,\ b_i = \frac{b_0 x_i}{x_0},$$

where x_0 is the mole fraction of the solvent, expressible both as a function of the molalities as well as a function of the other mole fractions:

$$x_0 = \left(1 + M_0 \sum_{j=1}^{n} b_j\right) = 1 - \sum_{j=1}^{n} x_j.$$

Molar Concentration (Molarity)

The conversions to and from the molar concentration, c, for one-solute solutions are

$$c = \frac{\rho b}{1 + bM},\ b = \frac{c}{\rho - cM}$$

where ρ is the mass density of the solution, b is the molality, and M is the molar mass of the solute.

For solutions with n solutes, the conversions are

$$c_i = c_0 M_0 b_i,\ b_i = \frac{b_0 c_i}{c_0},$$

where the molar concentration of the solvent c_0 is expressible both as a function of the molalities as well as a function of the molarities:

$$c_0 = \frac{\rho b_0}{1 + \sum_{j=1}^{n} b_j M_j} = \frac{\rho - \sum_{j=1}^{n} c_i M_i}{M_0}.$$

Mass Concentration

The conversions to and from the mass concentration, ρ_{solute}, of a single-solute solution are

$$\rho_{\text{solute}} = \frac{\rho b M}{1 + bM},\ b = \frac{\rho_{solute}}{M(\rho - \rho_{solute})},$$

where ρ is the mass density of the solution, b is the molality, and M is the molar mass of the solute.

For the general n-solute solution, the mass concentration of the i-th solute, ρ_i, is related to its molality, b_i, as follows:

$$\rho_i = \rho_0 b_i M_i,\ b_i = \frac{\rho_i}{\rho_0 M_i},$$

where the mass concentration of the solvent, ρ_0, is expressible both as a function of the molalities as well as a function of the mass concentrations:

$$\rho_0 = \frac{\rho}{1 + \sum_{j=1}^{n} b_j M_j} = \rho - \sum_{j=1}^{n} \rho_i$$

Equal Ratios

Alternatively, we may use just the last two equations given for the compositional property of the solvent in each of the preceding sections, together with the relationships given below, to derive the remainder of properties in that set:

$$\frac{b_i}{b_j} = \frac{x_i}{x_j} = \frac{c_i}{c_j} = \frac{\rho_i M_j}{\rho_i M_i} = \frac{w_i M_j}{w_i M_i},$$

where i and j are subscripts representing *all* the constituents, the n solutes plus the solvent.

Example of Conversion

An acid mixture consists of 0.76/0.04/0.20 mass fractions of (70% HNO_3) / (49% HF) /(H_2O), where the percentages refer to mass fractions of the bottled acids carrying a balance of H_2O. The first step is determining the mass fractions of the constituents:

$$w_{HNO_3} = 0.70 \times 0.76 = 0.532$$

$$w_{HF} = 0.49 \times 0.04 = 0.0196$$

$$w_{H_2O} = 1 - w_{HNO_3} - w_{HF} = 0.448$$

The approximate molar masses in kg/mol are

$$M_{HNO_3} = 0.063,\ M_{HF} = 0.020,\ M_{H_2O} = 0.018.$$

First derive the molality of the solvent, in mol/kg,

$$b_{H_2O} = \left(M_{H_20}\right)^{-1} = \frac{1}{0.018},$$

and use that to derive all the others by use of the equal ratios:

$$\frac{b_{HNO_3}}{bH_2O} = \frac{w_{HNO_3} M_{H_2O}}{w_{HNO_3}}$$

$$\therefore \quad b_{HNO_3} = 18.83$$

Actually, b_{H2O} cancels out, because it is not needed. In this case, there is a more direct equation: we use it to derive the molality of HF:

$$b_{HF} = \frac{W_{HF}}{W_{H_20} M_{HNO_3}} = 2.19.$$

The mole fractions may be derived from this result:

$$x_{H_2O} = \left[1 + M_{H_2O}\left(b_{HNO_3} + b_{HF}\right)\right]^{-1} = 0.726$$

$$\frac{x_{HNO_3}}{x_{H_2O}} = \frac{b_{HNO_3}}{b_{H_2O}}$$

$$\therefore \quad x_{HNO_3} = 0.246$$

$$x_{HF} = 1 - x_{HNO_3} - x_{H_2O} = 0.029.$$

Osmolality

Osmolality is a variation of molality that takes into account only solutes that contribute to a solution's osmotic pressure. It is measured in osmoles of the solute per kilogram of water. This unit is frequently used in medical laboratory results in place of osmolarity, because it can be measured simply by depression of the freezing point of a solution, orcryoscopy (see also: osmostat and colligative properties).

Relation to apparent (molar) properties

Molality appears in the expression of the apparent (molar) volume of a solute as a function of the molality b of that solute (and density of the solution and solvent):

$$\phi_{\tilde{V}_1} = \frac{1}{b}\left(\frac{1}{\rho} - \frac{1}{\rho_0^0}\right) + \frac{M_1}{\rho}$$

For multicomponent systems the relation is slightly modified by the sum of molalities of solutes.

$$\phi_{\tilde{V}_i} = \frac{1}{\Sigma b_j}\left(\frac{1}{\rho} - \frac{1}{\rho_0^0}\right) + \frac{\Sigma b_j M_j}{\Sigma b_j \rho}$$

Corrosionpedia Explains Molal Solution

A solution obtained by dissolving one gram of the solute in 1000 grams of solvent is known as a 1 molal solution. For example, when 60 g of NaOH are dissolved in 1000 g of solvent, the solution contains 1.5 moles of solute in 1 kg of solvent. Therefore, the molality is 1.5.

The factors needed to calculate molality are moles of solute and the mass of solvent in kilograms. The SI unit for molality is mol/kg. A solution with a molality of 3 mol/kg is often described as "3 molal" or "3 m."

The primary advantage of using molality to specify concentration is that unlike its volume, the mass of the solvent does not change with changes of temperature or pressure; molality remains constant under changing environment conditions. Molality, like mole fraction, is used in applications dealing with certain physical properties of solutions.

As the molality changes, it affects the boiling point and freezing point (also known as the melting point) of the solution. A higher molality increases the boiling point and decreases the freezing point of the solution. As molality is a more accurate measure of solutes in solution in dynamic conditions, it is often used in comparing and determining colligative properties of solution. Molality is a property of solutions. If the solvent is reactive, and one needs to know the stoichiometry between the solvent and the solute, knowing the molality can be very important. The mass-based nature of molality implies that it can be readily converted into a mass ratio.

As is Clear From its Name, Molality Involves Moles

The molality of a solution is calculated by taking the moles of solute and dividing by the kilograms of solvent.

$$\text{Molality} = \frac{\text{moles of solute}}{\text{kilograms of solvent}}$$

This is probably easiest to explain with examples.

Example 1: Suppose we had 1.00 mole of sucrose (it's about 342.3 grams) and proceeded to mix it into exactly 1.00 liter water. It would dissolve and make sugar water. We keep adding water, dissolving and stirring until the entire solid was gone. We then made sure everything was well-mixed.

What would be the molality of this solution? Notice that my one liter of water weighs 1000 grams (density of water = 1.00 g / mL and 1000 mL of water in a liter). 1000 g is 1.00 kg, so:

$$\text{Molaity} = \frac{1.00 \text{ mol}}{1.00 \text{ kg}}$$

The answer is 1.00 mol/kg. Notice that both the units of mol and kg remain. Neither cancels. A symbol for mol/kg is often used. It is a lower-case m and is often in italics, *m*. Some textbooks also put in a dash, like this: 1.00-*m*. However, if you write 1.00 m for the answer, without the italics, then that usually is correct because the context calls for a molality. Having said that, however, be aware that often m is used for mass, so be careful. (A lower-case m is also used for meter, but the context should be clear that m means molality.) Maybe including the dash would be wise if there might be a potential misunderstanding. When you say it out loud, say this: "one point oh molal." You don't have to say the dash. And never forget this: replace the m with mol/kg when you do calculations. The *m* is a symbol that stands for mol/kg. It is not the actual unit.

Example 2: Suppose you had 2.00 moles of solute dissolved into 1.00 L of solvent. What's the molality?

$$\text{Molaity} = \frac{2.00 \text{ mol}}{1.00 \text{ kg}}$$

The answer is 2.00 m.

Notice that no mention of a specific substance is mentioned at all. The molarity would be the same. It doesn't matter if it is sucrose, sodium chloride or any other substance. One mole of anything contains 6.022×10^{23} units.

Example 3: What is the molality when 0.75 mol is dissolved in 2.50 L of solvent?

$$\text{Molality} = \frac{0.75 \text{ mol}}{2.50 \text{ kg}}$$

The answer is 0.300 m.

Now, let's change from using moles to g. This is much more common. After all, chemists use balances to weigh things and balances give grams, NOT moles.

Example 4: Suppose you had 58.44 g of NaCl and you dissolved it in exactly 2.00 kg of pure water (the solvent). What would be the molality of the solution?

The solution to this problem involves two steps.

Step One: convert grams to moles.

Step Two: divide moles by kg of solvent to get molality.

In the above problem, 58.44 grams/mol is the molar mass of NaCl.

Step One: 58.44 g / 58.44 gr/mol = 1.00mol.

Step Two: 1.00 mol / 2.00 kg = 0.500 mol/kg (or 0.500 m).

Sometimes, a book will write out the word "molal," as in 0.500-molal.

Example 5: Calculate the molality of 25.0 grams of KBr dissolved in 750.0 mL pure water.

$$\frac{25.0\text{ g}}{119.0\text{ g/mol}} = 0.210\text{ mol}$$

$$\frac{0.210\text{ mol}}{0.750\text{ kg}} = 0.280\text{ m}$$

Example 6: 80.0 g of glucose ($C_6H_{12}O_6$, mol. wt = 180. g/mol) is dissolved in1.00 kg of water. Calculate the molality.

$$\frac{80.0\text{ g}}{180.0\text{ g/mol}} = 0.444\text{ mol}$$

$$\frac{0.444\text{ mol}}{1.00\text{ kg}} = 0.444\text{ m}$$

Example 7: Calculate the molality when 75.0 g of $MgCl_2$ is dissolved in 500.0 g of solvent.

$$\frac{75.0\text{ g}}{95.2\text{ g/mol}} = 0.788\text{ mol}$$

$$\frac{0.788\text{ mol}}{0.500\text{ g}} = 1.58\text{ m}$$

Example 8: 100.0 g of sucrose ($C_{12}H_{22}O_{11}$, mol. wt. = 342.3 g/mol) is dissolved in 1.50 L of water. What is the molality?

$$\frac{100.0\text{ g}}{342.3\text{ g/mol}} = 0.292\text{ mol}$$

$$\frac{0.292\text{ mol}}{1.50\text{ g}} = 0.195\text{ m}$$

Example 9: 49.8 g of KI is dissolved in 1.00 kg of solvent. What is the molality?

$$\frac{49.8\text{ g}}{166.0\text{ g/mol}} = 0.300\text{ mol}$$

$$\frac{0.300\text{ mol}}{1.00\text{ kg}} = 0.300\text{ m}$$

In the molarity tutorial the phrase "of solution" kept showing up. The molarity definition is based on the volume of the solution. This makes molarity a temperature dependent definition. However, the molality definition does not have a volume in it and so is independent of any temperature changes. This will make molality a very useful concentration unit in the area of colligative properties.

Lastly, it is very common for students to confuse the two definitions of molarity and molality. The words differ by only one letter and sometimes that small difference is overlooked.

Molality concentration is defined as the moles of solute divided by kiograms of solvent.

Molality = moles of solute / kg of solvent

We will use the molality term in taking about some colligative propertives. Here are a few types of problems involving the molal concentration term.

Determining Molal Concentration

Determine the molality of 3000 g of solution containing 37.3 g of Potassium Chloride (KCl).

1. Convert grams KCl to moles KCl using the molecular weight of KCl

   37.3 g KCl × 1 mole KCl / 74.6 g KCl =0.5 mole KCl
2. Determine the grams of pure solvent from the given grams of solution and solute

   Total grams = 3000 g = Mass of solute + Mass of solvent

   3000 grams = 37.3 + grams of pure solvent

   3000 - 37.3 = grams of pure solvent
3. Convert grams of solvent to kilograms

   2962.7 grams solvent × 1 kg / 1000 g = 2.9627 kg
4. Apply the definition for molality

   molality = moles of KCl / kg of solvent = 0.5 / 2.9627 = 0.169 m.

Determining Grams of Solvent in a Molal Solution

How many grams of water must be used to dissolve 100 g of Sucrose $C_{12}H_{22}O_{11}$ to prepare a .2 molal solution?

1. Determine moles of Sucrose in 100 g.

   100 grams $C_{12}H_{22}O_{11}$ X 1 mole $C_{12}H_{22}O_{11}$ / 342 g = 0.292 moles.
2. Determine kilograms of solvent water from given molal and moles of solute

   molality = moles of Sucrose / kilograms of solvent

   0.2 = 0.292 / kg of water

   kg of water = 0.292 / .2 = 1.46 kg of water
3. Convert kilograms into grams

   1.46 kg × 1000 g / 1 kg = 1460 g water

Determining the Amount of Solvent and Solute for a Given Molality

How would you prepare 5000 g of a 0.5 molal NaOH solution?

1. Determine grams of water in 1000 g solution

   In 0.5 molal there is .5 mole NaOH in 1000 g solvent

   0.5 mole NaOH × 40 grams / 1 mole = 20 g NaOH

   Total grams solution = grams of NaOH + g of solvent

   1000 grams solution = 20 grams + grams solvent

   grams of solvent = 1000 - 20 = 980 grams solvent per 1000 g solution

   5000 grams solution × 980 grams water / 1000 g solution = 4900 g water

   grams NaOH = Total grams of solution - grams of solvent

   grams NaOH = 5000 - 4900 = 100 g NaOH

4. Percentage Solution

Percent [weight/weight (w/w) or %]

This is the grams of pure analyte in 100 g of sample. For example, a 37% (w/w) solution of commercial concentrated HCl contains 37 g of pure HCl in 100 g of solution. The % (w/w) of an analyte in a sample is calculated using following equation:

$$\% \text{ (w/w)} = \frac{\text{g of analyte in sample}}{\text{g of sample}} \times 100\%$$

Percent (weight/volume or w/v)

This is the grams of pure analyte in 100 mL of solution. For example, a 10% (w/v) sucrose solution contains 109 of sucrose per 100 mL. The % (w/v) is calculated using following equation and the grams of pure analyte needed to prepare a solution with a given volume (mL) and percent concentration are calculated using following equation:

$$\% \text{ (w/v)} = \frac{\text{g of analyte in sample}}{\text{mL of sample}} \times 100\%$$

$$\text{g of analyte} = \frac{\% \text{(w/v)} \times \text{ mL sample}}{100\%}$$

Milligram percent (mg %)

This is the milligrams of pure analyte in 100 mL of solution. For example, a 20 mg % solution of NaCl contains 20 mg of NaCl in 100 mL of the solution. The mg % is calculated using following equation and the milligrams of pure analyte needed to prepare a solution with a given volume (mL) and mg % concentration is calculated using following equation:

$$\text{mg } \% = \frac{\text{g of analyte in sample}}{\text{mL of sample}} \times 100\%$$

$$\text{mg of analyte} = \frac{\text{mg \% x mL of sample}}{100\%} \times 100\%$$

A complete description of a solution states what the solute is and how much solute is dissolved in a given amount of solvent or solution. The quantitative relationship between solute and solvent is the concentration of the solution. This concentration may be expressed using several different methods, as discussed next.

A. Concentration by Mass

The concentration of a solution may be given as the mass of solute in a given amount of solution, as in the following statements: The northern part of the Pacific Ocean contains 35.9 g salt in each 1000 g seawater. The North Atlantic Ocean has a higher salt concentration, 37.9 g salt/1000 g seawater.

B. Concentration by Percent

The concentration of a solution is often expressed as percent concentration by mass or percent by volume of solute in solution. Percent by mass is calculated from the mass of solute in a given mass of solution. A 5%-by-mass aqueous solution of sodium chloride contains 5 g sodium chloride and 95 g water in each 100 g solution.

$$\text{Percent by mass} = \frac{\text{mass of solute}}{\text{mass of solution}} \times 100\%$$

"Percentage solution" is an ambiguous term which is used to describe a solution with the unit "%". It may refer to:

- Mass fraction (chemistry) if % mass/mass ("% w/w") is meant. Also known as wt.%.
- Mass concentration (chemistry) if mass/volume multiplied by 100 (improperly written "% w/v") is meant (see also usage in biology)
- Volume concentration if % volume/volume ("% v/v") is meant

In chemistry, the mass fraction w_i is the ratio of one substance with mass m_i to the mass of the total mixture w_{tot}, defined as

$$w_i = \frac{m_i}{m_{tot}}$$

The sum of all the mass fractions is equal to 1:

$$\sum_{i=1}^{N} m_i = m_{tot}; \sum_{i=1}^{N} w_i = 1$$

Mass fraction can also be expressed, with a denominator of 100, as percentage by mass (frequently, though erroneously, called percentage by weight, abbreviated *wt* %). It is one way of expressing the composition of a mixture in a dimensionless size; mole fraction (percentage by moles, mol%) and volume fraction (percentage by volume, vol%) are others.

For elemental analysis, mass fraction (or "mass percent composition") can also refer to the ratio of the mass of one element to the total mass of a compound. It can be calculated for any compound using its empirical formula or its chemical formula.

TERMINOLOGY

"Percent concentration" does not refer to this quantity. This improper name persists, especially in elementary textbooks. In biology, the unit "%" is sometimes (incorrectly) used to denote mass concentration, also called "mass/volume percentage." A solution with 1 g of solute dissolved in a final volume of 100 mL of solution would be labeled as "1 %" or "1 % m/v" (mass/volume). This is incorrect because the unit "%" can only be used for dimensionless quantities. Instead, the concentration should simply be given in units of g/mL. "Percent solution" or "percentage solution" are thus terms best reserved for "mass percent solutions" (m/m = m% = mass solute/mass total solution after mixing), or "volume percent solutions" (v/v = v% = volume solute per volume of total solution after mixing). The very ambiguous terms "percent solution" and "percentage solutions" with no other qualifiers continue to occasionally be encountered.

In thermal engineering vapor quality is used for the mass fraction of vapor in the steam. In alloys, especially those of noble metals, the term fineness is used for the mass fraction of the noble metal in the alloy.

In chemistry, the mass concentration ρ_i (or γ_i) is defined as the mass of a constituent m_i divided by the volume of the mixture V:

$$\rho_i = \frac{m_i}{V}.$$

For a pure chemical the mass concentration equals its density (mass divided by volume); thus the mass concentration of a component in a mixture can be called the density of a component in a mixture. This explains the usage of ρ (the lower case Greek letter rho), the symbol most often used for density.

Definition and Properties

The volume V in the definition refers to the volume of the solution, *not* the volume of the solvent. One liter of a solution usually contains either slightly more or slightly less than 1 liter of solvent because the process of dissolution causes volume of liquid to increase or decrease. Sometimes the mass concentration is called titer.

Notation

The notation common with mass density underlines the connection between the two quantities (the mass concentration being the mass density of a component in the solution), but it can be a source of confusion especially when they appear in the same formula undifferentiated by an additional symbol (like a star superscript, a bolded symbol or varrho).

Dependence on Volume

Mass concentration depends on the variation of the volume of the solution due mainly to thermal expansion. On small intervals of temperature the dependence is :

$$\rho_i = \frac{\rho_i T_0}{2 + \alpha \Delta T}$$

where ρ_i, T_0 is the mass concentration at a reference temperature, α is the thermal expansion coefficient of the mixture.

Sum of Mass Concentrations - Normalizing Relation

The sum of the mass concentrations of all components (including the solvent) gives the density ρ of the solution:

$$\rho = \sum_i \rho_i$$

Thus, for pure component the mass concentration equals the density of the pure component.

Sum of Products Mass Concentrations - Partial Specific Volumes

The sum of products between these quantities equals one.

$$\sum_i \rho_i \cdot \overline{v_i} = 1$$

Units

The SI-unit for mass concentration is kg/m^3 (kilogram/cubic meter). However, more commonly the unit g/100mL is used, which is identical to g/dL (gram/deciliter).

Usage in Biology

In biology, the unit "%" is sometimes incorrectly used to denote mass concentration, also called "mass/volume percentage." A solution with 1 g of solute dissolved in a final volume of 100 mL of solution would be labeled as "1 %" or "1 % m/v" (mass/volume). The notation is mathematically flawed because the unit "%" can only be used for dimensionless quantities. "Percent solution" or "percentage solution" are thus terms best reserved for "mass percent solutions" (m/m = m% = mass solute/mass total solution after mixing), or "volume percent solutions" (v/v = v% = volume solute per volume of total solution after mixing). The very ambiguous terms "percent solution" and "percentage solutions" with no other qualifiers continue to occasionally be encountered.

This common usage of % to mean m/v in biology is because of many biological solutions being dilute and water-based or an aqueous solution. Liquid water has a density of approximately 1 g/cm^3 (1 g/ml) (water density). Thus 100 ml of water is equal to approximately 100 g. Therefore, a solution with 1 g of solute dissolved in final volume of 100 ml aqueous solution may also be considered 1% m/m (1 g solute in 99 g water). This approximation breaks down as the solute concentration is increased. For an example, refer to the densities of water-NaCl mixtures (density of water with dissolved NaCl). High solute concentrations are often not physiologically relevant, but are occasionally encountered in pharmacology, where the mass per volume notation is still sometimes encountered. An extreme example is saturated solution of potassium iodide (SSKI) which attains 100 "%" m/v potassium iodide mass concentration (1 gram KI per mL solution) only because the solubility of the dense salt KI is extremely high in water, and the resulting solution is very dense (1.72 times as dense as water).

Although there are examples to the contrary, it should be stressed that the commonly used "units" of % w/v are grams/milliliters (g/ml). 1% m/v solutions are sometimes thought of as being gram/100 ml but this detracts from the fact that % m/v is g/ml; 1 g of water has a volume of approximately 1 ml (at standard temperature and pressure) and the mass concentration is said to be 100%. To make 10 ml of an aqueous 1% cholate solution, 0.1 grams of cholate are dissolved in 10 ml of water. Volumetric flasks are the most appropriate piece of glassware for this procedure as deviations from ideal solution behavior can occur with high solute concentrations.

In solutions, mass concentration is commonly encountered as the ratio of mass/[volume solution], or m/volume. In water solutions containing relatively small quantities of dissolved solute (as in biology), such figures may be "percentivized" by multiplying by 100 a ratio of grams solute per mL solution. The result is given as "mass/volume percentage". Such a convention expresses mass concentration of 1 gram of solute in 100 mL of solution, as "1 m/v %."

Related Quantities

Density of Pure Component

The relation between mass concentration and density of a pure component (mass concentration of single component mixtures) is:

$$\rho_i = \rho_i^* \frac{V_i}{V}$$

where ρ_i^* is the density of the pure component, V_i the volume of the pure component before mixing.

Specific Volume (Or Mass-Specific Volume)

Specific volume is the inverse of mass concentration only in the case of pure substances, for which mass concentration is the same as the density of the pure-substance:

$$v = \frac{V}{m} = \rho^{-1}$$

Molar Concentration

The conversion to molar concentration c_i is given by:

$$c_i = \frac{\rho_i}{M_i}$$

where M_i is the molar mass of constituent i.

Mass Fraction

The conversion to mass fraction w_i is given by:

$$w_i = \frac{\rho_i}{\rho}$$

Mole Fraction

The conversion to mole fraction x_i is given by:

$$x_i = \frac{\rho_i}{\rho} \cdot \frac{M}{M_i}$$

where M is the average molar mass of the mixture.

Molality

For binary mixtures, the conversion to molality b_i is given by:

$$b_i = \frac{\rho_i}{M_i(\rho - \rho_i)}$$

Spatial Variation and Gradient

The values of (mass and molar) concentration different in space trigger the phenomenon of diffusion.

Volume Fraction

In chemistry, the volume fraction ϕ_i is defined as the volume of a constituent V_i divided by the volume of all constituents of the mixture V prior to mixing:

$$\phi_i = \frac{V_i}{\Sigma_j V_j}$$

Being dimensionless, its unit is 1; it is expressed as a number, e.g., 0.18. It is the same concept as volume percent (vol %) except that the latter is expressed with a denominator of 100, *e.g.*, 18%.

The volume fraction coincides with the volume concentration in ideal solutions where the volumes of the constituents are additive (the volume of the solution is equal to the sum of the volumes of its ingredients).

The sum of all volume fractions of a mixture is equal to 1:

$$\sum_{i=1}^{N} V_i = V; \sum_{i=1}^{N} \phi_i = 1$$

The volume fraction (percentage by volume, vol %) is one way of expressing the composition of a mixture with a dimensionless quantity; mass fraction (percentage by weight, wt%) and mole fraction (percentage by moles, mol%) are others.

Percent (%) Solutions Calculations

Meant to be used in both the teaching and research laboratory, this calculator (see below) can be utilized to perform a number of different calculations for preparing percent (%)solutions when starting with the solid or liquid material. It is very common to express the concentration of solutions in terms of percentages. Percent means per 100 parts, where for solutions, part refers to a measure of mass (μg, mg, g, kg, *etc.*) or volume (μL, mL, L, *etc.*). In percent solutions, the amount (weight or volume) of a solute is expressed as a percentage of the total solution weight or volume. Percent solutions can take the form of weight/volume % (wt/vol % or w/v %), weight/weight % (wt/wt % or w/w %), or volume/volume % (vol/vol % or v/v %). In each case, the percentage concentration is calculated as the fraction of the weight or volume of the solute related to the total weight or volume of the solution.

Because percent solutions can be expressed in three different ways, it is imperative that the type of percent solution be explicitly stated. If this information is not provided, the end user is left to "guess" whether w/v %, w/w %, or v/v % was used. Each percent solution is appropriate for a number of different applications. For example, commercial aqueous reagents, such as concentrated acids and bases, are typically expressed as weight/weight % solutions. For example, commercially available concentrated hydrochloric acid (HCl) is 37% by weight (w/w %). On the other hand, many dilute solutions used for biological research are expressed as weight/volume % (e.g., 1% sodium dodecyl sulfate, SDS). Volume/volume % solutes are also common, and are used when pure solutes in liquid form are used. For example, a 70 % (v/v) solution of ethanol can be prepared by dissolving 70 mL of 100% (i.e., 200 proof) ethanol in a total solution volume of 100 mL.

Other factors may also be important when deciding on the type of percent solution to prepare. For example, if the percent solution under consideration is to be used at widely different temperatures, then it is better to prepare the solution as a weight/weight % solution because its concentration would be independent of variations in ambient temperature.

An important note is in order. Here, we have used "weight" instead of "mass" simply to be consistent with tradition and popular use. Thus, weight/volume % solutions should be correctly referred to as mass/volume %. Similarly, weight/weight % solutions should be referred to as mass/mass %, or simply mass %.

If you wish to perform dilution calculations for solutions with molarity or percent concentration units, use our Molarity, Percent Dilution Calculator.

Percent Solution Equations

$$\frac{\text{weight}}{\text{volume}}\% = \frac{\text{weight of solute}}{\text{volume of solution}} \times 100 \qquad \text{...Eq. 1}$$

$$\frac{\text{weight}}{\text{weight}}\% = \frac{\text{weight of solute}}{\text{weight of solution}} \times 100 \quad \text{...Eq. 2}$$

$$\frac{\text{volume}}{\text{volume}}\% = \frac{\text{volume of solute}}{\text{volume of solution}} \times 100 \quad \text{...Eq. 3}$$

As noted above, weight refers to mass (i.e., measured on a balance). When examining the equation for each of the percent solutions above, it is very important to note that in all cases the denominator refers to the solution mass or volume and not just the solvent mass or volume. Thus, solution mass is the combined mass of solute and solvent, and solution volume is the combined volume of solute and solvent.

A final note is necessary when considering volume/volume % solutions. When different volumes of an identical solution are added together, the final volume will always be exactly the sum of the individual portions added. For example, adding 50 mL of water to 50 mL of water will result in a total volume of 100 mL, and adding 75 mL of 100% ethanol to 75 mL of 100% ethanol will result in a total volume of 150 mL. However, when mixing miscible liquids (such as water and ethanol), the final volume of solution is not exactly equal to the sum of the individual volumes. For example, adding 50 mL of ethanol to 50 mL of water will result in a total volume that is less than 100 mL. It is actually closer to 96 mL. Therefore, when preparing volume/volume percent solutions, it is always better to dissolve the solute in solvent and then add additional solvent to bring the total solution volume to the desired final value.

Preparing Chemical Solutions

Glossary, Basic Terms to Understand...

Solute - The substance which dissolves in a solution

Solvent - The substance which dissolves another to form a solution. For example, in a sugar and water solution, water is the solvent; sugar is the solute.

Solution - A mixture of two or more pure substances. In a solution one pure substance is dissolved in another pure substance homogenously. For example, in a sugar and water solution, the solution has the same concentration throughout, i.e. it is homogenous.

Mole - A fundamental unit of mass (like a "dozen" to a baker) used by chemists. This term refers to a large number of elementary particles (atoms, molecules, ions, electrons, *etc.*) of any substance. 1 mole is 6.02×10^{23} molecules of that substance (Avogadro's number) M.

Introduction to Preparation of Solutions

Many experiments involving chemicals call for their use in solution form. That is, two or more substances are mixed together in known quantities. This may involve weighing a precise amount of dry material or measuring a precise amount of liquid. Preparing solutions accurately will improve an experiment's safety and chances for success.

Solution 1: Using Percentage By Weight (W/V)

Formula: The formula for weight percent (w/v) is: [Mass of solute (g) / Volume of solution (ml)] × 100

Example

A 10% NaCl solution has ten grams of sodium chloride dissolved in 100 ml of solution.

Procedure

Weigh 10g of sodium chloride. Pour it into a graduated cylinder or volumetric flask containing about 80ml of water. Once the sodium chloride has dissolved completely (swirl the flasks gently if necessary), add water to bring the volume up to the final 100 ml. Caution: Do not simply measure100ml of water and add 10g of sodium chloride. This will introduce error because adding the solid will change the final volume of the solution and throw off the final percentage.

Solution 2: Using Percentage by Volume (V/V)

When the solute is a liquid, it is sometimes convenient to express the solution concentration as a volume percent.

Formula: The formula for volume percent (v/v) is: [Volume of solute (ml) / Volume of solution (ml)] × 100

Example

Make 1000ml of a 5% by volume solution of ethylene glycol in water.

Procedure

First, express the percent of solute as a decimal: 5% = 0.05

Multiply this decimal by the total volume: 0.05 × 1000ml = 50ml (ethylene glycol needed).

Subtract the volume of solute (ethylene glycol) from the total solution volume:

1000ml (total solution volume) - 50ml (ethylene glycol volume) = 950ml (water needed).

Dissolve 50ml ethylene glycol in a little less than 950ml of water. Now bring final volume of solution up to 1000ml with the addition of more water. (This eliminates any error because the final volume of the solution may not equal the calculated sum of the individual components).

So, 50ml ethylene glycol / 1000ml solution x100 = 5% (v/v) ethylene glycol solution.

Solution 3: Molar Solutions

Molar solutions are the most useful in chemical reaction calculations because they directly relate the moles of solute to the volume of solution.

Formula: The formula for molarity (M) is: moles of solute / 1 liter of solution or gram-molecular masses of solute / 1 liter of solution.

Examples

The molecular weight of a sodium chloride molecule (NaCl) is 58.44, so one gram-molecular mass (=1 mole) is 58.44 g. We know this by looking at the periodic table. The atomic mass (or weight) of Na is 22.99, the atomic mass of Cl is 35.45, so 22.99 + 35.45 = 58.44.

If you dissolve 58.44g of NaCl in a final volume of 1 liter, you have made a 1M NaCl solution, a 1 molar solution.

Procedure

To make molar NaCl solutions of other concentrations dilute the mass of salt to 1000ml of solution as follows:

0.1M NaCl solution requires 0.1 × 58.44 g of NaCl = 5.844g

0.5M NaCl solution requires 0.5 × 58.44 g of NaCl = 29.22g

2M NaCl solution requires 2.0 × 58.44 g of NaCl = 116.88g

Example:

How many grams of glucose and water are in 500g of a 5.3% by mass glucose solution?

Solution:

We know that 5.3% of the solution is glucose:

$$\frac{5.3 \text{ g glucose}}{100 \text{ g solution}} \times 500 \text{ g solution} = 26.5 \text{ g glucose}$$

The remainder of the 500 g is water:

500 g – 26.5 g = 437.5 g water

If both solute and solvent are liquids, the concentration may be expressed as percent by volume. Both ethyl alcohol and water are liquids; the concentration of alcohol-water solutions is often given as percent by volume. For example, a 95% solution of ethyl alcohol contains 95 mL ethyl alcohol in each 100 mL solution.

$$\text{Percent by volume} = \frac{\text{volume of solute}}{\text{volume of solution}} \times 100\ \%$$

Example:

Rubbing alcohol is an aqueous solution containing 70% isopropyl alcohol by volume. How would you prepare 250mL rubbing alcohol from pure isopropyl alcohol?

Solution

We know that 70% of the volume is isopropyl alcohol:

$$\frac{70 \text{ mL isopropyl alcohol}}{100 \text{ mL solution}} \times 250 \text{ mL solution} = 175 \text{ mL is isopropyl alcohol}$$

To prepare the solution, enough water is added to 175 mL isopropyl alcohol to form 250 mL solution.

5. PARTS PER MILLION (PPM SOLUTION)

Concentration in parts per million (ppm) and parts per Billion (ppb). The terms (ppm) and parts per billion (ppb) are encountered more and more frequently as we become aware of the effects of substances present in trace amounts in water and air, and as we develop instruments sensitive enough to detect substances present in such low concentrations. In discussing mass, parts per million means concentration in grams per 10^6 grams, or micrograms per gram. In discussing volume, parts per million may mean milliliters per cubic meter, or the mixed designation of milligrams per cubic meter. For parts per billion, the general trend is toward the use of micrograms per liter when discussing water contaminants, micrograms per cubic meter for air, and micrograms per kilogram for soil concentrations.

PPM = parts per million

PPM is a term used in chemistry to denote a very, very low concentration of a solution. One gram in 1000 ml is 1000 ppm and one thousandth of a gram (0.001g) in 1000 ml is one ppm.

One thousand of a gram is one milligram and 1000 ml is one liter, so that 1 ppm = 1 mg per liter = mg/Liter.

PPM is derived from the fact that the density of water is taken as 1kg/L = 1,000,000 mg/L, and 1mg/L is 1mg/1,000,000mg or one part in one million.

Observe the Following Units

1 ppm = 1mg/l = 1ug /ml = 1000ug/L

ppm = ug/g =ug/ml = ng/mg = pg/ug = 10^{-6}

ppm = mg/litres of water

1 gram pure element disolved in 1000ml = 1000 ppm

PPB = Parts per billion = ug/L = ng/g = ng/ml = pg/mg = 10^{-9}

Making up 1000 ppm Solutions

1. From the pure metal : weigh out accurately 1.000g of metal, dissolve in 1 : 1 conc. nitric or hydrochloric acid, and make up to the mark in 1 liter volume deionised water.
2. From a salt of the metal: e.g. Make a 1000 ppm standard of Na using the salt NaCl.

   FW of salt = 58.44g.

   At. wt. of Na = 23

   1g Na in relation to FW of salt = 58.44 / 23 = 2.542g.

   Hence, weigh out 2.542g NaCl and dissolve in 1 liter volume to make a 1000 ppm Na standard
3. From an acidic radical of the salt: e.g. Make a 1000 ppm phosphate standard using the salt KH_2PO_4

   FW of salt = 136.09

   FW of radical PO_4 = 95

   1g PO_4 in relation to FW of salt = 136.09 / 95 = 1.432g.

   Hence, weigh out 1.432g KH_2PO_4 and dissolve in 1 liter volume to make a 1000 ppm PO_4 standard.

Dilution Formula = $M_1V_1 = M_2V_2$

req is the required value you want.

$$\frac{\text{req ppm} \times \text{req vol}}{\text{stock}} = \text{no of mls for req vol}$$

e.g. Make up 50 mls vol of 25 ppm from 100 ppm

25 × 50 / 100 = 12.5 mls. i.e. 12.5 mls of 100 ppm in 50 ml volume will give a 25 ppm solution.

Serial Dilutions

Making up 10^{-1} M to 10^{-5} M solutions from a 1M stock solution.

Pipette 10 ml of the 1M stock into a 100 ml volumetric flask and make up to the mark to give a 10^{-1} M solution.

Now, pipette 10 ml of this 10^{-1} M solution into another 100 ml flask and make up to the mark to give a 10^{-2} M solution.

Pipette again, 10 ml of this 10^{-2} M solution into yet another 100 ml flask and make up to mark to give a 10^{-3} M solution.

Pipette a 10 ml of this 10^{-3} M solution into another 100 ml flask and make up to mark to give a 10^{-4} M solution.

And from this 10^{-4} M solution pipette 10 ml into a 100 ml flask and make up to mark to give a final 10^{-5} M solution.

Molarity to ppm

Convert molar concentration to grams per liter (Molarity × Atomic mass of solute), then convert to milligrams per liter (ppm) by multiplying by 1000.

e.g. What is the ppm concentration of calcium ion in 0.01M $CaCO_3$?

Molarity (M) × Atomic mass(At Wt) = grams per liter(g/l)

Atomic Mass (Wt.) of Ca = 40

0.01M × 40 =0.40 g/l

0.40g/l × 1000 = 400 mg/l = 400ppm.

Note:

The FW of an ion species is equal to its concentration in ppm at 10^{3}M. Fluoride has a FW of 19, hence a 10^{-3}M concentration is equal to 19ppm, 1M is equal to 19,000 ppm and 1ppm is equal to 5.2×10^{-5}M.

PPM to Molarity

Convert ppm to gram based or milligram based concentration.

ppm = 1 mg solute per liter solution or

ppm = 0.001 gram per liter solution

e.g. What is the Molarity of 400ppm Ca ions in an aqueous $CaCO_3$ solution?

Using the 0.001g/l concentration: 400ppm × 0.001g/l = 0.4g/l.

or, Divide 400 mg by 1000 to get g/l = 0.4 g/l

Now divide by the At. Mass of Ca to get Molarity.

0.4g/l divided by 40g/mol =0.01M

Using the mg/l concentration, the 40g Ca must be converted to milligrams by multiplying by 1000 to give 40,000mg.

Hence Molarity = 400ppm divided by 40,000mg/mol = 0.01M.

ppm (parts per million) to % (parts per hundred)

Divide the ppm amount by 1,000,000 and multiply by 100 to get %. e.g.:

1 ppm = 1/1,000,000 = 0.000001 = 0.0001%

10 ppm = 10/1,000,000 = 0.00001 = 0.001%

100 ppm = 100/1,000,000 = 0.0001 = 0.01%

200 ppn = 200/1,000,000 = 0.0002 = 0.02%

5000 ppm = 5000/1,000,000 = 0.005 = 0.5%

10,000 ppm = 10000/1,000,000 = 0.01 = 1.0%

20,000 ppm = 20000/1,000,000 = 0.02 = 2.0%

(Parts per hundred) % to ppm

Divide the % value by 100 and multiply by 1,000,000 to get ppm. e.g.:

1% =0.01 × 1,000,000 = 10,000 ppm

0.5% =0.0.005 × 1,000,000 = 5,000 ppm

0.1% =0.001 × 1,000,000 = 1,000 ppm

0.01% = 0.0001 × 1,000,000 = 100 ppm

Parts Per Million (Weight/Weight or ppm w/w)

This is the grams of pure analyte in 10^6 g of sample. For example, if trace Na^+ in solid $MgCl_2$ is stated as 10 ppm, then 10 g of Na^+ is contained in every 10^6 g of $MgCl_2$.The ppm (w/w) is calculated using following equation:

$$\text{ppm (w/w)} = \frac{\text{g of analyte in sample}}{\text{mL of sample}} \times 10^6 \text{ ppm}$$

Parts Per Million (Weight/Volume or ppm w/v)

This is the grams of pure analyte in 10^6 mL of sample. If, for example, the concentration of Na^+ in a standard solution is stated as 1000 ppm, the solution contains 1000 g of $Na^+/10^6$ mL. The ppm (w/v) is calculated using following equation and the grams of pure analyte needed to prepare a solution with a given volume (mL) and ppm (w/v) concentration is calculated using following equation:

$$\text{ppm (w/v)} = \frac{\text{g of analyte in sample}}{\text{mL of sample}} \times 10^6 \text{ ppm}$$

$$\text{g of analyte} = \frac{\text{ppm (w/v)} \times \text{mL sample}}{10^6 \text{ppm}}$$

Parts Per Billion (Weight/Weight or ppb w/w)

This is the grams of pure analyte in 10^9 g of sample. Thus, if the concentration of trace Pb^{2+} in solid $CaCl_2$ is stated as 50 ppb, then 10^9 g of the $CaCl_2$ contains 50 g of Pb^{2+}. The ppb (w/w) is calculated using following equation:

$$\text{ppb (w/v)} = \frac{\text{g of analyte in sample}}{\text{g of sample}} \times 10^9 \text{ ppb}$$

Parts Per Billion (Weight/Volume) or ppb (w/v)

This is the grams of pure analyte in 10^9 mL. Thus, if the concentration of trace K^+ in concentrated H_2SO_4 is stated as 100 ppb, the solution contains 100 g of K^+ /10 mL. The ppb (w/v) is calculated using following equation.

$$\text{ppb (w/v)} = \frac{\text{g of analyte in sample}}{\text{mL of sample}} \times 10^9 \text{ ppb}$$

$$\text{g of analyte} = \frac{\text{ppb (w/v)} \times \text{mL of sample}}{10^9 \text{ ppb}}$$

Density (p) and Specific Gravity (sp gr)

Density is the quantity of mass per unit volume of a substance. It is calculated using following equation with weight used to approximate mass.

$$P = \frac{wt}{vol}$$

Specific gravity is the density of a fluid relative to that of H_2O.

$$Sp.\ gr. = \frac{P_{sample}}{P_{H2O}}$$

Sub stituting 1 g/mL for the density of H_2O at ^0C into following equation.

$$Sp.\ gr. = \frac{P_{sample}(g/mL)}{1\,(g/mL)}$$

Therefore, the specific gravity of a fluid is numerically equal to its density.

Specific Volume (sp vol)

This is the volume occupied by a unit weight of a solute when dissolved. It is calculated using following equation.

$$sp.\ vol = \frac{\text{vol of dissolved solute}}{\text{wt of solute}}$$

Therefore, the specific volume of a solute is equal to the inverse of its density.

Dilution Factor in Concentration and Volume Calculations

Often, one seeks the volume of a stock reagent that should be added to a known volume of diluents or assay medium to yield a desired concentration or the final concentration of the reagent after adding a known volume to the diluents or assay medium. An equation relating the various parameters is derived as follows: Let V_1 and C_1 respectively be the needed volume and the needed concentration of the stock reagent and V_2, C_2 the final volume and desired the needed concentration, respectively of the diluted reagent. Then the equation will be:

$$\text{dillution factor} = \frac{C_1}{C_2} = \frac{V_2}{V_1}$$

$$C_1 V_1 = C_2 V_2$$

or

$$C_1 V_1 = \frac{C_2 V_2}{C_1}$$

Any of the parameters in above equation may be calculated, provided that the other three are known. In the calculations C_1 and C_2 must have identical units; likewise, V_1 and V_2 must have identical units.

Molecular Weight and Equivalent Weights of Some of the Chemicals Which are Generally used in the Research Laboratory

Name of chemical	Formula	Molecular weight (g)	Equivalent weight (g)
Calcium hydroxide	$Ca(OH)_2$	74	37
Ferrous ammonium sulphate	$FeSO_{4,}(NH_4)_2SO_{4.}6H_2O$	392	392
Ferrous sulphate (anhydrous)	$FeSO_4$	152	152
Ferrous sulphate (hydrated)	$FeSO_{4.}7H_2O$	278	278
Hydrochloric acid	HCl	36.5	36.5
Iodine	I_2	254	127
Iron (Ferrous)	Fe	56	56
Nitric acid	HNO_3	63	63
Oxalic acid	$(COOH)_2.2H_2O$	126	63
Oxalic acid (anhydrous)	$(COOH)_2$	90	45
Potassium chloride	KCl	74.5	74.5
Potassium dichromate	$K_2Cr_2O_7$	294	49
Potassium hydroxide	KOH	56	56
Potassium permanganate	$KMnO_4$	158	31.6
Silver nitrate	$AgNO_3$	170	170
Sodium carbonate	Na_2CO_3	106	53
Sodium chloride	NaCl	58.5	58.5
Sodium hydroxide	NaOH	40	40
Sodium thiosulphate	$Na_2S_2O_3.5H_2O$	248	248
Sulphuric acid	H_2SO_4	98	49

Specific Characters of Some of the Acids Generally used in Research Laboratory

Name	Approximate per cent by weight	Specific gravity	Normality	Volume required to make 1 dm^3 of approximate 1N solution $(cm)^3$
Acetic acid	99.5	1.05	17.4	58
Aqueous ammonia (NH_3)	27	0.90	14.3	71
Hydrochloric acid	35	1.18	11.3	89
Hydrofluoric acid	46	1.15	26.5	38
Nitric acid	70	1.42	16.0	63
Perchloric acid	70	1.66	11.6	86
Phosphoric acid	85	1.69	41.1	23
Sulphuric acid	96	1.84	36.0	28

Approximate pH of Some Common Reagents at Room Temperature

Substance	Molarity	pH
Alum, potassium	0.1	4.2
Alum, ammonium	0.05	4.6
Ammonia chloride	0.1	4.6
Ammonia oxalate	0.1	6.4
Ammonia water	0.1	11.3
Ammonium phosphate, primary	0.1	4.0
Ammonium phosphate, secondary	0.1	7.9
Ammonium sulphate	0.1	5.5
Barbital sodium	0.1	9.4
Benzoic acid	Saturated	2-8
Borax	0.1	9.2
Boric acid	0.1	5.3
Calcium hydroxide	Saturated	12.4
Citric acid	0.1	2.1
Hydrochloric acid	0.1	1.1
Oxalic acid	0.1	1.3

Contd...

Substance	Molarity	pH
Potassium acetate	0.1	9.7
Potassium bicarboacetate	0.1	8.2
Potassium bioxalate	0.1	2.7
Potassium carbonate	0.1	11.7
Potassium phosphate (primary)	0.1	4.5
Salicylic acid	Saturated	2.4
Sodium acetate	0.1	8.9
Sodium benzoate	0.1	8.0
Sodium bicarbonate	0.1	8.3
Sodium bisulphate	0.1	1.4
Sodium carbonate	0.1	11.5
Sodium hydroxide	0.1	12.9
Sodium phosphate primary	0.1	4.5
Sodium phosphate secondary	0.1	9.2
Succinic acid	0.1	2.7
Tartaric acid	0.1	2.0
Tri-Chloroacetic acid	0.1	1.2

Density and Normality of Selected Acids

Acid	Density	Approximate normality (N)
Acetic acid	1.05	17
Hydrochloric acid	1.20	10
Nitric acid	1.42	16
Phosphoric acid	1.70	15
Sulphuric acid	1.84	36

Standardization of Normality of HCl for Various Chemical Reactions

Reagents Required

A. NaOH: 0.02 Normal,

B. HCl: 0.02 Normal,

C. Potassium hydrogen phthalate: 0.02N.

D. Phenolphthalein indicator solution.

A. Sodium Hydroxide (NaOH): Molecular Weight 40.00g

Weight of substance taken (g)	Volume made (ml)	Normality (N)
40	1000	1
4.0	1000	0.1
0.40	1000	0.01
0.80	1000	0.02
0.20	250	0.02
10.0	250	1

B. HCl: Molecular Weight 36.5g; sp.gr.1.18, Purity 36.0%

Volume required for 1 N = (Eq.wt. × 100) ÷ (sp.gr. × purity); (36.5 × 100) ÷ (1.18 × 36.0) = 85.92.

Volume of substance taken (ml)	Volume made (ml)	Normality (N)
85.92	1000	1
8.592	1000	0.1
0.8592	1000	0.01
1.7184	1000	0.02
0.4296	250	0.02
21.48	250	1

C. Potassium Hydrogen Phthalate: Molecular weight 204.23g ($C_8H_5KO_4$)

Weight of substance taken (g)	Volume made (ml)	Normality (N)
204.23	1000	1
20.423	1000	0.1
2.0423	1000	0.01
4.0846	1000	0.02
1.0211	250	0.02
51.06	250	1

Titrations of above reagents are given below:

1. Take 10ml of NaOH having 0.02 Normality in a 100ml in triplicate in volumetric flask and titrate against potassium hydrogen phthalate solution for neutralization and measure the quantity required for titration. (Suppose 1. 9.3ml; 2. 9.4ml and 3.9.9ml and average of three reading is 9.40ml.
2. Now again take 10ml of NaOH having 0.02 Normality in a 100ml in triplicate in volumetric flask and titrate against hydrochloric acid solution for neutralization and measure the quantity required for titration. (Suppose 1. 8.8ml; 2. 8.8ml and 3.8.7ml and average of three reading is 8.77ml.

3. NaOH = HCl

   $N_1 V_1 = N_2 V_2$

   $0.02 \times 9.40 = N_2 \times 8.77$

   $N_2 \times 8.77 = 0.02 \times 9.40$

   $N_2 = (0.02 \times 9.40) \div 8.77$

   $N_2 = 0.188 \div 8.77$

   $N_2 = 0.021$

The correct Normality of the HCl is 0.021N. This value can be used for further estimation of proteins from any unknown material or other calculations.

CHAPTER 5

Buffer Solution

DEFINITION/PRINCIPLES AND ABBREVIATIONS USED

The function of pH buffers is to neutralize small changes in H^+ and OH^- concentrations, thereby maintaining pH fairly constant. The basics of pH buffering and buffer calculations and preparation are discussed below. The necessary symbols and their meanings are as follows: A weak acid and its conjugate base are represented by HA and A^-, respectively; a weak base and its conjugate acid are represented by R-NH_2 and R-NH, respectively, because the most commonly used weak base buffers has NH_2 basic functional group(s). In aqueous solutions, H^+ is hydrated and, therefore, is written as Hp+ when necessary. Molar concentration is indicated by enclosing the substance of interest in square brackets; for example, $[H^+]$ represents the molar concentration of H^+.

Buffer a solution that resists pH change is an important for many reactions e.g., enzymatic methods of analysis, etc.

Buffer solutions are solutions that resist changes in pH (by resisting changes in hydronium ion and hydroxideion concentrations) upon addition of small amounts of acid or base, or upon dilution. They usually consist of a weak acid and its conjugate base, or, less commonly, a weak base and its conjugate acid.

Buffer solutions are used in industry for chemical manufacturing and fermentation processes, and to set the proper conditions for dyeing fabrics. In research laboratories, buffers are used for chemical analyses, syntheses, and calibration of pH meters. In living organisms, these solutions maintain the correct pH for many enzymes to work. Blood plasma contains a buffer (of carbonic acid and bicarbonate) to maintain a pH of approximately 7.4.

The main component of a buffer solution, such as a weak acid or weak base, may be used as a buffering agent. The function of a buffering agent is to drive an acidic or alkaline solution to a certain pH and maintain it at that pH. As pH managers, they are important in many applications, including agriculture, food processing, medicine, and photography.

How Buffers Work

The ability of a buffer solution to resist changes in pH is the result of the equilibrium between a weak acid (HA) and its conjugate base (A^-):

$$HA(aq) + H_2O(l) \rightarrow H_3O^+(aq) + A^-(aq)$$

Any alkali added to the solution is consumed by the hydronium ions. These ions are mostly regenerated as the equilibrium moves to the right and some of the acid dissociates into hydronium ions and the conjugate base. If a strong acid is added, the conjugate base is protonated, and the pH is almost entirely restored. This is an example of Le Chatelier's principle and the common ion effect.

This contrasts with solutions of strong acids or strong bases, where any additional strong acid or base can greatly change the pH. This may be easier to see by comparing two graphs: When a strong acid is titrated with a strong base, the curve will have a large gradient throughout, showing that a small addition of base/acid will have a large effect; by comparison, a weak acid/strong base titration curve will have a smaller gradient when the pH is close to the pKa value.

Applications

Given their resistance to changes in pH, buffer solutions are very useful for chemical manufacturing and essential for many biochemical processes. The ideal buffer for a particular pH has a pKa equal to the pH desired, since a solution of this buffer would contain equal amounts of acid and base and be in the middle of the range of buffering capacity.

Buffer solutions are necessary to keep the correct pH for enzymes in many organisms to work. Many enzymes work only under very precise conditions; if the pH strays too far out of the margin, the enzymes slow or stop working and can denature, thus permanently disabling its catalytic activity. A buffer of carbonic acid (H_2CO_3) and bicarbonate (HCO_3^-) is present in blood plasma, to maintain a pH between 7.35 and 7.45.

Industrially, buffer solutions are used in fermentation processes and in setting the appropriate conditions for dyeing fabrics. They are also used in chemical analyses and syntheses, and for the calibration of pH meters.

Buffering Agents

A buffering agent adjusts the pH of an acidic or alkaline solution and stabilizes it at that pH. Buffering agents have variable properties: some are acidic, others are basic; some are more soluble than others. They are useful for a variety of applications, including agriculture, food processing, medicine, and photography.

Buffering agents and buffer solutions are similar in that they both regulate the pH of a solution and resist changes in pH. They function based on the same chemical principles. They may, however, be distinguished by the following differences:

1. A buffer solution maintains the pH of a system, preventing large changes in it, whereas a buffering agent modifies the pH of what it is placed into.
2. A buffering agent is the active component of a buffer solution.

Examples

- Buffered aspirin has a buffering agent, such as magnesium oxide, that will maintain the pH of the aspirin as it passes through the patient's stomach.
- Buffering agents are also present in antacid tablets, which are used mainly to lower acidity in the stomach.
- Monopotassium phosphate (MKP) is a buffering agent with a mildly acidic reaction. When used as a fertilizer component with urea or diammonium phosphate, it minimizes pH fluctuations that can cause loss of nitrogen.

Preparing buffer solutions

The pH of the mobile phase (eluent) is adjusted to improve component separation and to extend the column life. This pH adjustment should involve not simply dripping in an acid or alkali but using buffer solutions, as much as possible. Good separation reproducibility (stability) may not be achieved if buffer solutions are not used.

A buffer solution is prepared as a combination of weak acids and their salts (sodium salts, etc.) or of weak alkalis and their salts. Common preparation methods include: 1) dripping an acid (or alkali) into an aqueous solution of a salt while measuring the pH with a pH meter and 2) making an aqueous solution of acid with the same concentration as the salt and mixing while measuring the pH with a pH meter. However, if the buffer solution is used as an HPLC mobile phase, even small errors in pH can lead to problems with separation reproducibility. Therefore, it is important to diligently inspect and calibrate any pH meter that is used. This page introduces a method that does not rely on a pH meter. The method involves weighing theoretically calculated fixed quantities of a salt and acid (or alkali) as shown in the table below. Consider the important points below.

Denoting Buffer Solutions

A buffer solution denoted 100 mM phosphoric acid (sodium) buffer solution pH = 2.1 for example, contains phosphoric acid as the acid, sodium as the counter ion, 100 mM total concentration of the phosphoric acid group, and a guaranteed buffer solution pH of 2.1.

Maximum Buffer Action Close to the Acid (Or Alkali) pKa

When an acetic acid (sodium) buffer solution is prepared from 1:1 acetic acid and sodium acetate, for example, the buffer solution pH is approximately 4.7 (near the acetic acid pKa), and this is where the maximum buffer action can be obtained.

Buffer Capacity Increases as Concentration Increases

The buffer capacity of an acetic acid (sodium) buffer solution is larger at 100 mM concentration than at 10 mM, for example. However, precipitation occurs more readily at higher concentrations.

Beware of Salt Solubility and Precipitation

The salt solubility depends on the type of salt, such as potassium salt or sodium salt. Salts precipitate out more readily when an organic solvent is mixed in.

In addition, avoid using buffer solutions based on organic acids (carboxylic acid) as much as possible for highly sensitive analysis at short UV wavelengths. Consider the various analytical conditions and use an appropriate buffer solution, such as an organic acid with a hydroxyl group at α position to restrict the effects of metal impurity ions.

Properties of Acids and Bases

For the purpose of this chapter, acids and bases are defined according to Bronsted-Lowry. An acid is a chemical compound that donates a H^+ and a base is a compound that accepts an H^+. When an acid is dissolved in H_2O, it donates its H^+ to an H_2O molecule which, in this case, acts as a base. When a base is dissolved, it accepts an H^+ from a H_2O molecule which, in this case, acts as an acid.

WHAT IS A BUFFER SOLUTION?

A buffer solution is one which resists changes in pH when small quantities of an acid or an alkali are added to it.

Acidic buffer solutions: An acidic buffer solution is simply one which has a pH less than 7. Acidic buffer solutions are commonly made from a weak acid and one of its salts often a sodium salt. A common example would be a mixture of ethanoic acid and sodium ethanoate in solution. In this case, if the solution contained equal molar concentrations of both the acid and the salt, it would have a pH of 4.76. It wouldn't matter what the concentrations were, as long as they were the same. You can change the pH of the buffer solution by changing the ratio of acid to salt, or by choosing a different acid and one of its salts.

Alkaline buffer solutions: An alkaline buffer solution has a pH greater than 7. Alkaline buffer solutions are commonly made from a weak base and one of its salts. A frequently used example is a mixture of ammonia solution and ammonium chloride solution. If these were mixed in equal molar proportions, the solution would have a pH of 9.25. Again, it doesn't matter what concentrations you choose as long as they are the same.

How Do Buffer Solutions Work?

A buffer solution has to contain things which will remove any hydrogen ions or hydroxide ions that you might add to it - otherwise the pH will change. Acidic and alkaline buffer solutions achieve this in different ways.

A buffer solution (more precisely, pH buffer or hydrogen ion buffer) is an aqueous solution consisting of a mixture of a weak acid and its conjugate base, or vice versa. Its pH changes very little when a small or moderate amount of strong acid or base is added to it and thus it is used to prevent changes in the pH of a solution. Buffer solutions are used as a means of keeping pH at a nearly constant value in a wide variety of chemical applications. Many life forms thrive only in a relatively small pH range so they utilize a buffer solution to maintain a constant pH. One example of a buffer solution found in nature is blood.

Principles of Buffering

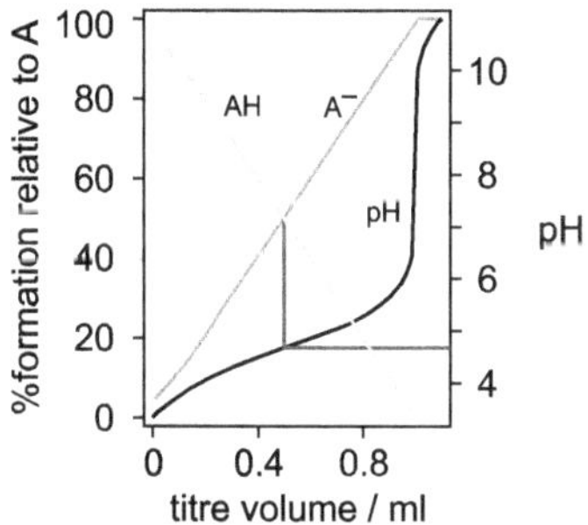

Simulated titration of an acidified solution of a weak acid ($pK_a = 4.7$) with alkali.

Buffer solutions achieve their resistance to pH change because of the presence of an equilibrium between the acid HA and its conjugate base A^-.

$$HA \rightleftharpoons H^+ + A^-$$

When some strong acid is added to an equilibrium mixture of the weak acid and its conjugate base, the equilibrium is shifted to the left, in accordance with Le Chatelier's principle. Because of this, the hydrogen ion concentration increases by less than the amount expected for the quantity of strong acid added. Similarly, if strong alkali is added to the mixture the hydrogen ion concentration decreases by less than the amount expected for the quantity of alkali added. The effect is illustrated by the simulated titration of a weak acid with $pK_a = 4.7$. The relative concentration of undissociated acid is shown in blue and of its conjugate base in red. The pH changes relatively slowly in the buffer region, $pH = pK_a \pm 1$, centered at pH = 4.7 where $[HA] = [A^-]$. The hydrogen ion concentration decreases by less than the amount expected because most of the added hydroxide ion is consumed in the reaction

$$OH^- + HA \rightarrow H_2O + A^-$$

and only a little is consumed in the neutralization reaction which results in an increase in pH.

$$OH^- + H^+ \rightarrow H_2O$$

Once the acid is more than 95% deprotonated the pH rises rapidly because most of the added alkali is consumed in the neutralization reaction.

Applications

Buffer solutions are necessary to keep the correct pH for enzymes in many organisms to work. Many enzymes work only under very precise conditions; if the pH moves outside of a narrow range, the enzymes slow or stop working and can denature. In many cases denaturation can permanently disable their catalytic activity. A buffer of carbonic acid (H_2CO_3) and bicarbonate (HCO_3^-) is present in blood plasma, to maintain a pH between 7.35 and 7.45.

Industrially, buffer solutions are used in fermentation processes and in setting the correct conditions for dyes used in colouring fabrics. They are also used in chemical analysis and calibration of pH meters. The majority of biological samples that are used in research are made in buffers, especially phosphate buffered saline (PBS) at pH 7.4.

Simple buffering agents

Buffering agent	pK_a	Useful pH range
Citric acid	3.13, 4.76, 6.40	2.1–7.4
Acetic acid	4.8	3.8–5.8
KH_2PO_4	7.2	6.2–8.2
CHES	9.3	8.3–10.3
Borate	9.24	8.25–10.25

For buffers in acid regions, the pH may be adjusted to a desired value by adding a strong acid such as hydrochloric acid to the buffering agent. For alkaline buffers, a strong base such as sodium hydroxide may be added. Alternatively, a buffer mixture can be made from a mixure of an acid and its conjugate base. For example, an acetate buffer can be made from a mixture of acetic acid and sodium acetate. Similarly an alkaline buffer can be made from a mixture of the base and its conjugate acid.

Universal Buffer Mixtures

By combining substances with pK_a values differing by only two or less and adjusting the pH, a wide range of buffers can be obtained. Citric acid is a useful component of a buffer mixture because it has three pK_a values, separated by less than two. The buffer range can be extended by adding other buffering agents. The following two-component mixtures (McIlvaine's buffer solutions) have a buffer range of pH 3 to 8.

0.2M Na_2HPO_4 /mL	0.1M Citric Acid /mL	pH
20.55	79.45	3.0
38.55	61.45	4.0
51.50	48.50	5.0
63.15	36.85	6.0
82.35	17.65	7.0
97.25	2.75	8.0

A mixture containing citric acid, monopotassium phosphate, boric acid, and diethyl barbituric acid can be made to cover the pH range 2.6 to 12.

Other universal buffers are Carmody buffer and Britton-Robinson buffer, developed in 1931.

Common Buffer Compounds Used in Biology

Common Name	pK_a at 25 °C	Buffer Range	Temp. Effect *d*pH/*d*T in (1/K)	Mol. Weight	Full Compound Name
TAPS	8.43	7.7–9.1	−0.018	243.3	3-{[tris (hydroxymethyl) methyl] amino} propanesulfonic acid
Bicine	8.35	7.6–9.0	−0.018	163.2	N,N-bis(2-hydroxyethyl) glycine
Tris	8.06	7.5–9.0	−0.028	121.14	tris(hydroxymethyl) methylamine
Tricine	8.05	7.4–8.8	−0.021	179.2	N-tris (hydroxymethyl) methylglycine
TAPSO	7.635	7.0-8.2		259.3	3-[N-Tris (hydroxymethyl) methylamino]-2-hydroxypropanesulfonic Acid
HEPES	7.48	6.8–8.2	−0.014	238.3	4-2-hydroxyethyl-1-piperazineethanesulfonic acid
TES	7.40	6.8–8.2	−0.020	229.20	2-{[tris (hydroxymethyl) methyl]amino}ethanesulfonic acid
MOPS	7.20	6.5–7.9	−0.015	209.3	3-(N-morpholino) propanesulfonic acid
PIPES	6.76	6.1–7.5	−0.008	302.4	piperazine-N,N′-bis(2-ethanesulfonic acid)
Cacodylate	6.27	5.0–7.4		138.0	dimethylarsinic acid
SSC	7.0	6.5-7.5		189.1	saline sodium citrate
MES	6.15	5.5–6.7	−0.011	195.2	2-(N-morpholino) ethanesulfonic acid
Succinic acid	7.4	7.4-7.5	-	118.1	2(R)-2-(methylamino)succinic acid

Biological buffers cover 1.9 to 11 pH range.

Buffer Capacity

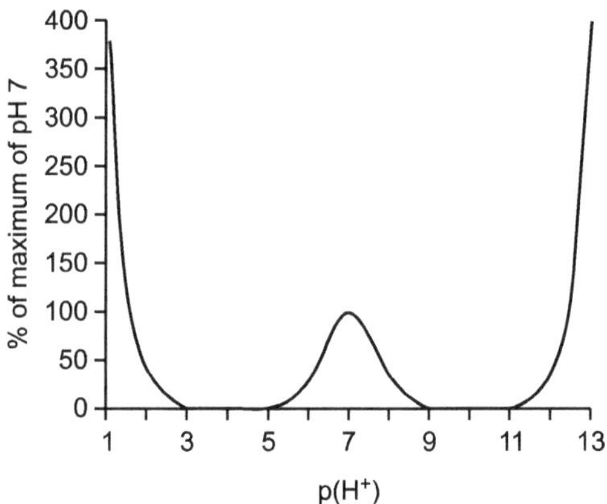

Buffer capacity for a 0.1 M solution of an acid with pK_a of 7

Buffer capacity, β, is a quantitative measure of the resistance of a buffer solution to pH change on addition of hydroxide ions. It can be defined as follows.

$$\beta = \frac{dn}{d(p[H+])}$$

where dn is an infinitesimal amount of added base and $d(p[H^+])$ is the resulting infinitesimal change in the cologarithm of the hydrogen ion concentration. With this definition the buffer capacity of a weak acid, with a dissociation constant K_a, can be expressed as

$$\frac{dn}{d(pH)} = 2.303\left([H^+] + \frac{C_A K_A [H^+]}{(K_a + [H^+])^2} + [OH^{-1}]\right)$$

where C_A is the analytical concentration of the acid. pH is defined as $-\log_{10}[H^+]$.

There are three regions of high buffer capacity.

- At very low $p[H^+]$ the first term predominates and β increases in proportion to the hydrogen ion concentration; buffer capacity rises exponentially with pH. This is independent of the presence or absence of buffering agents.
- In the region $p[H^+] = pK_a \pm 2$ the second term becomes important. Buffer capacity is proportional to the concentration of the buffering agent, C_A, so dilute solutions have little buffer capacity.
- At very high $p[H^+]$ the third term predominates and β increases in proportion to the hydroxide ion concentration; buffer capacity rises exponentially with pH. This is due to theself-ionization of water and is independent of the presence or absencc of buffering agents.

The buffer capacity of a buffering agent is at a local maximum when $p[H^+] = pK_a$. It falls to 33% of the maximum value at $p[H^+] = pK_a \pm 1$ and to 10% at $p[H^+] = pK_a \pm 1.5$. For this reason the useful range is approximately $pK_a \pm 1$.

Buffer capacity can be defined in many ways. You may find it defined as "maximum amount of either strong acid or strong base that can be added before a significant change in the pH will occur". This definition - instead of explaining anything - raises a question "what is a significant change?" – sometimes even change of 1 unit doesn't matter too much, sometimes - especially in biological systems - 0.1 unit change is a lot. Buffer capacity can be also defined as quantity of strong acid or base that must be added to change the pH of one liter of solution by one pH unit. Such definition - although have its practical applications - gives different values of buffer capacity for acid addition and for base addition (unless buffer is equimolar and its pH=pK_a). This contradicts intuition - for a given buffer solution its resistance should be identical regardless of whether acid or base is added.

Buffer capacity definition that takes this intuition into account is given by

$$\beta = \frac{dn}{dpH}$$

where n is number of equivalents of added strong base (per 1 L of the solution). Note that addition of dn moles of acid will change pH by exactly the same value but in opposite direction. We will derive formula connecting buffer capacity with pH, pK_a and buffer concentration. To make further calculations easier let's assume that the strong base added is monoprotic, we also assume volume of 1 which will allow us to treat concentration and number of moles interchangeably.

$$[A^-] + [OH^-] = [B^+] + [H^+]$$

$[B^+]$ is nothing else but concentration of the strong base present (or - as a volume is 1 - number of moles of strong base present) in the solution - thus it is n from 19.1 definition.

Total concentration of the buffer, C_{buf}, is given by

$$C_{buf} = [HA] + [A^-]$$

From dissociation constant definition we have

$$[HA] = \frac{[H^+][A^-]}{K_a}$$

so

$$C_{buf} = \frac{[H^+][A^-]}{K_a} + [A^-]$$

or

$$[A^-] = \frac{C_{buf} K_a}{K_a + [H^+]}$$

Above equations and water ionization constant definition when combined give us formula for the amount of the strong base:

$$n = \frac{K_W}{[H^+]} - [H^+] + \frac{C_{buf} K_a}{K_a + [H^+]}$$

Now we are ready to calculate derivative:

$$\beta = \frac{dn}{dpH} = \frac{dn}{d[H^+]} \frac{d[H^+]}{dpH}$$

$$\beta = \left(-\frac{K_W}{[H^+]^2}-1-\frac{C_{buf}K_a}{(K_a+[H^+])^2}\right)(-2.303[H^+])$$

So finally buffer capacity is given by

$$\beta = 2.303\left(\frac{K_W}{[H^+]}+[H^+]+\frac{C_{buf}K_a[H^+]}{(K_a+[H^+])^2}\right)$$

This equation can be easily generalized for buffer capacity of solutions containing several buffers:

$$\beta = 2.303\left(\frac{K_W}{[H^+]}+[H^+]+\sum\frac{C_{buf}K_a[H^+]}{K_a+[H^+]^2}\right)$$

Note that first two terms in the buffer capacity formula are not dependent on the buffer presence in the solution. They reflect the fact that solutions of high (or low) pH are resistant to pH changes. As it was already signaled in the buffer pH section, such solutions have high buffer capacity regardless of the presence (or lack of the presence) of a classic buffer. For table of example values of buffer capacities see buffer capacity discussion at buffer lectures.

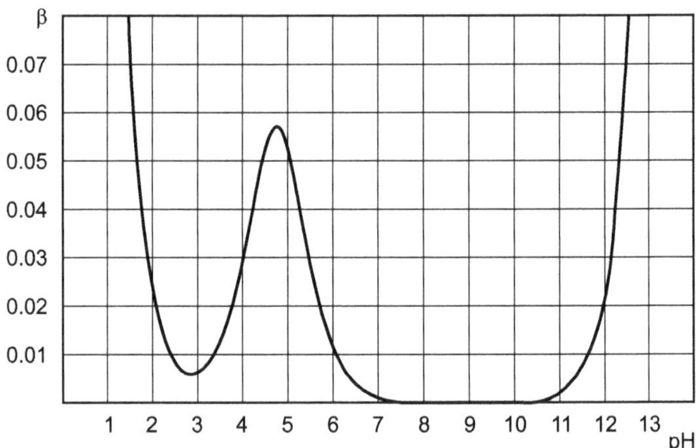

Above plot shows how the buffer capacity changes for the 0.1M solution of acetic buffer. As expected buffer exhibits the highest resistance to acid and base addition for the equimolar solution (when pH = pK_a). From the plot it is also obvious that buffer capacity has reasonably high values only for pH close to pK_a value. The further from the optimal value, the lower buffer capacity of the solution. Solution containing only conjugate base (pH 8-10) has buffer capacity of zero, for the higher pH presence of the strong base starts to play an important role. In the case of pure acetic acid solution (pH below 3) pH is already low enough to be resistant to changes due to the high concentration of H^+ cations.

Calculating Buffer pH

Monoprotic Acids

First write down the equilibrium expression.

$$HA \rightleftharpoons A^- + H^+$$

This shows that when the acid dissociates equal amounts of hydrogen ion and anion are produced. The equilibrium concentrations of these three components can be calculated in an ICE table.

ICE table for a monoprotic acid

	[HA]	[A⁻]	[H⁺]
I	C_0	0	y
C	-x	x	x
E	C_0-x	x	x+y

The first row, labelled I, lists the initial conditions: the concentration of acid is C_0, initially undissociated, so the concentrations of A^- and H^+ would be zero; y is the initial concentration of added strong acid, such as hydrochloric acid. If strong alkali, such as sodium hydroxide, is added y will have a negative sign because alkali removes hydrogen ions from the solution. The second row, labelled C for change, specifies the changes that occur when the acid dissociates. The acid concentration decreases by an amount $-x$ and the concentrations of A^- and H^+ both increase by an amount $+x$. This follows from the equilibrium expression. The third row, labelled E for equilibrium concentrations, adds together the first two rows and shows the concentrations at equilibrium.

To find x, use the formula for the equilibrium constant in terms of concentrations:

$$K_a = \frac{[H^+][A^-]}{[HA]}$$

Substitute the concentrations with the values found in the last row of the ICE table:

$$K_a = \frac{x(x+y)}{C_0 - x}$$

Simplify to:

$$x^2 + (K_a + Y)x - K_a C_0 = 0$$

With specific values for C_0, K_a and y this equation can be solved for x. Assuming that pH = $-\log_{10}[H^+]$ the pH can be calculated as pH = $-\log_{10}(x+y)$.

Polyprotic Acids

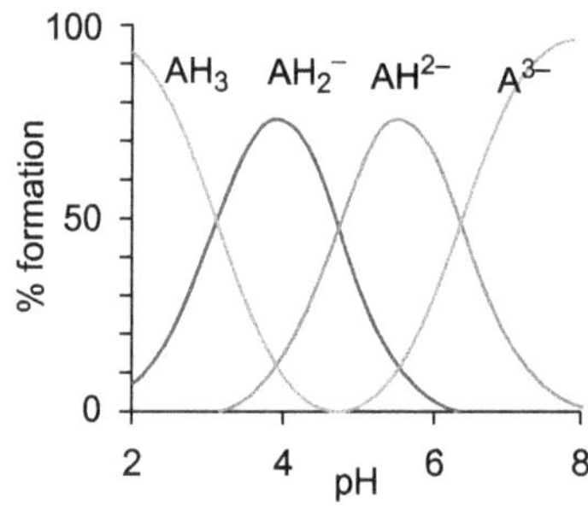

% species formation calculated for a 10 millimolar solution of citric acid.

Polyprotic acids are acids that can lose more than one proton. The constant for dissociation of the first proton may be denoted as K_{a1} and the constants for dissociation of successive protons as K_{a2}, etc. Citric acid, H_3A, is an example of a polyprotic acid as it can lose three protons.

Equilibrium	**pK_a value**
$H_3A \rightleftharpoons H_2A^- + H^+$	pK_{a1} = 3.13
$H_2A^- \rightleftharpoons HA^{2-} + H^+$	pK_{a2} = 4.76
$HA^{2-} \rightleftharpoons A^{3-} + H^+$	pK_{a3} = 6.40

When the difference between successive pK values is less than about three there is overlap between the pH range of existence of the species in equilibrium. The smaller the difference, the more the overlap. In the case of citric acid, the overlap is extensive and solutions of citric acid are buffered over the whole range of pH 2.5 to 7.5.

Calculation of the pH with a polyprotic acid requires a speciation calculation to be performed. In the case of citric acid, this entails the solution of the two equations of mass balance

$$C_A = [A^{3-}] + \beta_1 [A^{3-}][H^+] + \beta_2 [A^{3-}][H^+]^2 + \beta_3 [A^{3-}][H^+]^3$$

$$C_H = [H^+] + \beta_1 [A^{3-}][H^+] + 2\beta_2 [A^{3-}][H^+]^2 + 3\beta_3 [A^{3-}][H^+]^3 - K_w[H]^{-1}$$

C_A is the analytical concentration of the acid, C_H is the analytical concentration of added hydrogen ions, β_q are the cumulative association constants

$$log\ \beta_1 - pKa_3,\ log\ \beta_2 - pK_{a2} + pK_{a3},\ log\ \beta_3 - pK_{a1} + pK_{a2} + pK_{a3}$$

K_w is the constant for Self-ionization of water. There are two non-linear simultaneous equations in two unknown quantities $[A^{3-}]$ and $[H^+]$. Many computer programs are available to do this calculation. The speciation diagram for citric acid was produced with the program HySS.

HENDERSON–HASSELBALCH EQUATION

In chemistry, the Henderson–Hasselbalch equation describes the derivation of pH as a measure of acidity (using pK_a, the negative log of the acid dissociation constant) in biological and chemical systems. The equation is also useful for estimating the pH of a buffer solution and finding the equilibrium pH in acid-base reactions (it is widely used to calculate the isoelectric point of proteins).

The equation is given by:

$$pH = pK_a + \log_{10}\left(\frac{[A^-]}{[HA]}\right)$$

Here, [HA] is the molar concentration of the undissociated weak acid, $[A^-]$ is the molar concentration (molarity, M) of this acid's conjugate base and pK_a is $-\log_{10} K_a$ where Ka is the acid dissociation constant, that is:

$$pK_a = -\log_{10}(K_a) = -\log_{10}\left(\frac{[H_3O^+][A^-]}{[HA]}\right)$$

for the non-specific Brønsted acid-base reaction: $HA + H_2O \rightleftharpoons A^- + H_3O^+$

In these equations, A^- denotes the ionic form of the relevant acid. Bracketed quantities such as [base] and [acid] denote the molar concentration of the quantity enclosed.

For bases

For the standard base equation:

$B + H^+ \rightleftharpoons BH^+$

A second form of the equation, known as the Heylman Equation, expressed in terms of K_b where K_b is the base dissociation constant:

$$pK_a = -\log_{10}(K_b) = -\log_{10}\left(\frac{[OH^-][HA]}{[A^-]}\right)$$

In analogy to the above equations, the following equation is valid:

$$pOH = pK_b - \log_{10}\left(\frac{[BH^+]}{[B]}\right)$$

Where BH^+ denotes the conjugate acid of the corresponding base B. Using the properties of these terms at 25 degrees Celsius one can synthesise an equation for pH of basic solutions in terms of pK_a and pH:

$$pH = pK_a + \log_{10}\left(\frac{[B]}{[BH^+]}\right)$$

Derivation

The Henderson–Hasselbalch equation is derived from the acid dissociation constant equation by the following steps:

$$K_a = \frac{[H^+][A^-]}{[HA]}$$

Taking the log, to base ten, of both sides gives:

$$\log_{10} K_a = \log_{10} \frac{[H^+][A^-]}{[HA]}$$

Then, using the properties of logarithms:

$$\log_{10} K_a = \log_{10} [\mathrm{H}^+] + \log_{10}\left(\frac{[A^-]}{[HA]}\right)$$

Identifying the left-hand side of this equation as -pK_a and the $\log_{10}$[H$^+$] as pH:

$$-\mathrm{p}K_a = -\mathrm{pH} + \log_{10}\left(\frac{[A^-]}{[HA]}\right)$$

Adding pH and pK_a to both sides:

$$\mathrm{pH} = \mathrm{p}K_a + \log_{10}\left(\frac{[A^-]}{[HA]}\right)$$

The ratio [A$^-$]/[HA] is unitless, and as such, other ratios with other units may be used. For example, the mole ratio of the components, $n_A - /n_{HA}$ or the fractional concentrations $\alpha_A - /\alpha_{HA}$ where $\alpha_A - + /\alpha_{HA} = 1$ will yield the same answer. Sometimes these other units are more convenient to use.

History

Lawrence Joseph Henderson wrote an equation, in 1908, describing the use of carbonic acid as a buffer solution. Karl Albert Hasselbalch later re-expressed that formula inlogarithmic terms, resulting in the Henderson–Hasselbalch equation. Hasselbalch was using the formula to study metabolic acidosis.

Limitations

There are some significant approximations implicit in the Henderson–Hasselbalch equation. The most significant is the assumption that the concentration of the acid and its conjugate base at equilibrium will remain the same as the formal concentration. This neglects the dissociation of the acid and the binding of H+ to the base. The dissociation of water and relative water concentration itself is neglected as well. These approximations will fail when dealing with relatively strong acids or bases (pKa more than a couple units away from 7), dilute or very concentrated solutions (less than 1 mM or greater than 1M), or heavily skewed acid/base ratios (more than 100 to 1). In high buffer dilutions, where the concentration of protons arising from water become equally or more prevalent than the buffer species themselves (at pH 7, this means buffer component concentrations of $<10^{-5}$M formally, but practically much higher), the pKa of the 'buffer' system will tend towards neutrality.

Estimating Blood pH

The Henderson–Hasselbalch equation can be applied to relate the pH of blood to constituents of the bicarbonate buffering system:

$$pH = pK_a H_2CO_3 + \log_{10}\left(\frac{[HCO_3^-]}{[H_2CO_3]}\right)$$

where:

- $pK_{a\ H2CO3}$ is the cologarithm of the acid dissociation constant of carbonic acid. It is equal to 6.1.
- $[HCO_3^-]$ is the concentration of bicarbonate in the blood
- $[H_2CO_3]$ is the concentration of carbonic acid in the blood

This is useful in arterial blood gas, but these usually state p_{CO2}, that is, the partial pressure of carbon dioxide, rather than H_2CO_3. However, these are related by the equation.

$$[H_2CO_3] = K_H CO_2 \times pco_2,$$

where:

- $[H_2CO_3]$ is the concentration of carbonic acid in the blood
- $k_{H\ CO2}$ is the Henry's law constant for the solubility of carbon dioxide in blood. $k_{H\ CO2}$ is approximately 0.0307 mmol/(L-torr)
- p_{CO2} is the partial pressure of carbon dioxide in the blood

Taken together, the following equation can be used to relate the pH of blood to the concentration of bicarbonate and the partial pressure of carbon dioxide:

$$pH = 6.1 + \log 10 \left(\frac{[HCO_3^-]}{0.0307 \times pco_2}\right)$$

where:

- pH is the acidity in the blood
- $[HCO_3^-]$ is the concentration of bicarbonate in the blood
- PCO_2 is the partial pressure of carbon dioxide in the arterial blood

Acidic Buffer Solutions

We'll take a mixture of ethanoic acid and sodium ethanoate as typical. Ethanoic acid is a weak acid, and the position of this equilibrium will be well to the left:

$$CH_3COOH_{(aq)} \rightleftharpoons CH_3COO^-(aq) + H^+(aq)$$

Adding sodium ethanoate to this adds lots of extra ethanoate ions. According to Le Chatelier's Principle, that will tip the position of the equilibrium even further to the left.

The solution will therefore contain these important things:

- lots of un-ionized ethanoic acid;
- lots of ethanoate ions from the sodium ethanoate;
- enough hydrogen ions to make the solution acidic.

Other things (like water and sodium ions) which are present aren't important to the argument.

Adding an Acid to this Buffer Solution

The buffer solution must remove most of the new hydrogen ions otherwise the pH would drop markedly. Hydrogen ions combine with the ethanoate ions to make ethanoic acid. Although the reaction is reversible, since the ethanoic acid is a weak acid, most of the new hydrogen ions are removed in this way.

$$CH_3COO^-_{(aq)} + H^+_{(aq)} \rightleftharpoons CH_3COOH_{(aq)}$$

Since most of the new hydrogen ions are removed, the pH won't change very much - but because of the equilibria involved, it will fall a little bit.

Adding an Alkali to this Buffer Solution

Alkaline solutions contain hydroxide ions and the buffer solution removes most of these. This time the situation is a bit more complicated because there are two processes which can remove hydroxide ions. Removal by reacting with ethanoic acid.

The most likely acidic substance which a hydroxide ion is going to collide with is an ethanoic acid molecule. They will react to form ethanoate ions and water.

$$CH_3COOH_{(aq)} + OH^-_{(aq)} \rightleftharpoons CH_3COO^-_{(aq)} + H_2O_{(l)}$$

Because most of the new hydroxide ions are removed, the pH doesn't increase very much. Removal of the hydroxide ions by reacting with hydrogen ions Remember that there are some hydrogen ions present from the ionization of the ethanoic acid.

$$CH_3COOH_{(aq)} \rightleftharpoons CH_3COO^-_{(aq)} + H^+_{(aq)}$$

Hydroxide ions can combine with these to make water. As soon as this happens, the equilibrium tips to replace them. This keeps on happening until most of the hydroxide ions are removed.

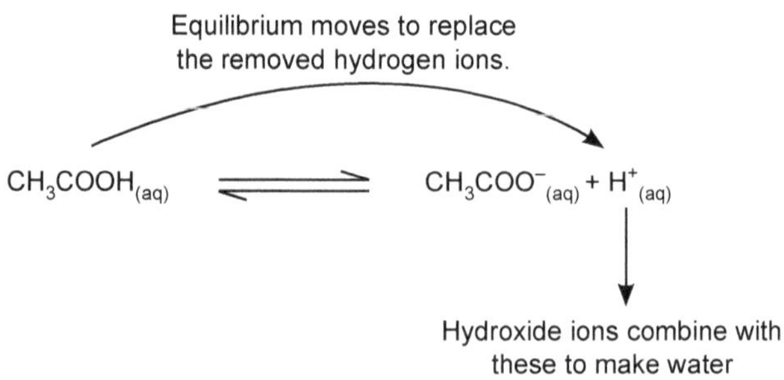

Again, because you have equilibria involved, not all of the hydroxide ions are removed - just most of them. The water formed re-ionizes to a very small extent to give a few hydrogen ions and hydroxide ions.

Alkaline Buffer Solutions

We'll take a mixture of ammonia and ammonium chloride solutions as typical. Ammonia is a weak base, and the position of this equilibrium will be well to the left:

$$NH_{3(aq)} + H_2O_{(l)} \rightleftharpoons NH_4^+{}_{(aq)} + OH^-{}_{(aq)}$$

Adding ammonium chloride to this adds lots of extra ammonium ions. According to Le Chatelier's Principle, that will tip the position of the equilibrium even further to the left. The solution will therefore contain these important things:

1. Lots of un reacted ammonia;
2. Lots of ammonium ions from the ammonium chloride;
3. Enough hydroxide ions to make the solution alkaline.
4. Other things (like water and chloride ions) which are present aren't important to the argument.

Adding an Acid to this Buffer Solution

There are two processes which can remove the hydrogen ions that you are adding.

Removal by Reacting with Ammonia

The most likely basic substance which a hydrogen ion is going to collide with is an ammonia molecule. They will react to form ammonium ions.

$$NH_{3(aq)} + H^+{}_{(aq)} \rightleftharpoons NH_4^+{}_{(aq)}$$

Most, but not all, of the hydrogen ions will be removed. The ammonium ion is weakly acidic, and so some of the hydrogen ions will be released again.

Removal of the Hydrogen Ions by Reacting with Hydroxide Ions

Remember that there are some hydroxide ions present from the reaction between the ammonia and the water.

$$NH_{3(aq)} + H_2O_{(l)} \rightleftharpoons NH_4^+{}_{(aq)}$$

Hydrogen ions can combine with these hydroxide ions to make water. As soon as this happens, the equilibrium tips to replace the hydroxide ions. This keeps on happening until most of the hydrogen ions are removed.

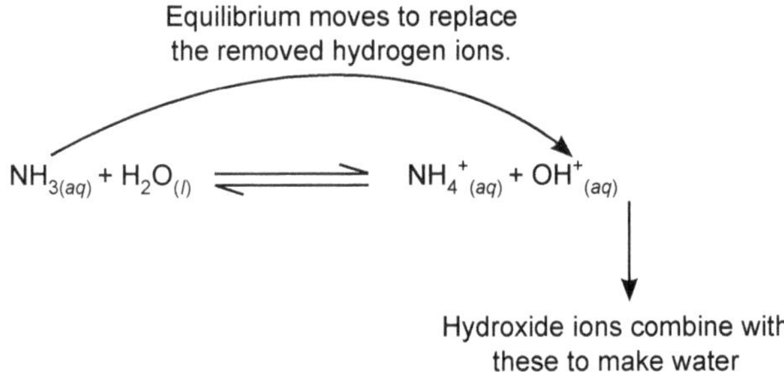

Again, because you have equilibria involved, not all of the hydrogen ions are removed - just most of them.

Adding an Alkali to this Buffer Solution

The hydroxide ions from the alkali are removed by a simple reaction with ammonium ions.

$$NH_4^+{}_{(aq)} + OH^-{}_{(aq)} \rightleftharpoons NH_{3(aq)} + H_2O_{(l)}$$

Because the ammonia formed is a weak base, it can react with the water - and so the reaction is slightly reversible. That means that, again, most (but not all) of the hydroxide ions are removed from the solution.

Calculations Involving Buffer Solutions

Acidic Buffer Solutions

This is easier to see with a specific example. Remember that an acid buffer can be made from a weak acid and one of its salts. Let's suppose that you had a buffer solution containing 0.10 mol dm^{-3} of ethanoic acid and 0.20 mol dm^{-3} of sodium ethanoate. How do you calculate its pH? In any solution containing a weak acid, there is equilibrium between the un-ionized acid and its ions. So for ethanoic acid, you have the equilibrium:

$$CH_3COOH_{(aq)} \rightleftharpoons CH_3COO^-{}_{(aq)} + H^+{}_{(aq)}$$

The presence of the ethanoate ions from the sodium ethanoate will have moved the equilibrium to the left, but the equilibrium still exists.

That means that you can write the equilibrium constant, K_a, for it:

$$K_a = \frac{[CH_3COO^-][H^+]}{[CH_3COOH]}$$

Where you have done calculations using this equation previously with a weak acid, you will have assumed that the concentrations of the hydrogen ions and ethanoate ions were the same. Every molecule of ethanoic acid that splits up gives one of each sort of ion.

That's no longer true for a buffer solution:

These two concentrations are no longer equal.

$$K_a = \frac{[CH_3COO^-][H^+]}{[CH_3COOH]}$$

If the equilibrium has been pushed even further to the left, the number of ethanoate ions coming from the ethanoic acid will be completely negligible compared to those from the sodium ethanoate. We therefore assume that the ethanoate ion concentration is the same as the concentration of the sodium ethanoate - in this case, 0.20 mol dm^{-3}. In a weak acid calculation, we normally assume that so little of the acid has ionized that the concentration of the acid at equilibrium is the same as the concentration of the acid we used. That is even more true now that the equilibrium has been moved even further to the left. So the assumptions we make for a buffer solution are:

Assume this is the same as the

concentration of the soldium ethanoate

$$K_a = \frac{[CH_3COO^-][H^+]}{[CH_3COOH]}$$

Assume this is the same as the
concentration of the original acid.

Now, if we know the value for K_a, we can calculate the hydrogen ion concentration and therefore the pH.

K_a for ethanoic acid is 1.74×10^{-5} mol dm^{-3}.

Remember that we want to calculate the pH of a buffer solution containing 0.10 mol dm^{-3} of ethanoic acid and 0.20 mol dm^{-3} of sodium ethanoate.

$$K_a = \frac{[CH_3COO^-][H^+]}{[CH_3COOH]}$$

$$1.74 \times 10^{-5} = \frac{0.20 \times [H^+]}{0.10}$$

$$[H^+] = 1.74 \times 10^{-5} \times \frac{0.10}{0.20}$$
$$= 8.7 \times 10^{-6} \text{ mol dm}^{-3}$$

Then all you have to do is to find the pH using the expression

$$pH = -\log_{10} [H^+]$$

You will still have the value for the hydrogen ion concentration on your calculator, so press the log button and ignore the negative sign (to allow for the minus sign in the pH expression). You should get an answer of 5.1 to two significant figures. You can't be more accurate than this, because your concentrations were only given to two figures. You could, of course, be asked to reverse this and calculate in what proportions you would have to mix ethanoic acid and sodium ethanoate to get a buffer solution of some desired pH. It is no more difficult than the calculation we have just looked at. Suppose you wanted a buffer with a pH of 4.46. If you un-log this to find the hydrogen ion concentration you need, you will find it is 3.47×10^{-5} mol dm^{-3}.

Feed that into the K_a expression.

$$K_a = \frac{[CH_3COO^-][H^+]}{[CH_3COOH]}$$

$$1.74 \times 10^{-5} = \frac{[CH_3COO^-] \times 3.47 \times 10^{-5}}{[CH_3COOH]}$$

$$\frac{[CH_3COO^-]}{[CH_3COOH]} = \frac{1.74 \times 10^{-5}}{3.47 \times 10^{-5}}$$

$$= 0.50$$

This entire means is that to get a solution of pH 4.46, the concentration of the ethanoate ions (from the sodium ethanoate) in the solution has to be 0.5 times that of the concentration of the acid. All that matters is that ratio. In other words, the concentration of the ethanoate has to be half that of the ethanoic acid. One way of getting this, for example, would be to mix together 10 cm^3 of 1.0 mol dm^{-3} sodium ethanoate solution with 20 cm^3 of 1.0 mol dm^{-3} ethanoic acid. Or 10 cm^3 of 1.0 mol dm^{-3} sodium ethanoate solution with 10 cm^3 of 2.0 mol dm^{-3} ethanoic acid. And there are all sorts of other possibilities.

Alkaline Buffer Solutions

We are talking here about a mixture of a weak base and one of its salts - for example, a solution containing ammonia and ammonium chloride. The modern, and easy, way of doing these calculations is to re-think them from the point of view of the ammonium ion rather than of the ammonia solution. Once you have taken this slightly different view-point, everything becomes much the same as before. So how would you find the pH of a solution containing 0.100 mol dm^{-3} of ammonia and 0.0500 mol dm^{-3} of ammonium chloride? The mixture will contain lots of unreacted ammonia molecules and lots of ammonium ions as the essential ingredients. The ammonium ions are weakly acidic, and this equilibrium is set up whenever they are in solution in water:

$$NH+4(aq) \rightleftharpoons NH_3(aq) + H^+(aq)$$

You can write a K_a expression for the ammonium ion, and make the same sort of assumptions as we did in the previous case:

Assume this is the same as the concentration of the original ammonia solution.

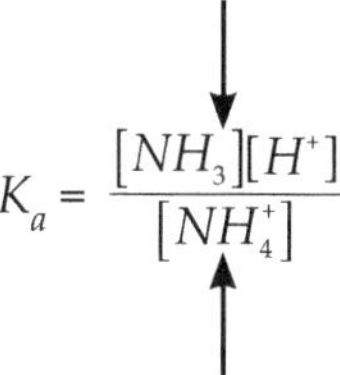

$$K_a = \frac{[NH_3][H^+]}{[NH_4^+]}$$

Assume this is the same as the concentration of the ammonia chloride.

The presence of the ammonia in the mixture forces the equilibrium far to the left. That means that you can assume that the ammonium ion concentration is what you started off with in the ammonium chloride, and that the ammonia concentration is all due to the added ammonia solution. The value for K_a for the ammonium ion is 5.62×10^{-10} mol dm^{-3}. Remember that we want to calculate the pH of a buffer solution containing 0.100 mol dm^{-3} of ammonia and 0.0500 mol dm^{-3} of ammonium chloride. Just put all these numbers in the K_a expression, and do the sum:

$$K_a = \frac{[NH_3][H^+]}{[NH_4^+]}$$

$$5.62 \times 10^{-10} = \frac{0.100 \times [H^+]}{0.0500}$$

$$[H^+] = \frac{1.74 \times 10^{-5}}{3.47 \times 10^{-5}}$$

$$= 2.81 \times 10^{-10}$$

$$pH = -\log_{10} [H^+]$$

$$= 9.55.$$

Preparation of Buffers and Related Solutions

Preparation of Buffers

Methods used to prepare buffers are based on the basic principle specified by the Henderson-Hasselbach equation: That the pH of a buffer is determined by the (conjugate base)/(conjugate acid) ratio, and vice versa. Preparing a buffer of a given pH, therefore, requires the preparation of a solution that contains the conjugate base and the conjugate acid at a ratio equal to the value predicted by the Henderson-Hasselbach equation. The appropriate ratio can be established by adding acid or base to a solution of one of the conjugates to adjust the pH to the desired value; or by dissolving pre calculated quantities of the conjugates. The following three methods are based on these principles.

Method 1: Simple pH Adjustment

- Calculate the weight of the buffer needed to prepare a solution of a given volume and molarity using equation 9 (use any of the conjugate forms of the buffer).
- Dissolve it in a volume of deionized H2O, which are about eight-tenths of the desired final volume.
- Adjust the pH to the desired value, and then add additional H2O to adjust the volume to the final value.

Method 2: Using Calculated Amounts of the Conjugate Forms

- Use the Henderson-Hasselbach equation to calculate the concentrations of the conjugate acid and base that will be present in the buffer at the given pH.
- Use equation 9 to calculate the weight corresponding to each of the concentrations in step 1.
- Dissolve these quantities as in step 2 of method 1, above.
- Adjust the volume to the target value by adding additional H_2O.
- Check the pH. It should be within ±O.2 units of the expected value.

Method 3: Mixing Proportionate Volumes of the Conjugate Forms

- For each conjugate, calculate the weight needed to prepare a solution at a concentration equal to that of the buffer.
- Calculate the ratio [A-]/[HA] or [R-NH_2]/[R-NH)+] at the given pH of the buffer.
- Use this ratio to calculate the volumes of both solutions which, when combined, yield a buffer with the given pH, concentration, and volume.
- Prepare the buffer by combining the measured volumes. Check the pH. It should be within ± 0.2 units of the expected value.

Preparation of Buffers for Use in Enzyme Studies

The buffers described below are suitable for use either in enzymatic or histochemical studies.

1. Acetate Buffer

Stock solutions

A. 0.2M solution of acetic acid (11.55g in 1000ml).

B. 0.2M solution of Sodium acetate (16.4g [$C_2H_3O_2Na$ or 27.2g of $C_2H_3O_2Na$. $3H_2O$] in 1000ml).

X ml of A + Y ml of B, diluted to a total of 100ml.

X	Y	pH	X	Y	pH
46.3	3.7	3.6	20.0	30.0	4.8
44.0	6.0	3.8	14.8	35.2	5.0
41.0	9.0	4.0	10.5	39.5	5.2
36.8	13.2	4.2	8.8	41.2	5.4
30.5	19.5	4.4	4.8	45.2	5.6
25.5	24.5	4.6			

2. Aconitate Buffer

Stock solutions

A. 0.5M solution of aconitic acid (87.05g in 1000ml).

B. 0.2M solution of NaOH (0.8g in 100ml).

20ml of A + X ml of B diluted to a total of 200ml.

X	pH	X	pH
15.0	2.5	83.0	4.3
21.0	2.7	90.0	4.5
28.0	2.9	97.0	4.7
36.0	3.1	103.0	4.9
44.0	3.3	108.0	5.1
52.0	3.5	113.0	5.3
60.0	3.7	119.0	5.5
68.0	3.9	126.0	5.7
76.0	4.1		

3. Barbital Buffer

Stock solutions

A. 0.2M solution of sodium barbital (veronal) (41.2g in 1000ml).

B. 0.2M solution of HCl (1.718ml in 100ml).

50ml of A + Xml of B, diluted to a total of 200ml.

X	pH	X	pH
1.5	9.2	17.5	8.0
2.5	9.0	22.5	7.8
4.0	8.8	32.5	7.4
6.0	8.6	39.0	7.2
9.0	8.4	43.0	7.0
12.7	8.2	45.0	6.8

4. Borax-NaOH Buffer

Stock solutions

A. 0.05M solution of borax (19.05g in 1000ml; 0.02M in terms of sodium borate).

B. 0.2M solution of NaOH (0.8g in 100ml).

50ml of A + Xml of B, diluted to a total of 200ml.

X	pH	X	pH
0.0	9.28	29.0	9.7
7.0	9.35	34.0	9.8
11.0	9.4	38.6	9.9
17.6	9.5	43.0	10.0
23.0	9.6	46.0	10.1

5. Boric Acid-Borax Buffer

Stock solutions

A. 0.2M solution of boric acid (12.4g in 1000ml).

B. 0.05M solution of borax (19.05g in 1000ml; 0.2M in terms of sodium borate).

50ml of A + Xml of B, diluted to a total of 200ml.

X	pH	X	pH
2.0	7.6	22.5	8.7
3.1	7.8	30.0	8.8
4.9	8.0	42.5	8.9
7.3	8.2	59.0	9.0
11.5	8.4	83.0	9.1
17.5	8.6	115.0	9.2

6. Carbonate-Bicarbonate Buffer

Stock solutions

A. 0.2M solution of anhydrous sodium carbonate (21.2g in 1000ml).

B. 0.2M solution of sodium bicarbonate (16.8g in 1000ml).

Xml of A + Xml of B, diluted to a total of 200ml.

X	Y	pH	X	Y	pH
4.0	46.0	9.2	27.5	22.5	10.0
7.5	42.5	9.3	30.0	20.0	10.1
9.5	40.5	9.4	33.0	17.0	10.2
13.0	37.0	9.5	35.5	14.5	10.3

Contd...

16.0	34.0	9.6	38.5	11.5	10.4
19.5	30.5	9.7	40.5	9.5	10.5
22.0	28.0	9.8	42.5	7.5	10.6
25.0	25.0	9.9	45.0	5.0	10.7

7. Cacodylate Buffer

Stock solutions

A. 0.2M solution of sodium cacodylate (42.8g of $Na(CH_3)_2$ $ASO_2.3H_2O$ in 1000ml).

B. 0.2M HCl solution (1.695ml in 100ml).

50ml of A + Xml of B, diluted to a total of 200ml.

X	pH	X	pH
2.7	7.4	29.6	6.0
4.2	7.2	34.8	5.8
6.3	7.0	39.2	5.6
9.3	6.8	43.0	5.4
13.3	6.6	45.0	5.2
18.3	6.4	47.0	5.0
23.8	6.2		

8. Cirate Buffer

Stock solutions

A. 0.1M solution of citric acid (21.01g in 1000ml).

B. 0.1M solution of Sodium citrate (29.41g [$C_6H_5O_7Na.2H_2O$] in 1000ml; the use of the salt with 51/2 H_2O is not recommended).

X ml of A + Y ml of B, diluted to a total of 100ml.

X	Y	pH	X	Y	pH
46.5	3.5	3.0	23.0	27.0	4.8
43.7	6.3	3.2	20.5	29.5	5.0
40.0	10.0	3.4	18.0	32.0	5.2
37.0	13.0	3.6	16.0	34.0	5.4
35.0	15.0	3.8	13.7	36.3	5.6
33.0	17.0	4.0	11.8	38.2	5.8
31.5	18.5	4.2	9.5	41.5	6.0
28.0	22.0	4.4	7.2	42.8	6.2
25.5	24.5	4.6			

9. Citrate-Phosphate Buffer

Stock solutions

A. 0.1M solution of citric acid (19.21g in 1000ml).

B. 0.1M solution of dibasic Sodium phosphate (53.65g [$Na_2HPO_4.7H_2O$ or 71.7g of $Na_2HPO_4.12H_2O$] in 1000ml).

X ml of A + Y ml of B, diluted to a total of 100ml.

X	Y	pH	X	Y	pH
44.6	5.4	2.6	24.3	25.7	5.0
42.2	7.8	2.8	23.3	26.7	5.2
39.8	10.2	3.0	22.2	27.8	5.4
37.7	12.3	3.2	21.0	29.0	5.6
35.9	14.1	3.4	19.7	30.3	5.8
33.9	16.1	3.6	17.9	32.1	6.0
32.3	17.7	3.8	16.9	33.1	6.2
30.7	19.3	4.0	15.4	34.6	6.4
29.4	20.6	4.2	13.6	36.4	6.6
27.8	22.2	4.4	9.1	40.9	6.8
26.7	23.3	4.6	6.5	43.5	7.0
25.2	24.8	4.8			

10. Glycine-HCl Buffer

Stock solutions

A. 0.2M solution of glycine (15.01g in 1000ml).

B. 0.2M solution of HCl (1.697ml in 100ml).

50ml of A + X ml of B diluted to a total of 200ml.

X	pH	X	pH
5.0	3.6	16.8	2.8
6.4	3.4	24.2	2.6
8.2	3.2	32.4	2.4
11.4	3.0	44.0	2.2

11. Glycine-NaOH Buffer

Stock solutions

A. 0.2M solution of glycine (15.01g in 1000ml).

B. 0.2M solution of NaOH (0.8g in 100ml).

50ml of A + Xml of B, diluted to a total of 200ml.

X	pH	X	pH
4.0	8.6	22.4	9.6
6.0	8.8	27.2	9.8
8.8	9.0	32.0	10.0
12.0	9.2	38.6	10.4
16.8	9.4	45.5	10.6

12. Hydrochloric Acid-Potassium Chloride Buffer

Stock Solutions

A. 0.2M Solution of KCl (14.91 g in 1000ml)

B. 0.2M Solution of HCl (1.718 ml in 1000ml)

50 ml of A + X ml of B diluted to a total of 200ml.

X	pH	X	pH
97.0	1.0	20.6	1.7
78.0	1.1	16.6	1.8
64.5	1.2	13.2	1.9
51.0	1.3	10.6	2.0
41.5	1.4	8.4	2.1
33.3	1.5	6.7	2.2
26.3	1.6		

13. Maleate Buffer

Stock solutions

A. 0.2M solution of sodium maleate acid (8.0g NaOH + 23.2g of maleic acid or 19.6g of maleic anhydride in 1000ml).

B. 0.2M solution of NaOH (0.8g in 100ml).

50ml of A + Xml of B, diluted to a total of 200ml.

X	pH	X	pH
7.2	5.2	33.0	6.2
10.5	5.4	38.0	6.4
15.3	5.6	41.6	6.6
20.8	5.8	44.4	6.8
26.9	6.0		

14. Phosphate Buffer

Stock solutions

A. 0.2M solution of monobasic sodium phosphate (27.8g in 1000ml).
B. 0.2M solution of dibasic sodium phosphate (53.65g of $Na_2HPO_4.7H_2O$ or 71.7g of $Na_2HPO_4.12H_2O$ in 1000ml).

Xml of A + Yml of B, diluted to a total of 200ml.

X	Y	pH	X	Y	pH
93.5	6.5	5.7	45.0	55.0	6.9
92.0	8.0	5.8	39.0	61.0	7.0
90.0	10.0	5.9	33.0	67.0	7.1
87.7	12.3	6.0	28.0	72.0	7.2
85.0	15.0	6.1	23.0	77.0	7.3
81.5	18.5	6.2	19.0	81.0	7.4
77.5	22.5	6.3	16.0	84.0	7.5
73.5	26.5	6.4	13.0	87.0	7.6
68.5	31.5	6.5	9.5	90.5	7.7
62.5	37.5	6.6	8.5	91.5	7.8
56.5	43.5	6.7	7.0	93.0	7.9
51.0	49.0	6.8	5.3	94.7	8.0

15. Phthalate-Hydrochloric Acid Buffer

Stock solutions

A. 0.2M solution of potassium acid phthalate (40.84g in 1000ml).
B. 0.2M solution of HCl (1.695ml in 100ml).

50ml of A + X ml of B diluted to a total of 200ml.

X	pH	X	pH
46.7	2.2	14.7	3.2
39.6	2.4	9.9	3.4
33.0	2.6	6.0	3.6
26.4	2.8	2.63	3.8
20.3	3.0		

16. Phthalate-Sodium Hydroxide Buffer

Stock solutions

A. 0.2M solution of potassium acid phthalate (40.84g in 100ml).
B. 0.2M solution of NaOH (0.8g in 100ml).

50ml of A + Xml of B, diluted to a total of 200ml.

X	pH	X	pH
3.7	4.2	30.0	5.2
7.5	4.4	35.5	5.4
12.2	4.6	39.8	5.6
17.7	4.8	43.0	5.8
23.9	5.0	45.5	6.0

17. Succinate Buffer

Stock solutions

A. 0.2M solution of succinic acid (23.6g in 1000ml).

B. 0.2M solution of NaOH (0.8g in 100ml).

25ml of A + Xml of B, diluted to a total of 100ml.

X	pH	X	pH
7.5	3.8	26.7	5.0
10.0	4.0	30.3	5.2
13.3	4.2	34.2	5.4
16.7	4.4	37.5	5.6
20.0	4.6	40.7	5.8
23.5	4.8	43.5	6.0

18. Tris (Hydroxymethyl) Amino Methane-Maleate (Tris-Maleate Buffer)

Stock solutions

A. 0.2M solution of Tris acid maleate (24.2g of tris (hydroxymethyl) aminomethane + 23.2g of maleic acid or 19.6g of maleic anhydride in 1000ml).

B. 0.2M solution of NaOH (0.8g in 100ml).

50ml of A + Xml of B, diluted to a total of 200ml.

X	pH	X	pH
7.0	5.2	48.0	7.0
10.8	5.4	51.0	7.2
15.5	5.6	54.0	7.4
20.5	5.8	58.0	7.6
26.0	6.0	63.5	7.8
31.5	6.2	69.0	8.0
37.0	6.4	75.0	8.2
42.0	6.6	81.0	8.4
45.0	6.8	86.5	8.6

19. Tris (Hydroxymethyl) Aminomethane (Tris) Buffer

Stock solutions

A. 0.2M solution of tris (hydroxymethyl) aminomethane (24.2g in 1000ml).

B. 0.2M solution of HCl (1.718ml in 100ml).

50ml of A + Xml of B, diluted to a total of 200ml.

X	pH	X	pH
5.0	9.0	26.8	8.0
8.1	8.8	32.5	7.8
12.2	8.6	38.4	7.6
16.5	8.4	41.4	7.4
21.9	8.2	44.2	7.2

20. 2-Amino-2-methyl-1, 3-Propanediol (Ammediol) Buffer

Stock solutions

A. 0.2M solution of 2-amino-2-methyl-1, 3-propanediol (21.03g in 1000ml).

B. 0.2M solution of HCl (1.718ml in 100ml).

50ml of A + Xml of B, diluted to a total of 200ml.

X	pH	X	pH
2.0	10.0	22.0	8.8
3.7	9.8	29.5	8.6
5.7	9.6	34.0	8.4
8.5	9.4	37.7	8.2
12.5	9.2	41.0	8.0
16.7	9.0	43.5	7.8

Other Examples to Prepare Buffer Solutions

Example 1:

100 mM phosphoric acid (sodium) buffer solution (pH=2.1)

Sodium dihydrogen phosphate dihydrate (M.W. = 156.01). 50 mmol (7.8 g)

Phosphoric acid (85 %, 14.7 mol/L)........................50 mmol (3.4 mL)

Add water to make up to 1 L.

Example 2:

10 mM phosphoric acid (sodium) buffer solution (pH=2.6)

Sodium dihydrogen phosphate dihydrate (M.W.=156.01)..5 mmol (0.78 g)

Phosphoric acid (85 %, 14.7 mol/L).........................5 mmol (0.34 mL)

Add water to make up to 1 L.

(Alternatively, dilute 100 mM phosphoric acid (sodium) buffer solution (pH=2.1) ten times).

Example 3:

50 mM phosphoric acid (sodium) buffer solution (pH=2.8)

Sodium dihydrogen phosphate dihydrate (M.W.=156.01)..40 mmol (6.24 g)

Phosphoric acid (85 %, 14.7 mol/L).........................10 mmol (0.68 mL)

Add water to make up to 1 L.

Example 4:

100 mM phosphoric acid (sodium) buffer solution (pH=6.8)

Sodium dihydrogen phosphate dihydrate (M.W.=156.01)..50 mmol (7.8 g)

Sodium dihydrogen phosphate 12-hydrate (M.W.=358.14)..50 mmol (17.9 g)

Add water to make up to 1 L.

Example 5:

10 mM phosphoric acid (sodium) buffer solution (pH=6.9)

Sodium dihydrogen phosphate dihydrate (M.W.=156.01)..5 mmol (0.78 g)

Sodium dihydrogen phosphate 12-hydrate (M.W.=358.14)..5 mmol (1.79 g)

Add water to make up to 1 L.

(Alternatively, dilute 100 mM phosphoric acid (sodium) buffer solution (pH=6.8) ten times).

Example 6:

20 mM citric acid (sodium) buffer solution (pH=3.1)

Citrate dihydrate (M.W.=210.14)...............16.7 mmol (3.51 g)

Sodium citrate dihydrate (M.W.=294.10)..3.3 mmol (0.97 g)

Add water to make up to 1 L.

Example 7:

20 mM citric acid (sodium) buffer solution (pH=4.6)

Citrate dihydrate (M.W.=210.14)...............10 mmol (2.1 g)

Sodium citrate dihydrate (M.W.=294.10)..10 mmol (2.94 g)

Add water to make up to 1 L.

Example 8:

10 mM tartaric acid (sodium) buffer solution (pH=2.9)

Tartaric acid (M.W.=150.09)...........................7.5 mmol (1.13 g)

Sodium tartrate dihydrate (M.W.=230.08)........2.5 mmol (0.58 g)

Add water to make up to 1 L.

Example 9:

10 mM tartaric acid (sodium) buffer solution (pH=4.2)

Tartaric acid (M.W.=150.09)...........................2.5 mmol (0.375 g)

Sodium tart rate dihydrate (M.W.=230.08)........7.5 mmol (1.726 g)

Add water to make up to 1 L.

Example 10:

20mM (acetic acid) ethanolamine buffer solution pH=9.6

Monoethanolamine (M.W.=61.87, d=1.017)...20 mmol (1.22 mL)

Acetic acid (glacial acetic acid, 17.4 mol/L)..................10 mmol (0.575 mL)

Add water to make up to 1 L.

Example 11:

100 mM acetic acid (sodium) buffer solution (pH=4.7)

Acetic acid (glacial acetic acid) (99.5 %, 17.4 mol/L)..................50 mmol (2.87 mL)

Sodium acetate trihydrate (M.W.=136.08)........50 mmol (6.80 g)

Add water to make up to 1 L.

Example 12:

100 mM boric acid (potassium) buffer solution (pH=9.1)

Boric acid (M.W.=61.83)...............100 mmol (6.18 g)

Potassium hydroxide (M.W.=56.11)...............50 mmol (2.81 g)

Add water to make up to 1 L.

Example 13:

100 mM boric acid (sodium) buffer solution (pH=9.1)

Boric acid (M.W.=61.83)...............100 mmol (6.18 g)

Sodium hydroxide (M.W.=40.00)...............50 mmol (2.00 g)

Add water to make up to 1 L.

CHAPTER 6

pH of the Solutions

An acid–base reaction is a chemical reaction that occurs between an acid and a base. Several theoretical frameworks provide alternative conceptions of the reaction mechanisms and their application in solving related problems. Their importance becomes apparent in analyzing acid–base reactions for gaseous or liquid species, or when acid or base character may be somewhat less apparent.

1. ACID AND BASE DEFINITIONS

The first scientific concept of acids and bases was provided by Lavoisier circa 1776. Since Lavoisier's knowledge of strong acids was mainly restricted to oxoacids, such as HNO_3 (nitric acid) and H_2SO_4 (sulfuric acid), which tend to contain central atoms in high oxidation states surrounded by oxygen, and since he was not aware of the true composition of the hydrohalic acids (HF, HCl, HBr, and HI), he defined acids in terms of their containing *oxygen*, which in fact he named from Greek words meaning acid-former meaning acid or sharp. The Lavoisier definition was held as absolute truth for over 30 years, until the 1810 article and subsequent lectures by Sir Humphry Davy in which he proved the lack of oxygen in H_2S, H_2Te, and the hydrohalic acids. However, Davy failed to develop a new theory, concluding that acidity does not depend upon any particular elementary substance, but upon peculiar arrangement of various substances. One notable modification of oxygen theory was provided by Berzelius, who stated that acids are oxides of nonmetals while bases are oxides of metals.

Brønsted–Lowry Definition

The Brønsted–Lowry definition, formulated in 1923, independently by Johannes Nicolaus Brønsted in Denmark and Martin Lowry in England, is based upon the idea of protonation of bases through the de-protonation of acids that is, the ability of acids to donate hydrogen ions (H^+) otherwise known as protons to bases, which "accept" them.

An acid–base reaction is, thus, the removal of a hydrogen ion from the acid and its addition to the base. The removal of a hydrogen ion from an acid produces its conjugate base, which is the acid with a hydrogen ion removed. The reception of a proton by a base produces its conjugate acid, which is the base with a hydrogen ion added.

Unlike the previous definitions, the Brønsted–Lowry definition does not refer to the formation of salt and solvent, but instead to the formation of conjugate acids and conjugate bases, produced by the transfer of a proton from the acid to the base. In this approach, acids and bases are fundamentally different in behavior from salts, which are seen as electrolytes, subject to the theories of Debye, Onsager, and others. An acid and a base react not to produce a salt and a solvent, but to form a new acid and a new base. The concept of neutralization is thus absent. Brønsted–Lowry acid–base behavior is formally independent of any solvent, making it more all-encompassing than the Arrhenius model.

The general formula for acid–base reactions according to the Brønsted–Lowry definition is:

$$HA + B \rightarrow BH^{+} + A^{-}$$

where HA represents the acid, B represents the base, BH^{+} represents the conjugate acid of B, and A^{-} represents the conjugate base of HA.

For example, a Brønsted-Lowry model for the dissociation of hydrochloric acid (HCl) in aqueous solution would be the following:

$$HCl + H_2O \rightleftharpoons H_3O^{+} + Cl^{-}$$

The removal of H^{+} from the HCl produces the chloride ion, Cl^{-}, the conjugate base of the acid. The addition of H^{+} to the H_2O (acting as a base) forms the hydronium ion, H_3O^{+}, the conjugate acid of the base.

Water is amphoteric that is, it can act as both an acid and a base. The Brønsted-Lowry model explains this, showing the dissociation of water into low concentrations of hydronium and hydroxide ions:

$$H_2O + H_2O \rightleftharpoons H_3O^{+} + OH^{-}$$

Here, one molecule of water acts as an acid, donating an H^{+} and forming the conjugate base, OH^{-}, and a second molecule of water acts as a base, accepting the H^{+} ion and forming the conjugate acid, H_3O^{+}.

2. ACID-BASE EQUILIBRIUM/CONCENTRATION

The reaction of a strong acid with a strong base is essentially a quantitative reaction. For example

$$HCl(aq) + Na(OH)(aq) \rightleftharpoons H_2O + NaCl(aq)$$

In this reaction both the sodium and chloride ions are spectators as the neutralization reaction,

$$H^{+} + OH^{-} \rightarrow H_2O$$

does not involve them. With weak bases addition of acid is not quantitative because a solution of a weak base is a buffer solution. A solution of a weak acid is also a buffer solution. When a weak acid reacts with a weak base an equilibrium mixture is produced. For example, adenine, written as AH can react with a hydrogen phosphate ion, HPO_4^{2-}

$$AH + HPO_4^{2-} \rightleftharpoons A^{-} + H_2PO_4^{-}$$

The equilibrium constant for this reaction can be derived from the acid dissociation constants of adenine and the hydrogen phosphate ion.

$[AH] = Ka_1[A^-][H^+]$

$[H_2PO_4^-] = Ka_2[HPO_4^{2-}][H^+]$

The notation [x] signifies concentration of x. When these two equations are combined by eliminating the hydrogen ion concentration, an expression for the equilibrium constant, K. is obtained.

$$[AH][HPO_4^{2-}] = K[A^-][H_2PO_4^-],\ K{=}Ka_1/Ka_2$$

Acid–Alkali Reaction

An acid–alkali reaction is a special case of an acid–base reaction, where the base used is also an alkali. When an acid reacts with an alkali it forms a metal salt and water. Acid alkali reactions are also a type of neutralization reaction.

In general, acid–alkali reactions can be simplified to

$$OH^-(aq) + H+(aq) \rightarrow H_2O$$

by omitting spectator ions.

Acids are in general pure substances that contain hydrogen ions (H+) or cause them to be produced in solutions. Hydrochloric acid (HCl) and sulfuric acid (H_2SO_4) are common examples. In water, these break apart into ions:

$HCl \rightarrow H+(aq) + Cl-(aq)$

$H_2SO_4 \rightarrow H+(aq) + HSO_{-4}(aq)$

To produce hydroxide ions in water, the alkali breaks apart into ions as below:

$NaOH \rightarrow Na+(aq) + OH-(aq)$

3. pH MEASUREMENT

pH

pH is defined as the decimal logarithm of the reciprocal of the hydrogen ion activity, a_H+, in a solution.

$$pH = -\log10\ (a_{H+}) = \log_{10}\left(\frac{1}{a_{H+}}\right)$$

This definition was adopted because ion-selective electrodes, which are used to measure pH, respond to activity. Ideally, electrode potential, E, follows the Nernst equation, which, for the hydrogen ion can be written as

$$E = E^0 + \frac{RT}{F} In(a_{H1}) = E^0 - \frac{2.303\ RT}{F} pH$$

where E is a measured potential, E^0 is the standard electrode potential, R is the gas constant, T is the temperature in Kelvin, F is the Faraday constant. For H^+ number of electrons transferred is one. It follows that electrode potential is proportional to pH when pH is defined in terms of activity. Precise measurement of pH is presented in International Standard ISO 31-8 as follows: A galvanic cell is set up to measure the electromotive force (e.m.f.) between a reference electrode and an electrode sensitive to the hydrogen ion activity when they are both immersed in the same aqueous solution. The reference electrode may be a silver chloride electrode or a calomel electrode. The hydrogen-ion selective electrode is a standard hydrogen electrode. Reference electrode | concentrated solution of KCl || test solution | H_2 | Pt.

Firstly, the cell is filled with a solution of known hydrogen ion activity and the e.m.f, E_S, is measured. Then the e.m.f, E_X, of the same cell containing the solution of unknown pH is measured.

$$\mathrm{pH(X)} = \mathrm{pH(S)} + \frac{E_S - E_X}{z}$$

The difference between the two measured e.m.f. values is proportional to pH. This method of calibration avoids the need to know the standard electrode potential. The proportionality constant, *1/z* is ideally equal to $\frac{1}{2.30RT/F}$ the Nernstian slope.

To apply this process in practice, a glass electrode is used rather than the cumbersome hydrogen electrode. A combined glass electrode has an in-built reference electrode. It is calibrated against buffer solutions of known hydrogen ion activity. IUPAC has proposed the use of a set of buffer solutions of known H^+ activity. Two or more buffer solutions are used in order to accommodate the fact that the "slope" may differ slightly from ideal. To implement this approach to calibration, the electrode is first immersed in a standard solution and the reading on a pH meter is adjusted to be equal to the standard buffer's value. The reading from a second standard buffer solution is then adjusted, using the "slope" control, to be equal to the pH for that solution. Further details, are given in the IUPAC recommendations. When more than two buffer solutions are used the electrode is calibrated by fitting observed pH values to a straight line with respect to standard buffer values. Commercial standard buffer solutions usually come with information on the value at 25 °C and a correction factor to be applied for other temperatures. The pH scale is logarithmic and therefore pH is a dimensionless quantity.

p[H]

This was the original definition of Sørensen, which was superseded in favor of pH in 1924. However, it is possible to measure the concentration of hydrogen ions directly, if the electrode is calibrated in terms of hydrogen ion concentrations. One way to do this, which has been used extensively, is to titrate a solution of known concentration of a strong acid with a solution of known concentration of strong alkaline in the presence of a relatively high concentration of background electrolyte. Since the concentrations of acid and alkaline are known, it is easy to calculate the concentration of hydrogen ions so that the measured potential can be correlated with concentrations. The calibration is usually carried out using a Gran plot. The calibration yields a value for the standard electrode potential, E^0, and a slope factor, *f*, so that the Nernst equation in the form

$$E = E_0 + f\frac{2.303RT}{F}\log[H^+]$$

can be used to derive hydrogen ion concentrations from experimental measurements of E. The slope factor, f, is usually slightly less than one. A slope factor of less than 0.95 indicates that the electrode is not functioning correctly. The presence of background electrolyte ensures that the hydrogen ion activity coefficient is effectively constant during the titration. As it is constant, its value can be set to one by defining the standard state as being the solution containing the background electrolyte. Thus, the effect of using this procedure is to make activity equal to the numerical value of concentration.

The glass electrode (and other ion selective electrodes) should be calibrated in a medium similar to the one being investigated. For instance, if one wishes to measure the pH of a seawater sample, the electrode should be calibrated in a solution resembling seawater in its chemical composition, as detailed below. The difference between p[H] and pH is quite small. It has been stated that pH = p[H] + 0.04. It is common practice to use the term "pH" for both types of measurement.

pH Indicators

Indicators may be used to measure pH, by making use of the fact that their color changes with pH. Visual comparison of the color of a test solution with a standard color chart provides a means to measure pH accurate to the nearest whole number. More precise measurements are possible if the color is measured spectrophotometrically, using a colorimeter of spectrophotometer. Universal indicator consists of a mixture of indicators such that there is a continuous color change from about pH 2 to pH 10. Universal indicator paper is made from absorbent paper that has been impregnated with universal indicator.

pOH

pOH is sometimes used as a measure of the concentration of hydroxide ions, OH^-, or alkalinity. pOH values are derived from pH measurements. The concentration of hydroxide ions in water is related to the concentration of hydrogen ions by

$$[OH^-] = \frac{K_W}{[H^+]}$$

where K_W is the self-ionisation constant of water. Taking logarithms

$$pOH = PK_W - pH$$

So, at room temperature pOH ≈ 14 – pH. However this relationship is not strictly valid in other circumstances, such as in measurements of soil alkalinity.

Extremes of pH

Measurement of pH below about 2.5 (ca. 0.003 mol dm^{-3} acid) and above about 10.5 (ca. 0.0003 mol dm^{-3} alkaline) requires special procedures because, when using the glass electrode, the Nernst law breaks down under those conditions. Various factors contribute to this. It cannot be assumed that liquid junction potentials are independent of pH. Also, extreme pH implies that the solution is concentrated, so electrode potentials are affected by ionic strength variation. At high pH the glass electrode may be affected by "alkaline error", because the electrode becomes sensitive to the concentration of cations such as Na^+ and K^+ in the solution. Specially constructed electrodes are available which partly overcome these problems. Runoff from mines or mine tailings can produce some very low pH values.

NON-AQUEOUS SOLUTIONS

Hydrogen ion concentrations (activities) can be measured in non-aqueous solvents. pH values based on these measurements belong to a different scale from aqueous pH values, because activities relate to different standard states. Hydrogen ion activity, a_H^+, can be defined as:

$$a_{H+} = \exp\left(\frac{\mu_{H+} - m^{\theta}_{H+}}{RT}\right)$$

where μ_H^+ is the chemical potential of the hydrogen ion, $\mu^{\sigma}{}_H^+$ is its chemical potential in the chosen standard state, R is the gas constant and T is the thermodynamic temperature. Therefore pH values on the different scales cannot be compared directly, requiring an inter solvent scale which involves the transfer activity coefficient of hydrolyonium ion. pH is an example of an acidity function. Other acidity functions can be defined. For example, the Hammett acidity function, H_0, has been developed in connection with super acids. The concept of "Unified pH scale" has been developed on the basis of the absolute chemical potential of the proton. This scale applies to liquids, gases and even solids.

CHAPTER 7

Spectrophotometry

BASIC PRINCIPLES

A spectrophotometer is employed to measure the amount of light that a sample absorbs. The instrument operates by passing a beam of light through a sample and measuring the intensity of light reaching a detector.

The beam of light consists of a stream of photons, represented by the purple balls in the simulation shown below. When a photon encounters an analyte molecule (the analyte is the molecule being studied), there is a chance the analyte will absorb the photon. This absorption reduces the number of photons in the beam of light, thereby reducing the intensity of the light beam. You can visualize this process by running the simulation shown below. Click on the Start button to start the simulation and the Stop button to stop the simulation. The light source is set to emit 10 photons per second. Watch the motion of the photons and observe how some of the photons are absorbed (removed) as the beam of light passes through the cell containing the sample solution. The intensity of the light reaching the detector is less than the intensity emitted by the light source.

COLOURIMETRY

- Many biochemical experiments involve the measurement of a compound or group of compounds present in a mixture. Probably the most widely used method for determining the concentration of biochemical compound is colourimetry.

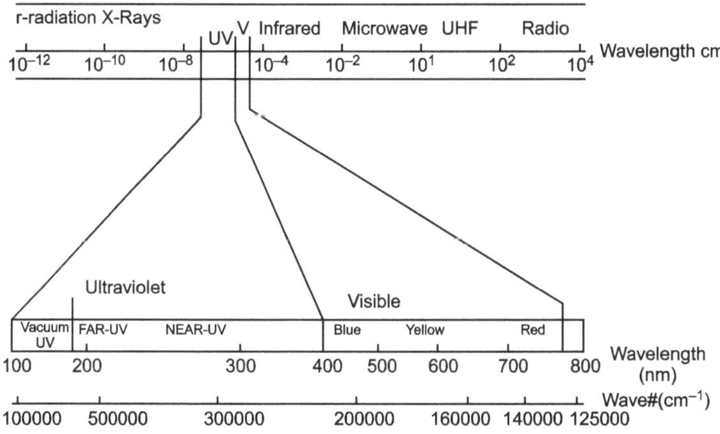

Figure 7.1: Spectral range of various regions.

Colorimetry

- It uses white light
- Coloured solution
- Suitable reagents
- Reactions are often fairly specific & very sensitive
- Quantitative (millimole per litter)
- Complete isolation of the compound is not necessary
- Depth of colour is directly proportional to the concentration of the compound
- Separation of individual compound from mixture of compounds
- Measure enzyme activity rate
- Simple, quick and less expensive

Light source:

1. Ultraviolet region → Deuterium lamp
2. Above 360 nm → Tungsten lamp

Photocell:

1. Blue photocell	400 → 625 nm
2. Red photocell	625 → 800 nm

Cuvette:

1. Glass cuvette	360 → 800 nm
2. Silica/Quartz	190 → 800 nm

Where Colorimerty can be Used

Determinations of:

- Sugars
- Amylose
- Cellulose
- Soluble proteins
- Minerals
- Pectic substances
- Pigments
- Phenolics
- Antinutritional factors
- Starch
- Inulin
- Hemicellulose
- Amino acids
- Vitamins
- Enzyme activity
- Hormones
- Tannins

Determination of Peroxidase Activity

1. Extraction of enzyme in 0.1 M Phosphate buffer
2. Reaction with Guaiacol/Pyrogallol and Hydrogen peroxide
3. Buffer + Guaiacol + enzyme extract + Hydrogen peroxide → Measure

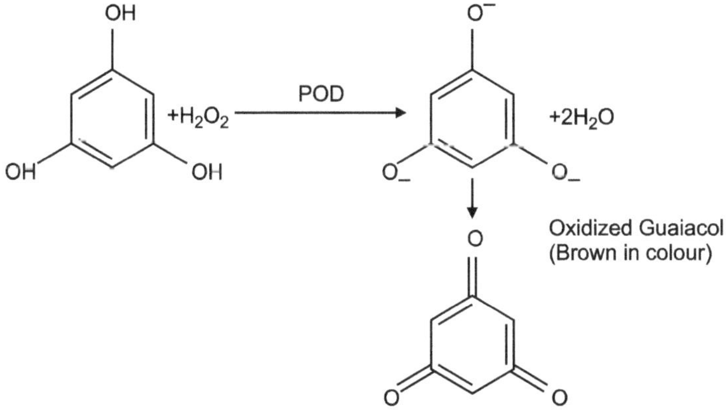

OH
$+H_2O_2$ POD → $+2H_2O$
OH OH O^- O^- O^-
O
Oxidized Guaiacol
(Brown in colour)
O O

The rate of formation of guaiacol dehydrogenation product is a measure of the peroxidase activity and can be assayed spectrophotometrically at 436mm.

Experimental Procedure

The following simulation illustrates the procedures for making Spectrophotometric measurements.

- First, the intensity of light (I_0) passing through a blank is measured. The intensity is the number of photons per second. The blank is a solution that is identical to the sample solution except that the blank does not contain the solute that absorbs light. This measurement is necessary, because the cell itself scatters some of the light.
- Second, the intensity of light (I) passing through the sample solution is measured. (In practice, instruments measure the power rather than the intensity of the light. The power is the energy per second, which is the product of the intensity (photons per second) and the energy per photon).
- Third, the experimental data is used to calculate two quantities: the transmittance (T) and the absorbance (A).

$$T = \frac{I}{I_0}$$

$$A = -\log_{10} T$$

The transmittance is simply the fraction of light in the original beam that passes through the sample and reaches the detector. The remainder of the light, 1 - T, is the fraction of the light absorbed by the sample. (Do not confuse the transmittance with the temperature, which often is given the symbol T).

In most applications, one wishes to relate the amount of light absorbed to the concentration of the absorbing molecule. It turns out that the absorbance rather than the transmittance is most useful for this purpose. If no light is absorbed, the absorbance is zero (100% transmittance). Each unit in absorbance corresponds with an order of magnitude in the fraction of light transmitted. For $A = 1$, 10% of the light is transmitted ($T = 0.10$) and 90% is absorbed by the sample. For $A = 2$, 1% of the light is transmitted and 99% is absorbed. For $A = 3$, 0.1% of the light is transmitted and 99.9% is absorbed.

Using the simulation below, perform the following steps:

- Measure the intensity of light passing through the blank.
- Measure the intensity of light passing through the sample.
- Calculate the transmittance.
- Calculate the absorbance.

Principles and Techniques

Spectrophotometry is the science of measuring the light absorption characteristics of substances for use in determining their concentration, identity, and other properties. This technique is possible because many substances absorb light of specific wavelengths within the ultraviolet (200-400 nm), visible (400-700 nm), and near-infrared (700-1000 nm) regions of the electromagnetic spectrum, and transmit the remainder. The wavelength of the transmitted (or reflected) light is what imparts a characteristic color to a substance: For example, a red wine appears red because it transmits red light (wavelength, 600-700 nm), and absorbs light of shorter wavelengths.

A measure of the amount of light absorbed by a substance is called absorbance or optical density (OD), and a measure of the amount transmitted is called transmittance. The wavelength at which a substance has maximum absorbance is characteristic of the substance and is used to identify the substance. If two substances contain the same light-absorbing prosthetic group (e.g., riboflavin and flavin adenine dinucleotide both contain flavin), they usually absorb maximally at about the same wavelength, but the absorbance per mole of each substance (molar extinction coefficient) is usually different. A recording of the absorbance of a substance as a function of wavelength is called the absorption spectrum. The peaks (absorption maxima) on an absorbance spectrum are the regions of high absorption, and the troughs (absorption minima) are the regions of low absorption.

QUANTITATIVE ASPECTS AND BASIC APPLICATIONS

The Beer-Lambert Law

The Beer–Lambert law, also known as Beer's law, the Lambert–Beer law, or the Beer–Lambert–Bouguer law relates the attenuation of light to the properties of the material through which the light is traveling. The law is commonly applied to chemical analysis measurements and used in understanding attenuation in physical optics, for photons, neutrons or rarefied gases. In mathematical physics, this law arises as a solution of the BGK equation.

Absorbance

Measuring the Absorbance of a Solution

If you have read the page about how an absorption spectrometer works, you will know that it passes a whole series of wavelengths of light through a solution of a substance (the sample cell) and also through an identical container (the reference cell) which only has solvent in it. For each wavelength of light passing through the spectrometer, the intensity of the light passing through the reference cell is measured. This is usually referred to as I_o - that's I for Intensity.

The intensity of the light passing through the sample cell is also measured for that wavelength - given the symbol, I. If I is less than I_o, then obviously the sample has absorbed some of the light. A simple bit of maths is then done in the computer to convert this into something called the absorbance of the sample - given the symbol, A. For reasons to do with the form of the Beer-Lambert Law (below), the relationship between A (the absorbance) and the two intensities are given by:

$$A = \log_{10} \frac{I_0}{I}$$

On most of the diagrams you will come across, the absorbance ranges from 0 to 1, but it can go higher than that.

An absorbance of 0 at some wavelength means that no light of that particular wavelength has been absorbed. The intensities of the sample and reference beam are both the same, so the ratio I_o/I is 1. Log_{10} of 1 is zero. An absorbance of 1 happens when 90% of the light at that wavelength has been absorbed - which means that the intensity is 10% of what it would otherwise be.

In that case, I_o/I is 100/I0 (=10) and $\log_{10}$ of 10 is 1.

Absorbance isn't Very Good for Making Comparisons

The Importance of Concentration

The proportion of the light absorbed will depend on how many molecules it interacts with. Suppose you have got a strongly coloured organic dye. If it is in a reasonably concentrated solution, it will have a very high absorbance because there are lots of molecules to interact with the light. However, in an incredibly dilute solution, it may be very difficult to see that it is coloured at all. The absorbance is going to be very low. Suppose then that you wanted to compare this dye with a different compound. Unless you took care to make allowance for the concentration, you couldn't make any sensible comparisons about which one absorbed the most light.

The Importance of the Container Shape

Suppose this time that you had a very dilute solution of the dye in a cube shaped container so that the light travelled 1 cm through it. The absorbance isn't likely to be very high. On the other hand, suppose you passed the light through a tube 100 cm long containing the same solution. More light would be absorbed because it interacts with more molecules. Again, if you want to draw sensible comparisons between solutions, you have to allow for the length of the solution the light is passing through. Both concentration and solution length are allowed for in the Beer-Lambert Law.

The Beer-Lambert Law

What the Law Looks Like

You will find that various different symbols are given for some of the terms in the equation - particularly for the concentration and the solution length. I'm going to use the obvious form.

Where the concentration of the solution is "c" and the length is "1".

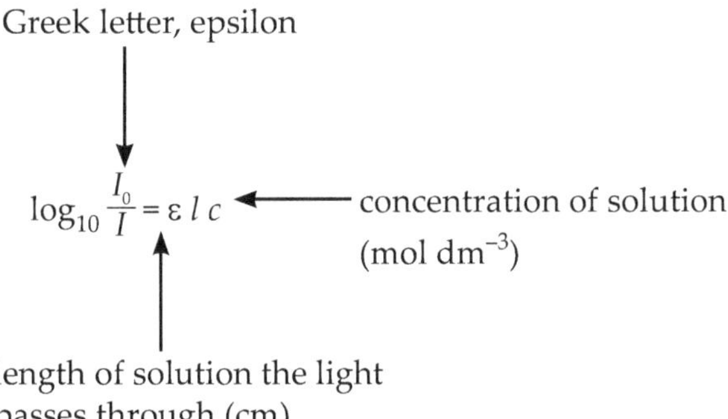

You should recognize the expression on the left of this equation as what we have just defined as the absorbance, A. You might also find the equation written in terms of A:

$$A = \varepsilon \mathrm{l} \mathrm{c}$$

That's obviously easier to remember than the first one, but you would still have to learn the equation for absorbance. It might be useful to learn it in the form:

$$A = \log_{10}\frac{I_0}{I} = \varepsilon\, l\, c$$

The Greek letter epsilon in these equations is called the molar absorptivity - or sometimes the molar absorption coefficient.

Molar Absorptivity

If you rearrange the simplest of the equations above to give an expression for epsilon (the molar absorptivity), you get:

$$\varepsilon = \frac{A}{lc}$$

Remember that the absorbance of a solution will vary as the concentration or the size of the container varies. Molar absorptivity compensates for this by dividing by both the concentration and the length of the solution that the light passes through. Essentially, it works out a value for what the absorbance would be under a standard set of conditions - the light travelling 1 cm through a solution of 1 mol dm^{-3}.

That means that you can then make comparisons between one compound and another without having to worry about the concentration or solution length.

Values for molar absorptivity can vary hugely. For example, ethanal has two absorption peaks in its UV-visible spectrum - both in the ultra-violet. One of these corresponds to an electron being promoted from a lone pair on the oxygen into a pi anti-bonding orbital; the other from a pi bonding orbital into a pi anti-bonding orbital.

By definition, the transmittance of material sample is related to its optical depth τ and to its absorbance A as

$$T = \frac{\Phi_e^i}{\Phi_p^i} = e^{-r} = 10^{-A} \; e^{-r} = 10^{-A}$$

where

- Φ_e^t is the radiant flux transmitted by that material sample;
- Φ_e^i is the radiant flux received by that material sample.

The Beer–Lambert law states that, for N attenuating species in the material sample,

$$T = e^{-\sum_{i=1}^{N} \sigma_1 \int_0^l n_i(n) dz} = 10^{-\sum_{i=1}^{N} \varepsilon_1 \int_0^E c_1(\approx) d\approx}$$

or equivalently that

$$\gamma = \sum_{i=1}^{N} \gamma_i = \sum_{i=1}^{N} \sigma_1 \int_0^l n_i(z) dz,$$

$$A = \sum_{i=1}^{N} A_i = \sum_{i=1}^{N} \varepsilon_i \int_0^l c_i(z) dz,,$$

where

- σ_i is the attenuation cross section of the attenuating specie i in the material sample;
- n_i is the number density of the attenuating specie i in the material sample;
- ε_i is the molar attenuation coefficient of the attenuating specie i in the material sample;
- c_i is the amount concentration of the attenuating specie i in the material sample;
- l is the path length of the beam of light through the material sample.

Attenuation cross section and molar attenuation coefficient are related by

$$\varepsilon_i = \frac{N_A}{In10}\sigma_i,$$

and number density and amount concentration by

$$c_i = \frac{n_i}{N_A},$$

where N_A is the Avogadro constant.

In case of *uniform* attenuation, these relations become

$$T = e^{-}\sum_{i=1}^{N}\sigma_i n_i l = 10^{-}\sum_{i=1}^{N}\varepsilon_i c_i l$$

or equivalently

$$r - \sum_{i=1}^{N}\sigma_2 n_i \ell,$$

$$A - \sum_{i=1}^{N}\varepsilon_i c_i \ell.$$

Cases of *non-uniform* attenuation occur in atmospheric science applications and radiation shielding theory for instance.

The law tends to break down at very high concentrations, especially if the material is highly scattering. If the radiation is especially intense, nonlinear optical processes can also cause variances. The main reason, however, is the following. At high concentrations, the molecules are closer to each other and begin to interact with each other. This interaction will change several properties of the molecule, and thus will change the attenuation.

Expression with Attenuation Coefficient

The Beer–Lambert law can be expressed in terms of attenuation coefficient, but in this case is better called Lambert's law since amount concentration, from Beer's law, is hidden inside the attenuation coefficient. The (Napierian) attenuation coefficient μ and the decadic attenuation coefficient $\mu_{10} = \mu/\ln 10$ of a material sample are related to its number densities and amount concentrations as

$$\mu(z) = \sum_{i=1}^{N}\mu_i(z) = \sum_{i=1}^{N}\sigma_i n_i(z),$$

$$\mu_{10}(z) = \sum_{i=1}^{N}\mu_{10,i}(z) = \sum_{i=1}^{N}\varepsilon_i c_i(z),$$

respectively, by definition of attenuation cross section and molar attenuation coefficient. Then the Beer–Lambert law becomes

$$T = e^{-\int_0^{\ell}\alpha(\ )d_2} = 10^{-\int_0^{\ell}\alpha_{10}(\ )d_2}$$

and

$$\tau = \int_0^{\ell}\mu(z)dz,$$

$$A = \int_0^{\ell} il_{10}(z)dz.$$

In case of *uniform* attenuation, these relations become

$$T = e^{-\mu l} = 10^{-\mu 10 \ell}$$

or equivalently

$$\tau = \mu \ell$$

$$A = \mu_{10} \ell$$

Derivation

In concept, the derivation of the Beer–Lambert law is straightforward. Assume that a beam of light enters a material sample. Define z as an axis parallel to the direction of the beam. Divide the material sample into thin slices, perpendicular to the beam of light; with thickness dz sufficiently small that one particle in a slice cannot obscure another particle in the same slice when viewed along the z direction. The radiant flux of the light that emerges from a slice is reduced, compared to that of the light that entered, by$d\Phi_e(z) = -\mu(z)\Phi_e(z)$ dz, where μ is the (Napierian) attenuation coefficient, which yields the following first-order linear ODE:

$$\frac{d\Phi}{dz}(z) = -\mu(z)\Phi_e(z)$$

The attenuation is caused by the photons that did not make it to the other side of the slice because of scattering or absorption. The solution to this differential equation is obtained by multiplying the integrating factor

$$e^{\int_0^\ell \mu(z')d_z}$$

throughout to obtain

$$\frac{d\Phi_e}{dz}(z)e^{\int_0^z \mu(z')dz'} + \mu(z)\Phi_e(z)e^{\int_0^z \mu(z')dz'} = 0$$

which simplifies due to the product rule (applied backwards) to

$$\frac{d}{dz}\left(\Phi_e(z)e^{\int_0^z \mu(z')dz'}\right) = 0$$

Integrating both sides and solving for Φ_e for a material of real thickness ℓ, with the incident radiant flux upon the slice $\Phi_e^i = \Phi_e(0)$ and the transmitted radiant flux $\Phi_e^t = \Phi_e(\ell)$ gives

$$\Phi_e^t = \Phi_e^i e^{-\int_0^z \mu(z')dz}$$

and finally

$$T = \frac{\Phi_e^t}{\Phi_e^i} = e^{-\int_0^\ell \mu(z)dz}$$

Since the decadic attenuation coefficient μ_{10} is related to the (Napierian) attenuation coefficient by $\mu_{10} = \mu/\ln 10$, one also have

$$T = e^{-\int_0^\ell la10\mu_{10}(z)dz} = \left(e^{-\int_0^\ell \mu_{10}(z)dz}\right)^{la10} = 10^{-\int_0^\ell \mu 10(z)dz}$$

To describe the attenuation coefficient in a way independent of the number densities n_i of the N attenuating species of the material sample, one introduces the attenuation cross section $\sigma_i = \mu_i(z)/n_i(z)$. σ_i has the dimension of an area; it expresses the likelihood of interaction between the particles of the beam and the particles of the specie i in the material sample:

$$T = e^{-\sum_{i=1}^{N} \sigma_1 \int_0^{\ell} n_i(z)dz}$$

One can also use the molar attenuation coefficients $\varepsilon_i = (N_A/\ln 10)\sigma_i$, where N_A is the Avogadro constant, to describe the attenuation coefficient in a way independent of the amount concentrations $c_i(z) = n_i(z)/N_A$ of the attenuating species of the material sample:

$$T = e^{-\sum_{i=1}^{N} \frac{In10}{N_A} \varepsilon_1 \int_0^{\ell} n_1(z)dz} = \left(e^{-\sum_{i=1}^{N} \varepsilon_i \int_0^{e} \frac{n_i(e)}{N_A} dz}\right)^{In10} = 10^{-\sum_{i=1}^{N} \varepsilon_i \int_0^{\ell} c_i(z)dz}$$

Validity

Under certain conditions Beer–Lambert law fails to maintain a linear relationship between attenuation and concentration of analyte. These deviations are classified into three categories:

1. Real fundamental deviations due to the limitations of the law itself.
2. Chemical deviations observed due to specific chemical species of the sample which is being analyzed.
3. Instrument deviations which occur due to how the attenuation measurements are made.

There are at least six conditions that need to be fulfilled in order for Beer–Lambert law to be valid. These are:

1. The attenuators must act independently of each other.
2. The attenuating medium must be homogeneous in the interaction volume.
3. The attenuating medium must not scatter the radiation no turbidity unless this is accounted for as in DOAS.
4. The incident radiation must consist of parallel rays, each traversing the same length in the absorbing medium.
5. The incident radiation should preferably be monochromatic, or have at least a width that is narrower than that of the attenuating transition. Otherwise a spectrometer as detector for the power is needed instead of a photodiode which has not selective wavelength dependence.
6. The incident flux must not influence the atoms or molecules; it should only act as a non-invasive probe of the species under study. In particular, this implies that the light should not cause optical saturation or optical pumping, since such effects will deplete the lower level and possibly give rise to stimulated emission.

If any of these conditions are not fulfilled, there will be deviations from Beer–Lambert law.

Chemical Analysis by Spectrophotometry

Beer–Lambert law can be applied to the analysis of a mixture by spectrophotometry, without the need for extensive pre-processing of the sample. An example is the determination of bilirubin in blood plasma samples. The spectrum of pure bilirubin is known, so the molar attenuation coefficient ε is known. Measurements of decadic attenuation coefficient μ_{10} are made at one wavelength λ that is nearly unique for bilirubin and at a second wavelength in order to correct for possible interferences. The amount concentration c is then given by

$$C = \frac{\mu_{10}(\lambda)}{\varepsilon(\lambda)}$$

For a more complicated example, consider a mixture in solution containing two species at amount concentrations c_1 and c_2. The decadic attenuation coefficient at any wave length λ is, given by

$$\mu_{10}(\lambda) = \varepsilon_1(\lambda)c_1 + \varepsilon_2(\lambda)c_2.$$

Therefore, measurements at two wavelengths yield two equations in two unknowns and will suffice to determine the amount concentrations c_1 and c_2 as long as the molar attenuation coefficient of the two components, ε_1 and ε_2 are known at both wavelengths. This two system equation can be solved using Cramer's rule. In practice it is better to use linear least squares to determine the two amount concentrations from measurements made at more than two wavelengths. Mixtures containing more than two components can be analyzed in the same way, using a minimum of N wavelengths for a mixture containing N components.

The law is used widely in infra-red spectroscopy and near-infrared spectroscopy for analysis of polymer degradation and oxidation (also in biological tissue). The carbonyl group attenuation at about 6 micrometres can be detected quite easily, and degree of oxidation of the polymer calculated.

Beer–Lambert Law in the Atmosphere

This law is also applied to describe the attenuation of solar or stellar radiation as it travels through the atmosphere. In this case, there is scattering of radiation as well as absorption. The optical depth for a slant path is $\tau' = m\tau$, where τ refers to a vertical path, m is called the relative air mass, and for a plane-parallel atmosphere it is determined as $m = \sec\theta$ where θ is the zenith angle corresponding to the given path. The Beer–Lambert law for the atmosphere is usually written

$$T = e^{-m\left(\tau_a + \tau_g - r_{RS} + r_{NO_2} + \tau_w + \tau_{O_3} + r_r + \ldots\right)}$$

where each τ_x is the optical depth whose subscript identifies the source of the absorption or scattering it describes:

- a refers to aerosols (that absorb and scatter);
- g are uniformly mixed gases (mainly carbon dioxide (CO_2) and molecular oxygen (O_2) which only absorb);
- NO_2 is nitrogen dioxide, mainly due to urban pollution (absorption only);

- RS are effects due to Raman scattering in the atmosphere;
- w is water vapour absorption;
- O_3 is ozone (absorption only);
- r is Rayleigh scattering from molecular oxygen (O_2) and nitrogen (N_2) (responsible for the blue color of the sky);
- the selection of the attenuators which have to be considered depends on the wavelength range and can include various other compounds. This can include tetra oxygen, HONO, formaldehyde, glyoxal, a series of halogen radicals and others.

m is the *optical mass* or *airmass factor*, a term approximately equal (for small and moderate values of θ) to $1/\cos\theta$, where θ is the observed object's zenith angle (the angle measured from the direction perpendicular to the Earth's surface at the observation site). This equation can be used to retrieve τ_a, the aerosol optical thickness, which is necessary for the correction of satellite images and also important in accounting for the role of aerosols in climate.

Calculating Concentrations

Non-Enzymatic Analytes

The Beer-Lambert law is used to calculate the concentration of substances using absorbance data. The calculation is handled in two ways:

1. Direct Calculation

This is applicable to substances that directly absorb light. To calculate the concentration of a sample, first measure its absorbance. Obtain *E* and l; if unknown, measure *E* as described above, and measure *t* as the length of the cuvette's light path (usually 1 cm).

2. Use of a Standard Curve to Calculate Concentration

The use of a standard curve is often necessary when analyzing substances that do not absorb light directly. These substances may be converted to light-absorbing species by either a chemical reaction or by coupling to other reactions in which a light absorber is being consumed or produced. Direct calculation of concentration in these cases is tedious and sometimes impossible because the extinction coefficients of the light-absorbing species are unknown. Standards of the pure substance are assayed along with the samples, and a standard curve is constructed by plotting the absorbance values for these standards against the corresponding concentrations. The concentration of the sample is then obtained by reading from this curve the concentration corresponding to the sample's absorbance. If the sample was diluted, the result is multiplied by the dilution factor. However, if the standards and the sample were diluted equally, the concentration of the sample should not be multiplied by the dilution factor since this factor was incorporated into the standard curve.

Alternatively, the absorbance and concentration of a single standard can be used to calculate the unknown concentration, provided that this standard is within the linear range of the assay.

A standard curve can also be used when several samples are being assayed simultaneously; reading the concentrations off the standard curve is faster than calculating them.

Analyzing Enzymes Spectrophotometrically

The concentration of an enzyme is usually measured as activity. Because activity is defined as the amount of substrate consumed or product liberated per unit time, the activity of an enzyme can be determined spectrophotometrically if the substrate or product absorbs light, or if it can be coupled to a reaction in which a light absorber is being consumed or produced. Enzymes that catalyze oxidation-reduction (redox) reactions (e.g., the cytochromes), contain light-absorbing prosthetic groups. Their redox transition activities are best assayed spectrophotometrically.

Notes: (a) The Beer-Lambert equation is linear and has zero intercept and a slope of *Et;* therefore, the standard curve should pass through the zero origin. (b) At higher concentrations, the curve usually becomes nonlinear mainly because of intermolecular interactions, depletion of light, light scattering, instrument limitations at low levels of transmitted light, and reagent depletion. Absorbance values above the linear limit do not give accurate concentrations. Therefore, (i) only the linear portion of a standard curve should be used to obtain the concentration of samples; samples with higher absorbance values should be diluted and reassayed. (ii) Except when a sophisticated spectrophotometer with high accuracy is used, absorbance values greater than about 1.5 should not be used for calculations; the sample should be diluted and reassayed.

Quantifying Nucleic Acids

Nucleic acids absorb UV light between 250 and 280 nm, with DNA and RNA absorbing optimally at 260 run (see Appendix E for specifics). As such, they can be quantified spectrophotometrically using equation A = ElC. However, molecular biologists usually quantify nucleic acids in absorbance units (AU) or optical density (OD) units. One AU or 0D unit of a substance (e.g., nucleic acid) is defined as the concentration that gives 1 AU at a given wavelength.

$$OD = ElC; C/OD = 1/E = 1AU$$

C/OD defines 1 AU or 1 OD unit. Thus, 1 AU is the inverse of the absorption coefficient. Above equation is used to obtain the value of 1 AU when the absorption coefficient is known, and vice versa. To calculate the concentration of nucleic acids (or other light-absorbing substances) using their AU and measured OD, the following equations can be used:

$$C/OD = 1AU; C = 1AU \times OD$$

If the sample was diluted before measuring the OD and DF is the dilution factor, then

$$C = 1AU \times OD \times DF$$

Note: The unit for concentration will be that of the AU, usually mg/ml.

Values for the AU and absorption coefficient for RNA and DNA are given in following Table.

Absorption constants for selected nucleic acids

Nucleic acid	$E^{1mg/ml}_{1cm}$ (260nm)	$1AU_{260}$ (μg/ml)
Double-strand DNA	20	50
Single-strand DNA or RNA	25	40
Single-strand oligos	30	33
Single-strand oligos	40	25

Base pairing and stacking decrease the absorbance of DNA and RNA. Thus, when double-stranded DNA melts, its absorbance increases [hyperchromic effect]. For this reason, double-stranded DNA (or RNA) has a lower absorption coefficient and a higher value for AU than the single-stranded forms.

The values for absorption coefficient and AU for short single-stranded oligonucleotides vary, depending on the length and base composition: The shorter the oligo, the higher the absorption coefficient.

When quantifying nucleic acids, take OD readings at 260 nm and 280 nm wavelengths. Calculate the concentration using the OD_{260} then calculate the OD_{260}/OD_{280} and use it to assess the purity of the sample: Pure DNA and RNA have OD_{260}/OD_{280} ratio of 1.8 and 2.0, respectively. If the ratios are significantly less than these values, then the samples are contaminated.

Identifying Substrates

All direct absorbers have characteristic absorption spectra. The spectrum may be regarded as an optical "fingerprint" which identifies the compound. Identification is made using important features of the spectrum: (i) The wavelengths at which the absorption peaks and troughs occur are characteristic of the substance, (ii) the excitation coefficients at the absorption maxima are also characteristic, and (iii) the ratio of the absorbance at two characteristic wavelengths is a constant. As an example, the spectrum of riboflavin shows absorption maxima at 450 and 375 nm, and an absorption minimum at 400 nm. The E^{1M}_{1cm} (450 and 374 nm) are always 1.22×10^4 and 1.06×10^4, respectively, and the A_{450}/A_{375} ratio is always 1.15 for pure riboflavin. Together, these characteristics distinguish riboflavin from other compounds, including flavin adenine dinucleotide (FAD) which also contains flavin the light-absorbing prosthetic group in riboflavin. Other compounds can be identified by converting them to light-absorbing analogues, and then recording and analyzing their spectra.

Characterizing Substances

Spectrophotometric techniques have been used to characterize biomolecules.

Examples include the determination of the pK_a of weak acids, oxidation-reduction transitions of heme proteins, ligand-receptor interactions including enzyme substrate interactions and transitions of DNA between single and double-stranded forms.

1. SPECTROPHOTOMETER

Spectrophotometry is the quantity based study of electromagnetic spectra. A spectrophotometer measures either the amount of light reflected from a sample object or the amount of light that is absorbed by the sample object.

- A spectrophotometer is a sophisticated type of colorimeter where monochromatic light is provided· by a grating or prism.
- A spectrophometer is needed when the two peaks can be selected on the monochromator.
- Many compounds have characteristic absorption spectra in the Ultraviolet and Visible region so that identification of these materials in a mixture is possible by spectrophotometer.

Compound	Wavelength needed for absorption
1. Proteins	280 nm
2. Pyridine nucleotide	340 nm
3. Nucleic acid	260 nm

- When molecule absorbs energy at ground state and goes too excited state → absorption spectrum
- When molecule gives its excess energy and goes back to the ground state → emission spectrum

Design

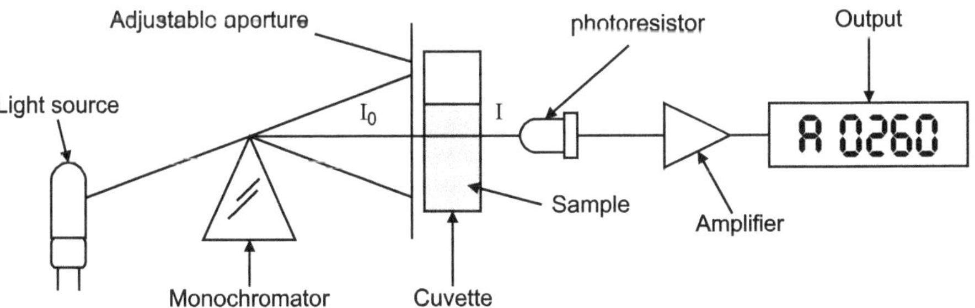

Figure 7.2: Single beam spectrophotometer

In short, the sequence of events in a modern spectrophotometer is as follows:

1. The light source shines on the sample.
2. A fraction of the light is transmitted or reflected from the sample
3. The light from the sample is directed to the entrance slit of the monochromator
4. The monochromator separates the wavelengths of light and focuses each of them onto the photodetector sequentially.

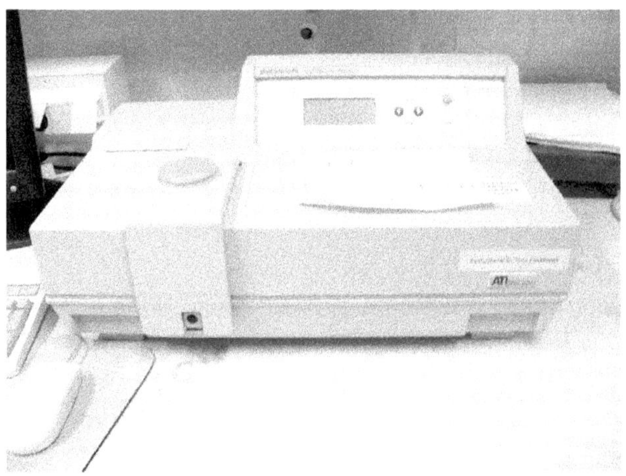

Figure 7.3: Spectrophotometer machine.

There are two kinds of spectrophotometers: single beam and double beam. A double beam spectrophotometer compares the light intensity between two light paths. One path containing a reference sample. The other path for the test sample. A single beam spectrophotometer measures the relative light intensity of the beam before and after a test sample is inserted. A double beam machine makes comparison readings easier and more stable. But a single beam machine can have measure a wider range of light frequencies. Single beam machines have simple optical systems and are more compact. When the spectrophotometer is built into another device (like microscopes or telescopes) only single beam machines will work.

Many older spectrophotometers must be calibrated by a procedure known as "zeroing." The absorbancy of a reference substance is set as a baseline value, so the absorbancies of all other substances are recorded relative to the initial "zeroed" substance. The spectrophotometer then displays % absorbancy (the amount of light absorbed relative to the initial substance).

Spectrophotometers can also measure luminescence. For example, the machine can shine ultraviolet light of one frequency on the sample. This will excite the sample and make it glow. The detectors can then measure the light glowing from the sample at a different frequency.

Electromagnetic Spectrum

The electromagnetic (EM) spectrum is the range of all possible electromagnetic radiation. Electromagnetic radiation can be divided into octaves as sound waves are adding up to eighty-one octaves. Physicists have studied electromagnetic radiation with wavelengths from thousands of kilometres down to fractions of the size of an atom. It is commonly said that EM waves beyond these limits are uncommon, although this is not known to be true. The short wavelength limit is likely to be the Planck length, and the long wavelength limit is the size of the universe itself, though in principle the spectrum is infinite.

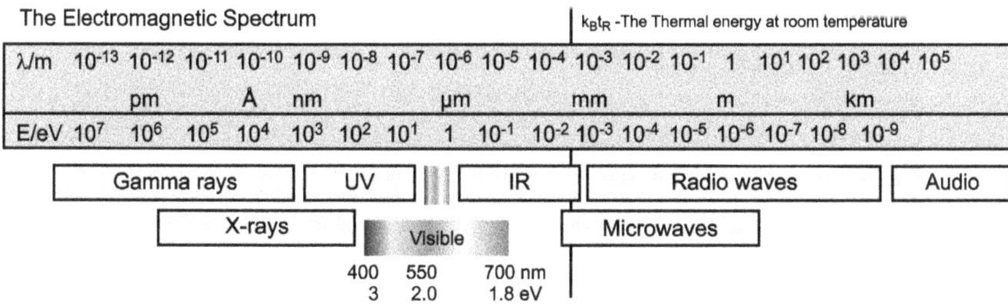

Spectra of Objects

Nearly all objects in the universe emit, reflect or transmit some light. (One hypothetical exception may be dark matter.) The distribution of this light along the electromagnetic spectrum (called the spectrum of the object) is determined by the object's composition. Several types of spectra can be distinguished depending upon the nature of the radiation coming from an object.

Spectroscopy is the branch of physics that studies matter by its emitted or reflected spectra.

NOTE: The AUDIO entry in this graphic is there for comparison only. Sound waves and light are two different things entirely.

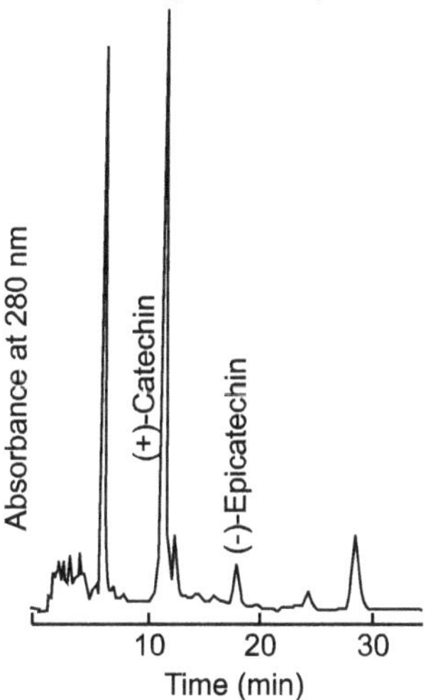

Figure 7.4: Chromatogram of the fraction from Sephadex LH20, Vinillin +ve at 500nm.

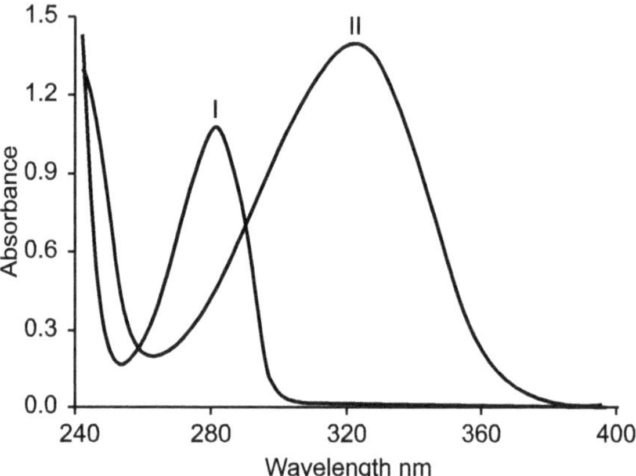

Figure 7.5: Comparative standard UV Spectral chromatogram of Catechin and Sinapic acid (I) Catechin maxima at 280 nm and (II) Sinapic acid maxima at 322 nm.

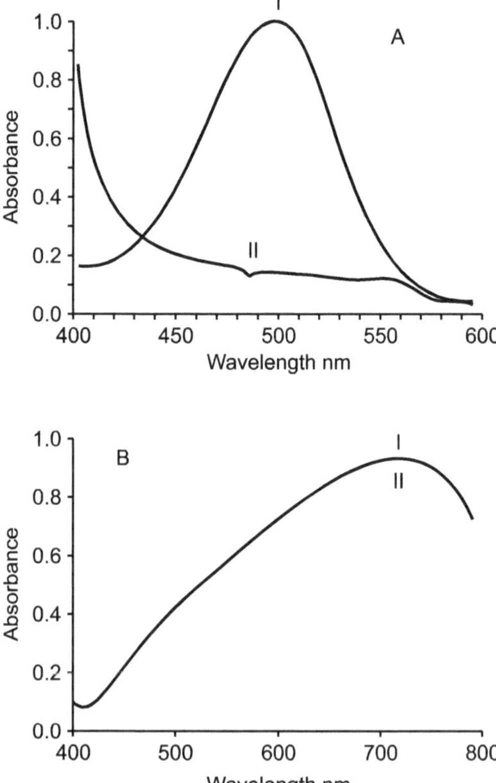

Figure 7.6: UV spectral chromatogram for total phenolic compounds and condensed tannins.

A: (I) Catechin + Vanillin gives +Ve test, maxima at 500 nm.

(II) Sinapic acid + Vanillin -Ve test, no maxima.

B: Total phenolic compounds with Folin-Denis gives maxima at 725 nm, (I) Standard & (II) Sample.

2. SPECTROSCOPY

Spectroscopy is the study of light as a function of length of the wave that has been emitted, reflected or shone through a solid, liquid, or gas. Many times it is analyzed when the chemical is heated, because it makes a special colour of flame. Most chemicals make a different colour or spectrum than other chemicals. This can be used to see what chemicals are in a substance. Spectroscopy allows scientists to investigate and explore things that are too small to be seen through a microscope, such as molecules, and the even smaller subatomic particles like protons, neutrons and electrons. There are special instruments to measure and analyse these light waves.

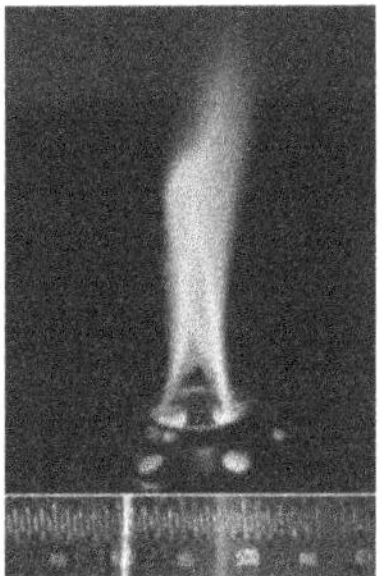

Figure 7.7: Alcohol flame and its spectrum

METHODS

Infrared spectroscopy measures light in the infrared electromagnetic spectrum. The highlight of IR spectroscopy is that it is very useful in identifying functional groups of organic molecules. The absorption of infrared light by organic molecules causes molecular vibrations. The vibrational frequencies are unique to the individual functional groups. IR spectra is given graphically by transmittance (%) vs. wavenumber (cm^{-1}).

X-ray crystallography can look at the structure of a crystalline molecule. The electron cloud of each atom diffracts the X-rays thus revealing the positions of the atoms. Various inorganic and organic molecules can be crystallized and used in this method including DNA, proteins, salts and metals. The sample used for analysis is not destroyed.

Ultraviolet–visible spectroscopy uses visible and ultraviolet light to look at how much of a chemical is in a liquid. The colour of the solution is the basis for how UV-Vis works. The colour of the solution we are working with is coloured because of its chemical composition. So the solution absorbs some light colours and reflects other colours, the light it reflects is the colour of the solution. UV-Vis spectroscopy works by passing light through a sample of your solution then determining how much light gets absorbed by the solution.

Nuclear magnetic resonance can look at nuclei. It uses the magnetic properties of certain nuclei, the most common being ^{13}C and ^{1}H. The NMR instrument generates a large magnetic field that makes the nuclei act like tiny bar magnets. The nuclei either align with the instruments magnetic field or against it. At this point we have two possible orientations the nuclei could be in α or β. Next the nuclei are exposed to radio waves that make α go to the β orientation. When this change occurs energy is given off and detected. The data is interpreted graphically (Intensity vs. chemical shifts in ppm) by a computer system. NMR does not destroy the sample you use for analysis. Below is a 900 MHz NMR system.

Types of Spectroscopy

- Absorption spectroscopy
- Astronomical spectroscopy
- Time-domain spectroscopy
- Auger electron spectroscopy

Types

Other types of spectroscopy are distinguished by specific applications or implementations:

- Acoustic resonance spectroscopy is based on sound waves primarily in the audible and ultrasonic regions.
- Auger spectroscopy is a method used to study surfaces of materials on a micro-scale. It is often used in connection with electron microscopy.
- Cavity ring down spectroscopy.
- Circular Dichroism spectroscopy.
- Coherent anti-Stokes Raman spectroscopy (CARS) is a recent technique that has high sensitivity and powerful applications for *in vivo* spectroscopy and imaging.
- Cold vapour atomic fluorescence spectroscopy.
- Correlation spectroscopy encompasses several types of two-dimensional NMR spectroscopy.
- Deep-level transient spectroscopy measures concentration and analyzes parameters of electrically active defects in semiconducting materials.
- Dual polarisation interferometry measures the real and imaginary components of the complex refractive index.

- Electron phenomenological spectroscopy measures physicochemical properties and characteristics of electronic structure of multicomponent and complex molecular systems.
- EPR spectroscopy.
- Force spectroscopy.
- Fourier transform spectroscopy is an efficient method for processing spectra data obtained using interferometers. Fourier transform infrared spectroscopy (FTIR) is a common implementation of infrared spectroscopy. NMR also employs Fourier transforms.
- Hadron spectroscopy studies the energy/mass spectrum of hadrons according to spin, parity, and other particle properties. Baryon spectroscopy and meson spectroscopy are both types of hadron spectroscopy.
- Hyperspectral imaging is a method to create a complete picture of the environment or various objects, each pixel containing a full visible, VNIR, NIR, or infrared spectrum.
- Inelastic electron tunneling spectroscopy (IETS) uses the changes in current due to inelastic electron-vibration interaction at specific energies that can also measure optically forbidden transitions.
- Inelastic neutron scattering is similar to Raman spectroscopy, but uses neutrons instead of photons.
- Laser-Induced Breakdown Spectroscopy (LIBS), also called Laser-induced plasma spectrometry (LIPS).
- Laser spectroscopy uses tunable lasers and other types of coherent emission sources, such as optical parametric oscillators, for selective excitation of atomic or molecular species.
- Mass spectroscopy is an historical term used to refer to mass spectrometry. Current recommendations are to use the latter term. Use of the term mass spectroscopy originated in the use of phosphor screens to detect ions.
- Mössbauer spectroscopy probes the properties of specific isotopic nuclei in different atomic environments by analyzing the resonant absorption of gamma-rays. See alsoMössbauer effect.
- Neutron spin echo spectroscopy measures internal dynamics in proteins and other soft matter systems.
- Photoacoustic spectroscopy measures the sound waves produced upon the absorption of radiation.
- Photoemission spectroscopy.
- Photothermal spectroscopy measures heat evolved upon absorption of radiation.
- Pump-probe spectroscopy can use ultrafast laser pulses to measure reaction intermediates in the femtosecond timescale.

- Raman optical activity spectroscopy exploits Raman scattering and optical activity effects to reveal detailed information on chiral centers in molecules.
- Raman spectroscopy.
- Saturated spectroscopy.
- Scanning tunneling spectroscopy.
- Spectrophotometry.
- Time-resolved spectroscopy measures the decay rate(s) of excited states using various spectroscopic methods.
- Time-Stretch Spectroscopy.
- Thermal infrared spectroscopy measures thermal radiation emitted from materials and surfaces and is used to determine the type of bonds present in a sample as well as their lattice environment. The techniques are widely used by organic chemists, mineralogists, and planetary scientists.
- Ultraviolet photoelectron spectroscopy (UPS).
- Video spectroscopy.
- Vibrational circular dichroism spectroscopy.
- X-ray photoelectron spectroscopy (XPS).

A. Absorption Spectroscopy

Atomic absorption spectroscopy (AAS) is a spectroanalytical procedure for the quantitative determination of chemical elements using the absorption of optical radiation (light) by free atoms in the gaseous state.

In analytical chemistry the technique is used for determining the concentration of a particular element (the analyte) in a sample to be analyzed. AAS can be used to determine over 70 different elements in solution or directly in solid samples used in pharmacology, biophysics and toxicology research.

Atomic absorption spectroscopy was first used as an analytical technique, and the underlying principles were established in the second half of the 19th century by Robert Wilhelm Bunsen and Gustav Robert Kirchhoff, both professors at the University of Heidelberg, Germany.

The modern form of AAS was largely developed during the 1950s by a team of Australian chemists. They were led by Sir Alan Walsh at the Commonwealth Scientific and Industrial Research Organisation (CSIRO), Division of Chemical Physics, in Melbourne, Australia.

Atomic absorption spectrometry has many uses in different areas of chemistry such as:

- Clinical analysis: Analyzing metals in biological fluids and tissues such as whole blood, plasma, urine, saliva, brain tissue, liver, muscle tissue, semen
- Pharmaceuticals: In some pharmaceutical manufacturing processes, minute quantities of a catalyst that remain in the final drug product
- Water analysis: Analyzing water for its metal content.

Principles

The technique makes use of absorption spectrometry to assess the concentration of an analyte in a sample. It requires standards with known analyte content to establish the relation between the measured absorbance and the analyte concentration and relies therefore on the Beer-Lambert Law.

In short, the electrons of the atoms in the atomizer can be promoted to higher orbitals (excited state) for a short period of time (nanoseconds) by absorbing a defined quantity of energy (radiation of a given wavelength). This amount of energy, i.e., wavelength, is specific to a particular electron transition in a particular element. In general, each wavelength corresponds to only one element, and the width of an absorption line is only of the order of a few picometers (pm), which gives the technique its elemental selectivity. Theradiation flux without a sample and with a sample in the atomizer is measured using a detector, and the ratio between the two values (the absorbance) is converted to analyte concentration or mass using the Beer-Lambert Law.

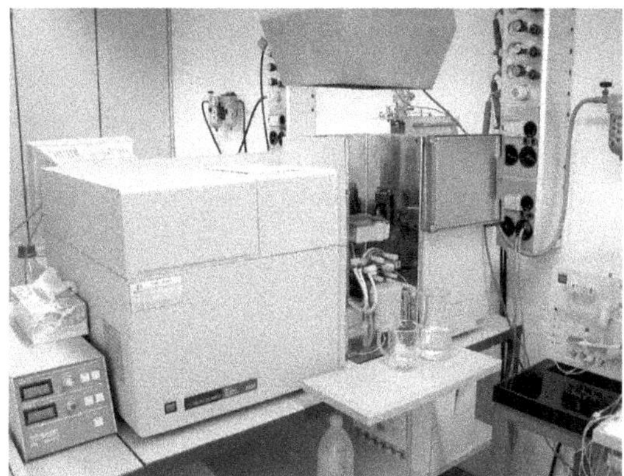

Figure 7.8: Flame atomic absorption spectroscopy instrument

Instrumentation

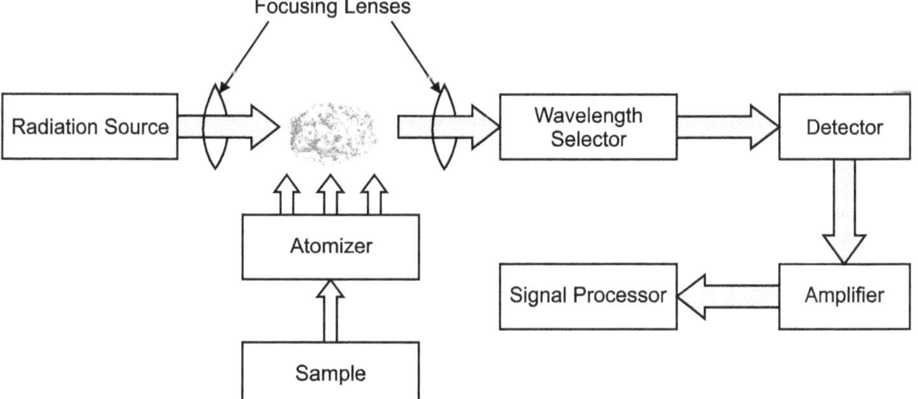

Figure 7.9: Atomic absorption spectrometer block diagram

In order to analyze a sample for its atomic constituents, it has to be atomized. The atomizers most commonly used nowadays are flames and electrothermal (graphite tube) atomizers. The atoms should then be irradiated by optical radiation, and the radiation source could be an element-specific line radiation source or a continuum radiation source. The radiation then passes through amonochromator in order to separate the element-specific radiation from any other radiation emitted by the radiation source, which is finally measured by a detector.

Atomizers

The atomizers most commonly used nowadays are (spectroscopic) flames and electrothermal (graphite tube) atomizers. Other atomizers, such as glow-discharge atomization, hydride atomization, or cold-vapor atomization might be used for special purposes.

Flame Atomizers

The oldest and most commonly used atomizers in AAS are flames, principally the air-acetylene flame with a temperature of about 2300 °C and the nitrous oxide system (N_2O)-acetylene flame with a temperature of about 2700 °C. The latter flame, in addition, offers a more reducing environment, being ideally suited for analytes with high affinity to oxygen.

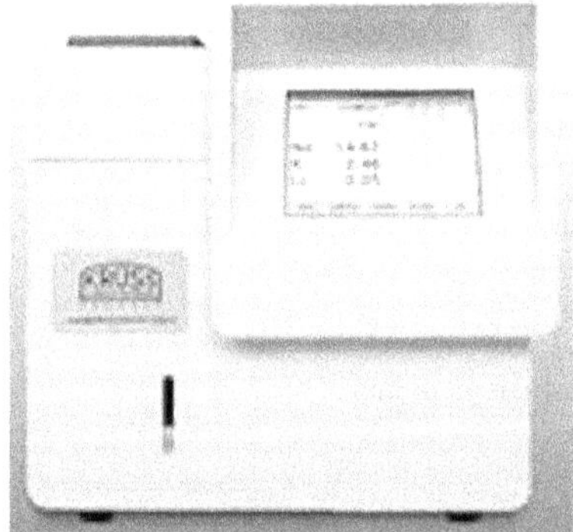

Figure 7.10: A laboratory flame photometer that uses propane operated flame atomizer

Liquid or dissolved samples are typically used with flame atomizers. The sample solution is aspirated by a pneumatic analytical nebulizer, transformed into an aerosol, which is introduced into a spray chamber, where it is mixed with the flame gases and conditioned in a way that only the finest aerosol droplets (< 10 µm) enter the flame. This conditioning process is responsible that only about 5% of the aspirated sample solution reaches the flame, but it also guarantees a relatively high freedom from interference.

On top of the spray chamber is a burner head that produces a flame that is laterally long (usually 5–10 cm) and only a few mm deep. The radiation beam passes through this flame at its longest axis, and the flame gas flow-rates may be adjusted to produce the highest concentration of free atoms. The burner height may also be adjusted, so that the radiation beam passes through the zone of highest atom cloud density in the flame, resulting in the highest sensitivity.

The processes in a flame include the following stages:

- Desolvation (drying) – the solvent is evaporated and the dry sample nano-particles remain;
- Vaporization (transfer to the gaseous phase) – the solid particles are converted into gaseous molecules;
- Atomization – the molecules are dissociated into free atoms;
- Ionization – depending on the ionization potential of the analyte atoms and the energy available in a particular flame, atoms might be in part converted to gaseous ions.

Each of these stages includes the risk of interference in case the degree of phase transfer is different for the analyte in the calibration standard and in the sample. Ionization is generally undesirable, as it reduces the number of atoms that are available for measurement, i.e., the sensitivity.

In flame AAS a steady-state signal is generated during the time period when the sample is aspirated. This technique is typically used for determinations in the mg L^{-1} range, and may be extended down to a few µg L^{-1} for some elements.

Electrothermal Atomizers

Elements in Graphite-Furnace-AAS Overview (GFAA Method Development)

Element	Preferred Tube Type	Modifier	Pyrolysis Tempera-ture	Pyrolysis T. w/o modifier	Atomiza-tion Tempera-ture	Remarks
Ag	Platform	$PdMg(NO_3)_2$	800	250	1700	Absorption effects at various materials possible complexing reagents might be used.
Al	Platform	$Mg(NO_3)_2$	1200	1000	2400	Danger of confirmation via flask materials or environment.
As	Platform	$PdMg(NO_3)_2$	1100	300	2100	

Contd...

Element	Preferred Tube Type	Modifier	Pyrolysis Tempera -ture	Pyrolysis T. w/o modifier	Atomiza -tion Tempera -ture	Remarks
Aj	Platform	$PdMg(NO_3)_2$	800	250	1700	Absorption effects at various materials possible complexing reagents might be used
B	Wall	$Ca(NO_3)_2$	1200	1000	2500	
Ba	Wall	$Ca(NO_3)_2$	1200	1000	2500	
Be	Platform	$Mg(NO_3)_2$	1200	1000	2300	
Bi	Platform	$PdMg(NO_3)_2$	1100	400	1900	
Ca	Wall		1100	1000	2500	High risk of contraction
Cd	Platform	$NH_4H_2PO_4$	700	250	1400	
		$PdMg(NO_3)_2$	800	250	1700	Supports evaporation of chlorides
Co	Platform	$Mg(NO_3)_2$	1200	1000	2200	
Cr	Platform	$Mg(NO_3)_2$	1400	1000	2300	
Cu	Platform	$PdMg(NO_3)_2$	1200	900	2100	
Fe	Platform	$Mg(NO_3)_2$	1200	900	2100	
K	Platform		900		1500	High risk of concentration
Mn	Platform	$PdMg(NO_3)_2$	1200	800	2000	
Mo	Wall		1200	1000	2450	
Na	Platform			850	1500	High risk of concentration
Ni	Platform	$Mg(NO_3)_2$	1200	1000	2300	
Pb	Platform	$NH_4H_2PO_4$	800	300	1700	
		$PdMg(NO_3)_2$	900	300	1900	Supports evaporation of chlorides
Sb	Platform	$PdMg(NO_3)_2$	1200	300	2100	
Se	Platform	$PdMg(NO_3)_2$	1200	300	2100	
Si	Platform	$PdMg(NO_3)_2$	1200	1000	2400	
Su	Platform	$PdMg(NO_3)_2$	1200	700	2300	

Contd...

Element	Preferred Tube Type	Modifier	Pyrolysis Tempera -ture	Pyrolysis T. w/o modifier	Atomiza -tion Tempera -ture	Remarks
Te	Platform	$PdMg(NO_3)_2$	1000	300	2000	
Ti	Wall		1300	1200	2500	
n	Platform	$PdMg(NO_3)_2$	700	300	1700	Evaporates in chloric materials at 200 ^{0}C
V	Wall		1300	1200	2500	

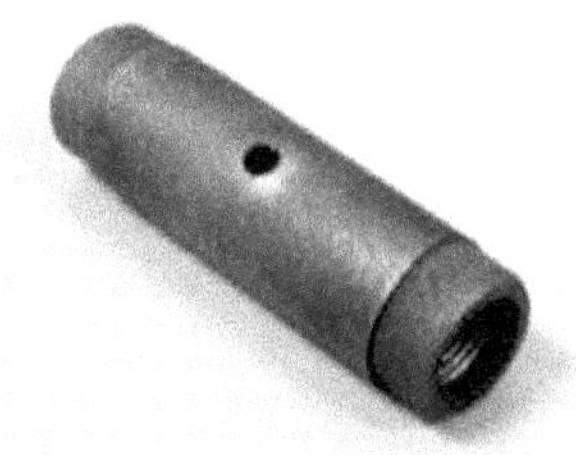

Figure 7.11: Graphite tube

Electrothermal AAS (ET AAS) using graphite tube atomizers was pioneered by Boris V. L'vov at the Saint Petersburg Polytechnical Institute, Russia, since the late 1950s, and investigated in parallel by Hans Massmann at the Institute of Spectrochemistry and Applied Spectroscopy (ISAS) in Dortmund, Germany.

Although a wide variety of graphite tube designs have been used over the years, the dimensions nowadays are typically 20–25 mm in length and 5–6 mm inner diameter. With this technique liquid/dissolved, solid and gaseous samples may be analyzed directly. A measured volume (typically 10–50 μL) or a weighed mass (typically around 1 mg) of a solid sample are introduced into the graphite tube and subject to a temperature program. This typically consists of stages, such as:

- Drying – the solvent is evaporated
- Pyrolysis – the majority of the matrix constituents are removed
- Atomization – the analyte element is released to the gaseous phase
- Cleaning – eventual residues in the graphite tube are removed at high temperature.

The graphite tubes are heated via their ohmic resistance using a low-voltage high-current power supply; the temperature in the individual stages can be controlled very closely, and temperature ramps between the individual stages facilitate separation of sample components. Tubes may be heated transversely or longitudinally, where the former ones have the advantage of a more homogeneous temperature distribution over their length. The so-called stabilized temperature platform furnace (STPF) concept, proposed by Walter Slavin, based on research of Boris L'vov, makes ET AAS essentially free from interference. The major components of this concept are:

- Atomization of the sample from a graphite platform inserted into the graphite tube (L'vov platform) instead of from the tube wall in order to delay atomization until the gas phase in the atomizer has reached a stable temperature;
- Use of a chemical modifier in order to stabilize the analyte to a pyrolysis temperature that is sufficient to remove the majority of the matrix components;
- Integration of the absorbance over the time of the transient absorption signal instead of using peak height absorbance for quantification.

In ET AAS a transient signal is generated, the area of which is directly proportional to the mass of analyte (not its concentration) introduced into the graphite tube. This technique has the advantage that any kind of sample, solid, liquid or gaseous, can be analyzed directly. Its sensitivity is 2–3 orders of magnitude higher than that of flame AAS, so that determinations in the low $\mu g\ L^{-1}$ range (for a typical sample volume of 20 μL) and $ng\ g^{-1}$ range (for a typical sample mass of 1 mg) can be carried out. It shows a very high degree of freedom from interferences, so that ET AAS might be considered the most robust technique available nowadays for the determination of trace elements in complex matrices.

Specialized Atomization Techniques

While flame and electrothermal vaporizers are the most common atomization techniques, several other atomization methods are utilized for specialized use.

Glow-Discharge Atomization

A glow-discharge (GD) device serves as a versatile source, as it can simultaneously introduce and atomize the sample. The glow discharge occurs in a low-pressure argon gas atmosphere between 1 and 10 torr. In this atmosphere lies a pair of electrodes applying a DC voltage of 250 to 1000 V to break down the argon gas into positively charged ions and electrons. These ions, under the influence of the electric field, are accelerated into the cathode surface containing the sample, bombarding the sample and causing neutral sample atom ejection through the process known as sputtering. The atomic vapor produced by this discharge is composed of ions, ground state atoms, and fraction of excited atoms. When the excited atoms relax back into their ground state, a low-intensity glow is emitted, giving the technique its name.

The requirement for samples of glow discharge atomizers is that they are electrical conductors. Consequently, atomizers are most commonly used in the analysis of metals and other conducting samples. However, with proper modifications, it can be utilized to analyze liquid samples as well as nonconducting materials by mixing them with a conductor (e.g. graphite).

Hydride Atomization

Hydride generation techniques are specialized in solutions of specific elements. The technique provides a means of introducing samples containing arsenic, antimony, tin, selenium, bismuth, and lead into an atomizer in the gas phase. With these elements, hydride atomization enhances detection limits by a factor of 10 to 100 compared to alternative methods. Hydride generation occurs by adding an acidified aqueous solution of the sample to a 1% aqueous solution of sodium borohydride, all of which is contained in a glass vessel. The volatile hydride generated by the reaction that occurs is swept into the atomization chamber by an inert gas, where it undergoes decomposition. This process forms an atomized form of the analyte, which can then be measured by absorption or emission spectrometry.

Cold-Vapor Atomization

The cold-vapor technique an atomization method limited to only the determination of mercury, due to it being the only metallic element to have a large enough vapor pressure at ambient temperature. Because of this, it has an important use in determining organic mercury compounds in samples and their distribution in the environment. The method initiates by converting mercury into Hg^{2+} by oxidation from nitric and sulfuric acids, followed by a reduction of Hg^{2+} with tin(II) chloride. The mercury, is then swept into a long-pass absorption tube by bubbling a stream of inert gas through the reaction mixture. The concentration is determined by measuring the absorbance of this gas at 253.7 nm. Detection limits for this technique are in the parts-per-billion range making it an excellent mercury detection atomization method.

Radiation Sources

We have to distinguish between line source AAS (LS AAS) and continuum source AAS (CS AAS). In classical LS AAS, as it has been proposed by Alan Walsh, the high spectral resolution required for AAS measurements is provided by the radiation source itself that emits the spectrum of the analyte in the form of lines that are narrower than the absorption lines. Continuum sources, such as deuterium lamps, are only used for background correction purposes. The advantage of this technique is that only a medium-resolution monochromator is necessary for measuring AAS; however, it has the disadvantage that usually a separate lamp is required for each element that has to be determined. In CS AAS, in contrast, a single lamp, emitting a continuum spectrum over the entire spectral range of interest is used for all elements. Obviously, a high-resolution monochromator is required for this technique, as will be discussed later.

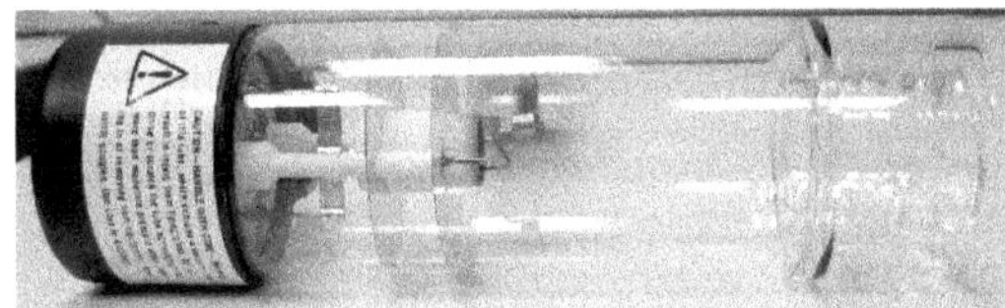

Figure 7.12: Hollow cathode lamp (HCL)

Hollow Cathode Lamps

Hollow cathode lamps (HCL) are the most common radiation source in LS AAS. Inside the sealed lamp, filled with argon or neon gas at low pressure, is a cylindrical metal cathode containing the element of interest and an anode. A high voltage is applied across the anode and cathode, resulting in an ionization of the fill gas. The gas ions are accelerated towards the cathode and, upon impact on the cathode, sputter cathode material that is excited in the glow discharge to emit the radiation of the sputtered material, i.e., the element of interest. Most lamps will handle a handful of elements, *i.e.* 5-8. A typical machine will have two lamps, one will take care of five elements and the other will handle four elements for a total of nine elements analyzed.

Electrodeless Discharge Lamps

Electrodeless discharge lamps (EDL) contain a small quantity of the analyte as a metal or a salt in a quartz bulb together with an inert gas, typically argon, at low pressure. The bulb is inserted into a coil that is generating an electromagnetic radio frequency field, resulting in a low-pressure inductively coupled discharge in the lamp. The emission from an EDL is higher than that from an HCL, and the line width is generally narrower, but EDLs need a separate power supply and might need a longer time to stabilize.

Deuterium Lamps

Deuterium HCL or even hydrogen HCL and deuterium discharge lamps are used in LS AAS for background correction purposes. The radiation intensity emitted by these lamps decreases significantly with increasing wavelength, so that they can be only used in the wavelength range between 190 and about 320 nm.

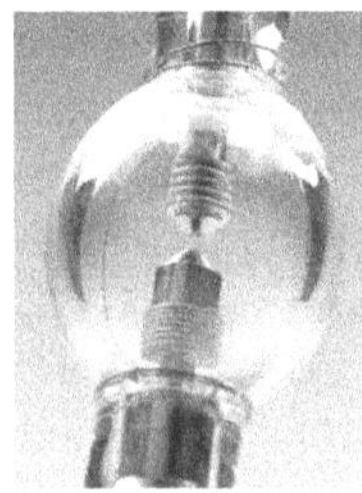

Figure 7.13: Xenon lamp as a continuous radiation source

Continuum Sources

When a continuum radiation source is used for AAS, it is necessary to use a high-resolution monochromator, as will be discussed later. In addition, it is necessary that the lamp emits radiation of intensity at least an order of magnitude above that of a typical HCL over the entire wavelength range from 190 nm to 900 nm. A special high-pressure xenon short arc lamp, operating in a hot-spot mode has been developed to fulfill these requirements.

Spectrometer

As already pointed out above, there is a difference between medium-resolution spectrometers that are used for LS AAS and high-resolution spectrometers that are designed for CS AAS. The spectrometer includes the spectral sorting device (monochromator) and the detector.

Spectrometers for LS AAS

In LS AAS the high resolution that is required for the measurement of atomic absorption is provided by the narrow line emission of the radiation source, and the monochromator simply has to resolve the analytical line from other radiation emitted by the lamp. This can usually be accomplished with a band pass between 0.2 and 2 nm, i.e., a medium-resolution monochromator. Another feature to make LS AAS element-specific is modulation of the primary radiation and the use of a selective amplifier that is tuned to the same modulation frequency, as already postulated by Alan Walsh. This way any (unmodulated) radiation emitted for example by the atomizer can be excluded, which is imperative for LS AAS. Simple monochromators of the Littrow or (better) the Czerny-Turner design are typically used for LS AAS. Photomultiplier tubes are the most frequently used detectors in LS AAS, although solid state detectors might be preferred because of their better signal-to-noise ratio.

Spectrometers for CS AAS

When a continuum radiation source is used for AAS measurement it is indispensable to work with a high-resolution monochromator. The resolution has to be equal to or better than the half width of an atomic absorption line (about 2 pm) in order to avoid losses of sensitivity and linearity of the calibration graph. The research with high-resolution (HR) CS AAS was pioneered by the groups of O'Haver and Harnly in the USA, who also developed the (up until now) only simultaneous multi-element spectrometer for this technique. The break-through, however, came when the group of Becker-Ross in Berlin, Germany, built a spectrometer entirely designed for HR-CS AAS. The first commercial equipment for HR-CS AAS was introduced by Analytik Jena (Jena, Germany) at the beginning of the 21st century, based on the design proposed by Becker-Ross and Florek. These spectrometers use a compact double monochromator with a prism pre-monochromator and an echelle grating monochromator for high resolution. A linear charge coupled device (CCD) array with 200 pixels is used as the detector. The second monochromator does not have an exit slit; hence the spectral environment at both sides of the analytical line becomes visible at high resolution. As typically only 3–5 pixels are used to measure the atomic absorption, the other pixels are available for correction purposes. One of these corrections is that for lamp flicker noise, which is independent of wavelength, resulting in measurements with very low noise level; other corrections are those for background absorption, as will be discussed later.

Background Absorption and Background Correction

The relatively small number of atomic absorption lines (compared to atomic emission lines) and their narrow width (a few pm) make spectral overlap rare; there are only very few examples known that an absorption line from one element will overlap with another. Molecular absorption, in contrast, is much broader, so that it is more likely that some molecular absorption band will overlap with an atomic line. This kind of absorption might be caused by un-dissociated molecules of concomitant elements of the sample or by flame gases. We have to distinguish between the spectra of di-atomic molecules, which exhibit a pronounced fine structure, and those of larger (usually tri-atomic) molecules that don't show such fine structure. Another source of background absorption, particularly in ET AAS, is scattering of the primary radiation at particles that are generated in the atomization stage, when the matrix could not be removed sufficiently in the pyrolysis stage.

All these phenomena, molecular absorption and radiation scattering, can result in artificially high absorption and an improperly high (erroneous) calculation for the concentration or mass of the analyte in the sample. There are several techniques available to correct for background absorption, and they are significantly different for LS AAS and HR-CS AAS.

Background Correction Techniques in LS AAS

In LS AAS background absorption can only be corrected using instrumental techniques, and all of them are based on two sequential measurements, firstly, total absorption (atomic plus background), secondly, background absorption only, and the difference of the two measurements gives the net atomic absorption. Because of this, and because of the use of additional devices in the spectrometer, the signal-to-noise ratio of background-corrected signals is always significantly inferior compared to uncorrected signals. It should also be pointed out that in LS AAS there is no way to correct for (the rare case of) a direct overlap of two atomic lines. In essence there are three techniques used for background correction in LS AAS:

Deuterium Background Correction

This is the oldest and still most commonly used technique, particularly for flame AAS. In this case, a separate source (a deuterium lamp) with broad emission is used to measure the background absorption over the entire width of the exit slit of the spectrometer. The use of a separate lamp makes this technique the least accurate one, as it cannot correct for any structured background. It also cannot be used at wavelengths above about 320 nm, as the emission intensity of the deuterium lamp becomes very weak. The use of deuterium HCL is preferable compared to an arc lamp due to the better fit of the image of the former lamp with that of the analyte HCL.

Smith-Hieftje Background Correction

This technique (named after their inventors) is based on the line-broadening and self-reversal of emission lines from HCL when high current is applied. Total absorption is measured with normal lamp current, i.e., with a narrow emission line, and background absorption after application of a high-current pulse with the profile of the self-reversed line, which has little emission at the original wavelength, but strong emission on both sides of the analytical line. The advantage of this technique is that only one radiation source is used; among the disadvantages are that the high-current pulses reduce lamp lifetime, and that the technique can only be used for relatively volatile elements, as only those exhibit sufficient self-reversal to avoid dramatic loss of sensitivity. Another problem is that background is not measured at the same wavelength as total absorption, making the technique unsuitable for correcting structured background.

Zeeman-Effect Background Correction

An alternating magnetic field is applied at the atomizer (graphite furnace) to split the absorption line into three components, the π component, which remains at the same position as the original absorption line, and two σ components, which are moved to higher and lower wavelengths, respectively (see Zeeman Effect). Total absorption is measured without magnetic field and background absorption with the magnetic field on. The π component has to be removed in this case, e.g. using a polarizer, and the σ components do not overlap with the emission profile of the lamp, so that only the background absorption is measured. The advantages of this technique are:

1. that total and background absorption are measured with the same emission profile of the same lamp, so that any kind of background, including background with fine structure can be corrected accurately, unless the molecule responsible for the background is also affected by the magnetic field
2. using a chopper as a polariser reduces the signal to noise ratio. While the disadvantages are the increased complexity of the spectrometer and power supply needed for running the powerful magnet needed to split the absorption line.

Background Correction Techniques in HR-CS AAS

In HR-CS AAS background correction is carried out mathematically in the software using information from detector pixels that are not used for measuring atomic absorption; hence, in contrast to LS AAS, no additional components are required for background correction.

Background Correction using Correction Pixels

It has already been mentioned that in HR-CS AAS lamp flicker noise is eliminated using correction pixels. In fact, any increase or decrease in radiation intensity that is observed to the same extent at all pixels chosen for correction is eliminated by the correction algorithm. This obviously also includes a reduction of the measured intensity due to radiation scattering or molecular absorption, which is corrected in the same way. As measurement of total and background absorption, and correction for the latter, are strictly simultaneous (in contrast to LS AAS), even the fastest changes of background absorption, as they may be observed in ET AAS, do not cause any problem. In addition, as the same algorithm is used for background correction and elimination of lamp noise, the background corrected signals show a much better signal-to-noise ratio compared to the uncorrected signals, which is also in contrast to LS AAS.

Background Correction using a Least-Squares Algorithm

The above technique can obviously not correct for a background with fine structure, as in this case the absorbance will be different at each of the correction pixels. In this case HR-CS AAS is offering the possibility to measure correction spectra of the molecule(s) that is (are) responsible for the background and store them in the computer. These spectra are then multiplied with a factor to match the intensity of the sample spectrum and subtracted pixel by pixel and spectrum by spectrum from the sample spectrum using a least-squares algorithm. This might sound complex, but first of all the number of di-atomic molecules that can exist at the temperatures of the atomizers used in AAS is relatively small, and second, the correction is performed by the computer within a few seconds. The same algorithm can actually also be used to correct for direct line overlap of two atomic absorption lines, making HR-CS AAS the only AAS technique that can correct for this kind of spectral interference.

B. Astronomical Spectroscopy

Astronomical spectroscopy is the study of astronomy using the techniques of spectroscopy to measure the spectrum of electromagnetic radiation, including visible light, which radiates from stars and other hot celestial objects. Spectroscopy can be used to derive many properties of distant stars and galaxies, such as their chemical composition, temperature, density, mass, distance, luminosity, and relative motion using Doppler shift measurements.

Background

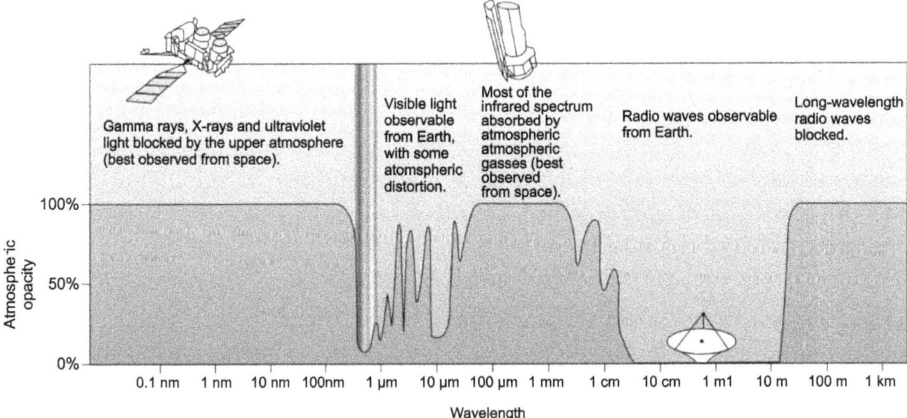

Figure 7.14: Electromagnetic transmittance, or opacity, of the Earth's atmosphere

Astronomical spectroscopy is used to measure three major bands of radiation: optical, radio, and X-ray. While all spectroscopy looks at specific areas of the spectrum, different methods are required to acquire the signal depending on the frequency. Ozone (O_3) and molecular oxygen (O_2) absorb light with wavelengths under 300 nm, meaning that X-ray and ultraviolet spectroscopy require the use of a satellite telescope or rocket mounted detectors. Radio signals have much longer wavelengths than optical signals, and require the use of antennas or radio dishes. Infrared light is absorbed by atmospheric water and carbon dioxide, so while the equipment is similar to that used in optical spectroscopy, satellites are required to record much of the infrared spectrum.

Optical Spectroscopy

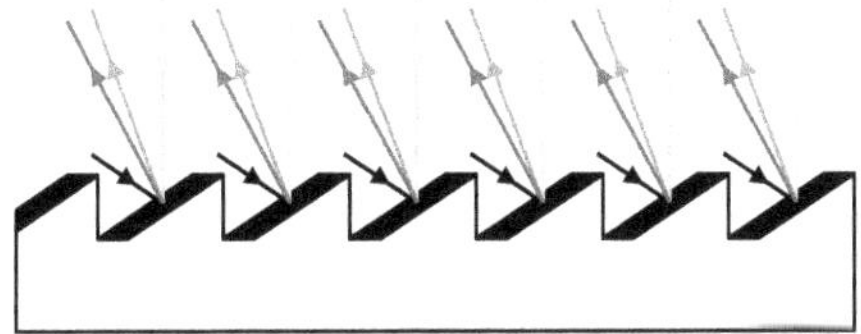

Figure 7.15: Incident light reflects at the same angle (black lines), but a small portion of the light is refracted as coloured light (red and blue lines).

Physicists have been looking at the solar spectrum since Isaac Newton first used a simple prism to observe the refractive properties of light. In the early 1800s Joseph von Fraunhofer used his skills as a glass maker to create very pure prisms, which allowed him to observe 574 dark lines in a seemingly continuous spectrum. Soon after he combined telescope and prism to observe the spectrum ofVenus, the Moon, Mars, and various stars such as Betelgeuse; his company continued to manufacture and sell high-quality refracting telescopes based on his original designs until its closure in 1884.

The resolution of a prism is limited by its size; a larger prism will provide a more detailed spectrum, but the increase in mass makes it unsuitable for highly detailed work. This issue was resolved in the early 1900s with the development of high-quality reflection gratings byJ.S. Plaskett at the Dominion Observatory in Ottawa, Canada. Light striking a mirror will reflect at the same angle, however a small portion of the light will be refracted at a different angle; this is dependent upon the indices of refraction of the materials and the wavelength of the light. By creating a "blazed" grating which utilizes a large number of parallel mirrors, the small portion of light can be focused and visualized. These new spectroscopes were more detailed than a prism, required less light, and could be focused on a specific region of the spectrum by tilting the grating.

The limitation to a blazed grating is the width of the mirrors, which can only be ground a finite amount before focus is lost; the maximum is around 1000 lines/mm. In order to overcome this limitation holographic gratings were developed. Volume phase holographic gratings use a thin film of dichromated gelatin on a glass surface, which is subsequently exposed to a wave pattern created by an interferometer. This wave pattern sets up a reflection pattern similar to the blazed gratings but utilizing Bragg diffraction, a process where the angle of reflection is dependent on the arrangement of the atoms in the gelatin. The holographic gratings can have up to 6000 lines/mm and can be up to twice as efficient in collecting light as blazed gratings. Because they are sealed between two sheets of glass, the holographic gratings are very versatile, potentially lasting decades before needing replacement.

Radio Spectroscopy

Radio astronomy was founded with the work of Karl Jansky in the early 1930s, while working for Bell Labs. He built a radio antenna to look at potential sources of interference for transatlantic radio transmissions. One of the sources of noise discovered came not from Earth, but from the center of the Milky Way, in the constellation Sagittarius. In 1942, JS Hey captured the sun's radio frequency using military radar receivers.

Radio interferometry was pioneered in 1946, when Joseph Lade Pawsey, Ruby Payne-Scott and Lindsay McCready used a single antenna atop a sea cliff to observe 200 MHz solar radiation. Two incident beams, one directly from the sun and the other reflected from the sea surface, generated the necessary interference. The first multi-receiver interferometer was built in the same year by Martin Ryle and Vonberg. In 1960, Ryle and Antony Hewish published the technique of aperture synthesis to analyze interferometer data. The aperture synthesis process, which involves autocorrelating and discrete Fourier transforming the incoming signal, recovers both the spatial and frequency variation in flux. The result is a 3D image whose third axis is frequency. For this work, Ryle and Hewish were jointly awarded the 1974 Nobel Prize in Physics.

X-Ray Spectroscopy

Stars and their Properties

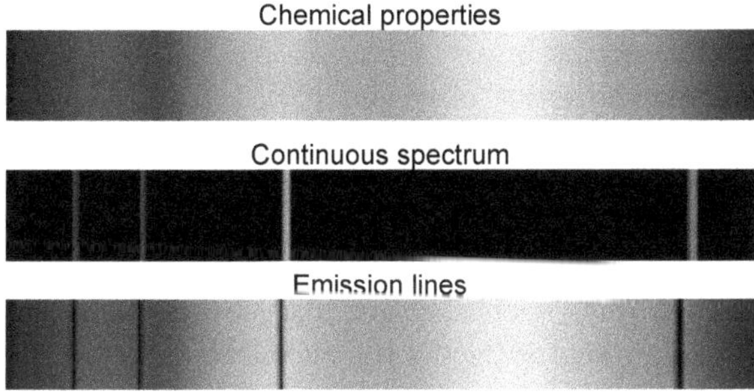

Newton used a prism to split white light into a spectrum of color, and Fraunhofer's high-quality prisms allowed scientists to see dark lines of an unknown origin. It was not until the 1850s that Gustav Kirchhoff and Robert Bunsen would describe the phenomena behind these dark lines hot solid objects produce light with a continuous spectrum, hot gasses emit light at specific wavelengths, and hot solid objects surrounded by cooler gasses will show a near-continuous spectrum with dark lines corresponding to the emission lines of the gasses. By comparing the absorption lines of the sun with emission spectra of known gasses, the chemical composition of stars can be determined.

The major Fraunhofer lines, and the elements they are associated with, are shown in the following table. Designations from the earlyBalmer Series are in parentheses.

Designation	Element	Wavelength (nm)	Designation	Element	Wavelength (nm)
Y	O_2	898.765	c	Fe	495.761
Z	O_2	822.696	F (Hβ)	H	486.134
A	O_2	759.370	d	Fe	466.814
B	O_2	686.719	e	Fe	438.355
C (Hα)	H	656.281	G′ (Hγ)	H	434.047
A	O_2	627.661	G	Fe	430.790
D_1	Na	589.592	G	Ca	430.774
D_2	Na	588.995	h (Hδ)	H	410.175
D_3 or d	He	587.5618	H	Ca^+	396.847
E	Hg	546.073	K	Ca^+	393.368
E_2	Fe	527.039	L	Fe	38.044
b_1	Mg	518.362	N	Fe	358.121
b_2	Mg	517.270	P	Ti^+	336.112
b_3	Fe	516.891	T	Fe	302.108
b_4	Mg	516.733	t	Ni	299.444

Not all of the elements in the sun were immediately identified. Two examples are listed below.

- In 1868 Norman Lockyer and Pierre Janssen independently observed a line next to the sodium doublet (D_1 and D_2) which Lockyer determined to be a new element. He named it Helium, but it wasn't until 1895 the element was found on Earth.
- In 1869 the astronomers Charles Augustus Young and William Harkness independently observed a novel green emission line in the Sun's corona during an eclipse. This "new" element was incorrectly named coronium, as it was only found in the corona. It was not until the 1930s that Walter Grotrian and Bengt Edlén discovered that the spectral line at 530.3 nm was due to highly ionized iron (Fe^{13+}). Other unusual lines in the coronal spectrum are also caused by highly charged ions, such as nickel andcalcium, the high ionization being due to the extreme temperature of the solar corona.

To date more than 20 000 absorption lines have been listed for the Sun between 293.5 and 877.0 nm, yet only approximately 75% of these lines have been linked to elemental absorption.

By analyzing the width of each spectral line in an emission spectrum, both the elements present in a star and their relative abundances can be determined. Using this information stars can be categorized into stellar populations; Population I stars are the youngest stars and have the highest metal content (our Sun is a Pop I star), while Population III stars are the oldest stars with a very low metal content.

Temperature and Size

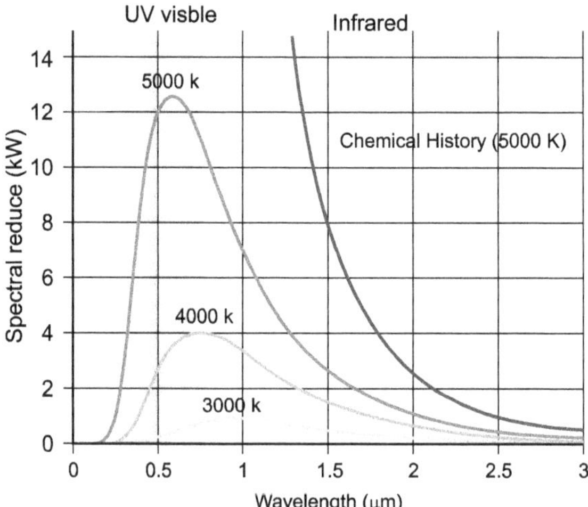

Figure 7.16: Black body curves for various temperatures.

In 1860 Gustav Kirchhoff proposed the idea of a black body, a material that emits electromagnetic radiation at all wavelengths. In 1894 Wilhelm Wien derived an expression relating the temperature (T) of a black body to its peak emission wavelength (λ_{max}).

$$\lambda_{max}T = b$$

b is a constant of proportionality called *Wien's displacement constant,* equal to $2.8977721(26)\times10^{-3}$ m K. This equation is calledWien's Law. By measuring the peak wavelength of a star, the surface temperature can be determined. For example, if the peak wavelength of a star is 502 nm the corresponding temperature will be 5778 Kelvin.

The luminosity of a star is a measure of the electromagnetic energy output in a given amount of time. Luminosity (L) can be related to the temperature (T) of a star by

$$L = R\pi R^2\sigma T^4$$

where R is the radius of the star and σ is the Stefan–Boltzmann constant, with a value of $5.670373(21)\times10^{-8}$ W m^{-2} K^{-4}. Thus, when both luminosity and temperature are known (via direct measurement and calculation) the radius of a star can be determined.

Galaxies

The spectra of galaxies look similar to stellar spectra, as they consist of the combined light of millions of stars.

Doppler shift studies of galaxy clusters by Fritz Zwicky in 1937 found that most galaxies were moving much faster than seemed to be possible from what was known about the mass of the cluster. Zwicky hypothesized that there must be a great deal of non-luminous matter in the galaxy clusters, which became known as dark matter. Since his discovery, astronomers have determined that a large portion of galaxies (and most of the universe) is made up of dark matter. In 2003, however, four galaxies (NGC 821, NGC 3379, NGC 4494, and NGC 4697) were found to have little to no dark matter influencing the motion of the stars contained within them; the reason behind the lack of dark matter is unknown.

In the 1950s, strong radio sources were found to be associated with very dim, very red objects. When the first spectrum of one of these objects was taken there were absorption lines at wavelengths where none were expected. It was soon realised that what was observed was a normal galactic spectrum, but highly red shifted. These were named *quasi-stellar radio sources,* or quasars, by Hong-Yee Chiu in 1964. Quasars are now thought to be galaxies formed in the early years of our universe, with their extreme energy output powered by super-massive black holes.

The properties of a galaxy can also be determined by analyzing the stars found within them. NGC 4550, a galaxy in the Virgo Cluster, has a large portion of its stars rotating in the opposite direction as the other portion. It is believed that the galaxy is the combination of two smaller galaxies that were rotating in opposite directions to each other. Bright stars in galaxies can also help determine the distance to a galaxy, which may be a more accurate method than parallax or standard candles.

Interstellar Medium

The interstellar medium is matter that occupies the space between star systems in a galaxy. 99% of this matter is gaseous - hydrogen, helium, and smaller quantities of other ionized elements such as oxygen. The other 1% is dust particles, thought to be mainly graphite, silicates, and ices. Clouds of the dust and gas are referred to as nebulae.

Therearethreemaintypesofnebula:absorption,reflection,andemissionnebulae. Absorption (or dark) nebulae are made of dust and gas in such quantities that they obscure the starlight behind them, making photometry difficult. Reflection nebulae, as their name suggest, reflect the light of nearby stars. Their spectra are the same as the stars surrounding them, though the light is bluer; shorter wavelengths scatter better than longer wavelengths. Emission nebulae emit light at specific wavelengths depending on their chemical composition.

Gaseous Emission Nebulae

In the early years of astronomical spectroscopy, scientists were puzzled by the spectrum of gaseous nebulae. In 1864 William Huggins noticed that many nebulae showed only emission lines rather than a full spectrum like stars. From the work of Kirchhoff, he concluded that nebulae must contain "enormous masses of luminous gas or vapour."[34]However, there were several emission lines that could not be linked to any terrestrial element, brightest among them lines at 495.9 nm and 500.7 nm. These lines were attributed to a new element, nebulium, until Ira Bowen determined in 1927 that the emission lines were from highly ionised oxygen (O^{+2}). These emission lines could not be replicated in a laboratory because they are forbidden lines; the low density of a nebula (one atom per cubic centimetre) allows for metastable ions to decay via forbidden line emission rather than collisions with other atoms.

Not all emission nebulae are found around or near stars where solar heating causes ionisation. The majority of gaseous emission nebulae are formed of neutral hydrogen. In theground state neutral hydrogen has two possible spin states: the electron has either the same spin or the opposite spin of the proton. When the atom transitions between these two states, it releases an emission or absorption line of 21 cm. This line is within the radio range and allows for very precise measurements:

- Velocity of the cloud can be measured via Doppler shift
- The intensity of the 21 cm line gives the density and number of atoms in the cloud
- The temperature of the cloud can be calculated

Using this information the shape of the Milky Way has been determined to be a spiral galaxy, though the exact number and position of the spiral arms is the subject of on-going research.

Complex Molecules

Dust and molecules in the interstellar medium not only obscures photometry, but also causes absorption lines in spectroscopy. Their spectral features are generated by transitions of component electrons between different energy levels, or by rotational or vibrational spectra. Detection usually occurs in radio, microwave, or infrared portions of the spectrum. The chemical reactions that form these molecules can happen in cold, diffuse clouds or in the hot ejecta around a white dwarf star from a nova or supernova.[41]Polycyclic aromatic hydrocarbons such as acetylene (C_2H_2) generally group together to form graphites or other sooty material, but other organic molecules such as acetone ($(CH_3)_2CO$) and buckminsterfullerenes (C_{60} and C_{70}) have been discovered.

Motion in the Universe

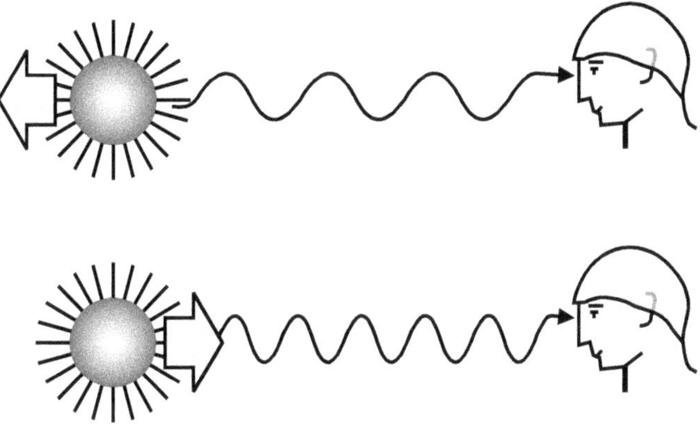

Figure 7.17: Redshift and blueshift

Stars and interstellar gas are bound by gravity to form galaxies, and groups of galaxies can be bound by gravity in galaxy clusters. With the exception of stars in the Milky Way and the galaxies in the Local Group, almost all galaxies are moving away from us due to theexpansion of the universe.

Doppler Effect and Redshift

The motion of stellar objects can be determined by looking at their spectrum. Because of the Doppler Effect, objects moving towards us are blueshifted, and objects moving away are redshifted. The wavelength of redshifted light is longer, appearing redder than the source. Conversely, the wavelength of blueshifted light is shorter, appearing bluer than the source light:

$$\frac{\lambda - \lambda_0}{\lambda_0} = \frac{v_0}{c}$$

where λ_0 is the emitted wavelength, v_0 is the velocity of the object, and λ is the observed wavelength. Note that $v<0$ corresponds to $\lambda < \lambda_0$, a blueshifted wavelength. A redshifted absorption or emission line will appear more towards the red end of the spectrum than a stationary line. In 1913 Vesto Slipher determined the Andromeda Galaxy was blueshifted, meaning it was moving towards the Milky Way. He recorded the spectra of 20 other galaxies all but 4 of which were redshifted and was able to calculate their velocities relative to the Earth. Edwin Hubble would later use this information, as well as his own observations, to define Hubble's law: The further a galaxy is from the Earth, the faster it is moving away from us. Hubble's law can be generalised to

$$v = H_0 d$$

where v is the velocity (or Hubble Flow), H_0 is the Hubble Constant, and d is the distance from Earth.

Redshift (z) can be expressed by the following equations:

Calculation of redshift, z

Based on wavelength	Based on frequency
$z = \frac{\lambda_{obav} - \lambda_{emit}}{\lambda_{emit}}$	$z = \frac{f_{emit} - f_{obsv}}{f_{obav}}$
$1 + z = \frac{\lambda_{obav}}{\lambda_{emit}}$	$1 + z = \frac{f_{emit}}{f_{obav}}$

In these equations, frequency is denoted by f and wavelength by λ. The larger the value of z, the more redshifted the light and the farther away the object is from the Earth. As of January 2013, the largest galaxy redshift of z~12 was found using the Hubble Ultra-Deep Field, corresponding to an age of over 13 billion years (the universe is approximately 13.82 billion years old).

The Doppler effect and Hubble's law can be combined to form the equation $z = \frac{v_{Hubble}}{C}$, where c is the speed of light.

Peculiar Motion

Objects that are gravitationally bound will rotate around a common center of mass. For stellar bodies, this motion is known as peculiar velocity, and can alter the Hubble Flow. Thus, an extra term for the peculiar motion needs to be added to Hubble's law:

$$v_{total} = H_0 d + v_{pec}$$

This motion can cause confusion when looking at a solar or galactic spectrum, because the expected redshift based on the simple Hubble law will be obscured by the peculiar motion. For example, the shape and size of the Virgo Cluster has been a matter of great scientific scrutiny due to the very large peculiar velocities of the galaxies in the cluster.

Binary Stars

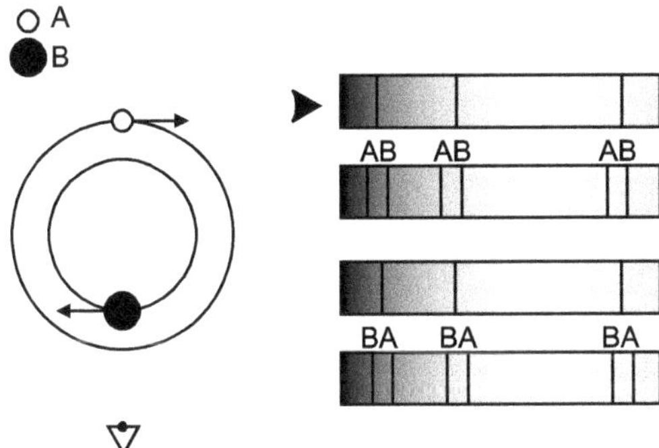

Figure 7.18: Two stars of different size orbiting the center of mass. The spectrum can be seen to split depending on the position and velocity of the stars.

Just as planets can be gravitationally bound to stars, pairs of stars can orbit each other. Some binary stars are visual binaries, meaning they can be observed orbiting each other through a telescope. Some binary stars, however, are too close together to be resolved. These two stars, when viewed through a spectrometer, will show a composite spectrum: the spectrum of each star will be added together. This composite spectrum becomes easier to detect when the stars are of similar luminosity and of different spectral class.

Spectroscopic binaries can be also detected due to their radial velocity; as they orbit around each other one star may be moving towards the Earth whilst the other moves away, causing a Doppler shifts in the composite spectrum. The orbital plane of the system determines the magnitude of the observed shift: if the observer is looking perpendicular to the orbital plane there will be no observed radial velocity. For example, if you look at a carousel from the side, you will see the animals moving toward and away from you, whereas if you look from directly above they will only be moving in the horizontal plane.

Planets, Asteroids, and Comets

Planets and asteroids shine only by the reflected light of their parent star, while comets both absorb and emit light at various wavelengths.

Planets

The reflected light of a planet contains absorption bands due to minerals in the rocks present for rocky bodies, or due to the elements and molecules present in the atmospheres of gas giants. To date almost 1000 exo-planets have been discovered. These include so-called Hot Jupiter's, as well as Earth-like planets. Using spectroscopy, compounds such as alkali metals, water vapour, carbon monoxide, carbon dioxide, and methane have all been discovered.

Asteroids

Asteroids can be classified into three major types according to their spectra. The original categories were created by Clark R. Chapman, David Morrison, and Ben Zellner in 1975, and further expanded by David J. Tholen in 1984. In what is now known as the Tholen classification, the C-types are made of carbonaceous material, S-types consist mainly ofsilicates, and X-types are 'metallic'. There are other classifications for unusual asteroids. C- and S-type asteroids are the most common asteroids. In 2002 the Tholen classification was further "evolved" into the SMASS classification, expanding the number of categories from 14 to 26 to account for more precise spectroscopic analysis of the asteroids.

Comets

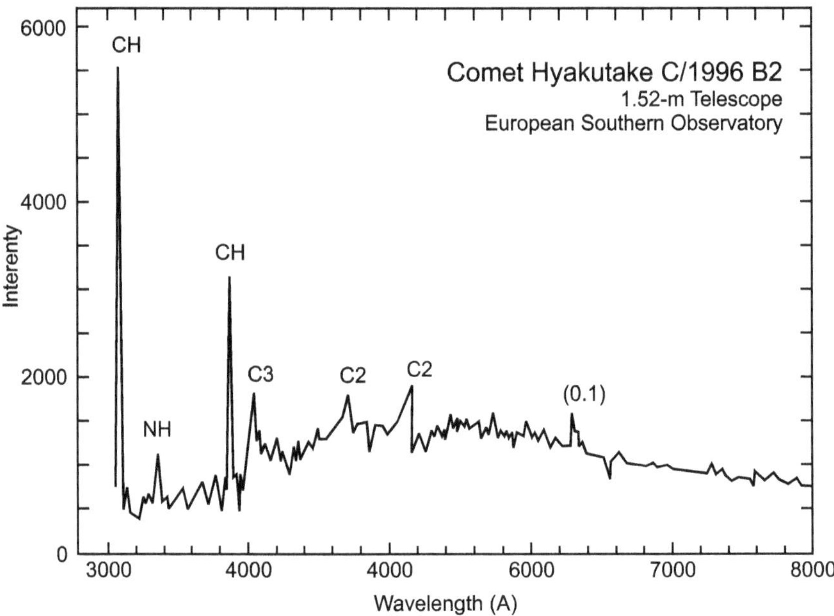

Figure 7.19: Optical spectrum of Comet Hyakutake.

The spectra of comets consist of a reflected solar spectrum from the dusty clouds surrounding the comet, as well as emission lines from gaseous atoms and molecules excited to fluorescence by sunlight and/or chemical reactions. For example, the chemical composition of Comet ISON was determined by spectroscopy due to the prominent emission lines of cyanogen (CN), as well as two- and three-carbon atoms (C_2 and C_3). Nearby comets can even be seen in X-ray as solar wind ions flying to the coma are neutralized. The come tary X-ray spectra therefore reflect the state of the solar wind rather than that of the comet.

C. Time-Domain Spectroscopy

In physics, terahertz time-domain spectroscopy (THz-TDS) is a spectroscopic technique in which the properties of a material are probed with short pulses of terahertz radiation. The generation and detection scheme is sensitive to the sample material's effect on both the amplitude and the phase of the terahertz radiation. In this respect, the technique can provide more information than conventional Fourier-transform spectroscopy, which is only sensitive to the amplitude.

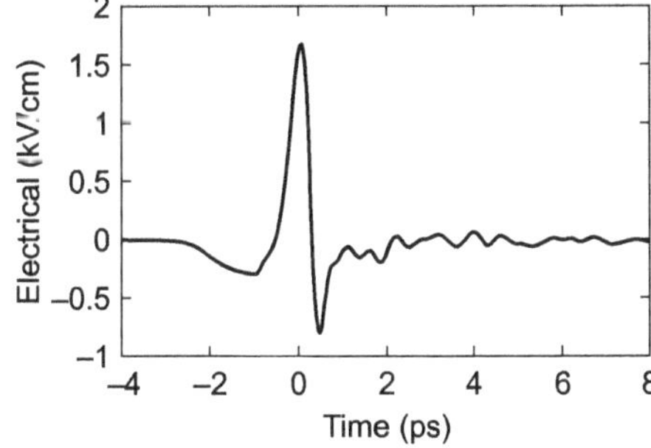

Figure 7.20: Typical pulse as measured with THz-TDS.

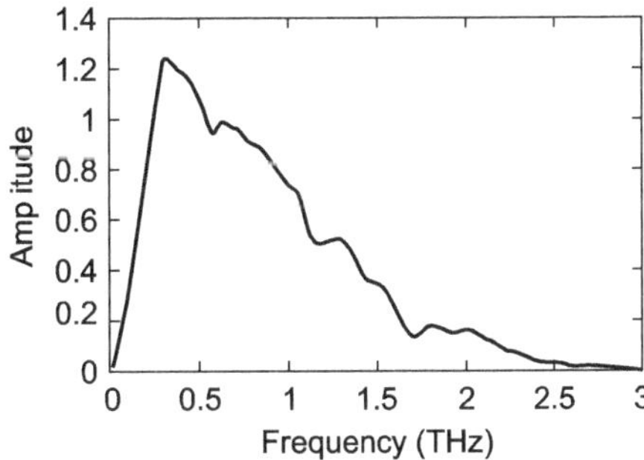

Figure 7.21: Fourier transform of the above pulse.

Explanation

Typically, the terahertz pulses are generated by an ultra-ultra-laser and last only a few picoseconds. A single pulse can contain frequency components covering the whole terahertz range from 0.05 to 4 THz. For detection, the electrical field of the terahertz pulse is sampled and digitized, conceptually similar to the way an audio card transforms electrical voltage levels in an audio signal into numbers that describe the audio waveform. In THz-TDS, the electrical field of the THz pulse interacts in the detector with a much-shorter laser pulse (e.g. 0.1 picoseconds) in a way that produces an electrical signal that is proportional to the electric field of the THz pulse at the time the laser pulse gates the detector on. By repeating this procedure and varying the timing of the gating laser pulse, it is possible to scan the THz pulse and construct its electric field as a function of time. Subsequently, a Fourier transform is used to extract the frequency spectrum from the time-domain data.

Advantages of THz radiation

THz radiation has several distinct advantages over other forms of spectroscopy: many materials are transparent to THz, THz radiation is safe for biological tissues because it isnon-ionizing (unlike for example X-rays), and images formed with terahertz radiation can have relatively good resolution (less than 1 mm). Also, many interesting materials have unique spectral fingerprints in the terahertz range, which means that terahertz radiation can be used to identify them. Examples which have been demonstrated include several different types of explosives, polymorphic forms of many compounds used as Active

Pharmaceutical Ingredients (API) in commercial medications as well as several illegal narcotic substances. Since many materials are transparent to THz radiation, these items of interest can be observed through visually opaque intervening layers, such as packaging and clothing. Though not strictly a spectroscopic technique, the ultra-short width of the THz radiation pulses allows for measurements (e.g., thickness, density, defect location) on difficult to probe materials (e.g., foam). The measurement capability shares many similarities to that observed with pulsed ultrasonic systems. Reflections from buried interfaces and defects can be found and precisely imaged. THz measurements are non-contact however.

Generation

There are three widely used techniques for generating terahertz pulses, all based on ultra-short pulses from titanium-sapphire lasers or mode-locked fibber lasers.

Surface Emitters

When an ultra-short (100 femtoseconds or shorter) optical pulse illuminates a semiconductor and its wavelength (energy) is above the energy band-gap of the material, it photogenerates mobile carriers. Given that absorption of the pulse is an exponential process most of the carriers are generated near the surface (typically within 1 micrometre). The presence of the surface has two main effects. Firstly it generates a band bending which has the effect of accelerating carriers of different signs in opposite directions (normal to the surface) creating a dipole, this effect is known as surface field emission. Secondly, the presence of the surface itself creates a break of symmetry which results carriers being able move (in average) only into the bulk of the semiconductor, this phenomenon combined with the difference of mobilities of electrons and holes also produces a dipole, this is known as photo-Dember effect and it is particularly strong in high-mobility semiconductors such as InAs.

Photoconductive Emitters

In a photoconductive emitter, the optical laser pulse (100 femtoseconds or shorter) creates carriers (electron-hole pairs) in a semiconductor material. Effectively, the semiconductor changes abruptly from being an insulator into being a conductor. This conduction leads to a sudden electric current across a biased antenna patterned on the semiconductor. This changing current emits terahertz radiation, similar to what happens in the antenna of a radio transmitter. Typically the two antenna electrodes are patterned on a low temperature gallium arsenide (LT-GaAs), semi-insulating gallium arsenide (SI-GaAs), or other semiconductor (such as InP) substrate. In a commonly used scheme, the electrodes are formed into the shape of a simple dipole antenna with a gap of a few micrometers and have a bias voltage up to 40 V between them. The ultrafast (100 fs) laser pulse must have a wavelength that is short enough to excite electrons across the bandgap of the semiconductor substrate. This scheme is suitable for illumination with aTi:sapphire oscillator laser with pulse energies of about 10 nJ. For use with amplified Ti:sapphire lasers with pulse energies of about 1 mJ, the electrode gap can be increased to several centimeters with a bias voltage of up to 200 kV.

More recent advances towards cost-efficient and compact THz-TDS systems are based on mode-locked fibber scources emitting at a center wavelength of 1550 nm. Therefore, the photoconductive emitters have to be based on semiconductor materials with smaller band gaps of approximately 0.74 eV such as Fe-doped indium gallium arsenide [1] or indium gallium arsenide/indium aluminum arsenide heterostructures .

The short duration of THz pulses generated (typically ~2 ps) are primarily due to the rapid rise of the photo-induced current in the semiconductor and the short carrier lifetime semiconductor materials (e.g., LT-GaAs). This current may persist for only a few hundred femtoseconds, up to several nanoseconds, depending on the material of which the substrate is composed. This is not the only means of generation, but is currently (as of 2008) the most common.

Pulses produced by this method have average power levels on the order of several tens of microwatts. The peak power during the pulses can be many orders of magnitude higher due to the low duty cycle of mostly >1%, which is dependent on the repetition rate of the laser scource. The maximum bandwidth of the resulting THz pulse is primarily limited by the duration of the laser pulse, while the frequency position of the maximum of the Fourier spectrum is determined by the carrier lifetime of the semiconductor.

Optical Rectification

In optical rectification, a high-intensity ultrashort laser pulse passes through a transparent crystal material that emits a terahertz pulse without any applied voltages. It is anonlinear-optical process, where an appropriate crystal material is quickly electrically polarized at high optical intensities. This changing electrical polarization emits terahertz radiation.

Because of the high laser intensities that are necessary, this technique is mostly used with amplified Ti: sapphire lasers. Typical crystal materials are zinc telluride, gallium phosphide, and gallium selenide.

The bandwidth of pulses generated by optical rectification is limited by the laser pulse duration, terahertz absorption in the crystal material, the thickness of the crystal, and a mismatch between the propagation speed of the laser pulse and the terahertz pulse inside the crystal. Typically, a thicker crystal will generate higher intensities, but lower THz frequencies. With this technique, it is possible to boost the generated frequencies to 40 THz (7.5 μm) or higher, although 2 THz (150 μm) is more commonly used since it requires less complex optical setups.

Detection

The electrical field of the terahertz pulses is measured in a detector that is simultaneously illuminated with an ultrashort laser pulse. Two common detection schemes are used in THz-TDS: photoconductive sampling and electro-optical sampling. THz pulses can also be detected by bolometers, heat detectors cooled to liquid-helium temperatures. Since bolometers can only measure the total energy of a terahertz pulse, rather than its electrical field over time, it is not suitable for use in THz-TDS.

In both THz-TDS detection methods, a part (called the *detection pulse*) of the same ultrashort laser pulse that was used to generate the terahertz pulse is fed to the detector, where it arrives simultaneously with the terahertz pulse. The detector will produce a different electrical signal depending on whether the detection pulse arrives when the electric field of the THz pulse is low or high. An optical delay line is used to vary the timing of the detection pulse.

Because the measurement technique is coherent, it naturally rejects incoherent radiation. Additionally, because the time slice of the measurement is extremely narrow, the noise contribution to the measurement is extremely low.

The signal-to-noise ratio (S/N) of the resulting time-domain waveform obviously depends on experimental conditions (e.g., averaging time), however due to the coherent sampling techniques described, high S/N values (>70 dB) are routinely seen with 1 minute averaging times.

Photoconductive Detection

Photoconductive detection is similar to photoconductive generation. Here, the bias electrical field across the antenna leads is generated by the electric field of the THz pulse focused onto the antenna, rather than being applied externally. The presence of the THz electric field generates current across the antenna leads, which is usually amplified using a low-bandwidth amplifier. This amplified current is the measured parameter which corresponds to the THz field strength. Again, the carriers in the semiconductor substrate have an extremely short lifetime. Thus, the THz electric field strength is only sampled for an extremely narrow slice (femtoseconds) of the entire electric field waveform.

Electro-Optical Sampling

The materials used for generation of terahertz radiation by optical rectification can also be used for its detection by using the Pockels effect, where certain crystalline materials become birefringent in the presence of an electric field. The birefringence caused by the electric field of a terahertz pulse leads to a change in the optical polarization of the detection pulse, proportional to the terahertz electric-field strength. With the help of polarizers and photodiodes, this polarization change is measured.

As with the generation, the bandwidth of the detection is dependent on the laser pulse duration, material properties, and crystal thickness.

D. Auger Electron Spectroscopy

Auger electron spectroscopy is a common analytical technique used specifically in the study of surfaces and, more generally, in the area of materials science. Underlying the spectroscopic technique is the Auger effect, as it has come to be called, which is based on the analysis of energetic electrons emitted from an excited atom after a series of internal relaxation events. The Auger effect was discovered independently by both Lise Meitner and Pierre Auger in the 1920s. Though the discovery was made by Meitner and initially reported in the journal Zeitschrift für Physik in 1922, Auger is credited with the discovery in most of the scientific community. Until the early 1950s Auger transitions were considered nuisance effects by spectroscopists, not containing much relevant material information, but studied so as to explain anomalies in x-ray spectroscopy data. Since 1953 however, AES has become a practical and straightforward characterization technique for probing chemical and compositional surface environments and has found applications in metallurgy, gas-phase chemistry, and throughout the microelectronics industry.

Electron Transitions and the Auger Effect

The Auger effect is an electronic process at the heart of AES resulting from the inter- and intrastate transitions of electrons in an excited atom. When an atom is probed by an external mechanism, such as a photon or a beam of electrons with energies in the range of several eV to 50 keV, a core state electron can be removed leaving behind a hole. As this is an unstable state, the core hole can be filled by an outer shell electron, whereby the electron moving to the lower energy level loses an amount of energy equal to the difference in orbital energies. The transition energy can be coupled to a second outer shell electron, which will be emitted from the atom if the transferred energy is greater than the orbital binding energy. An emitted electron will have a kinetic energy of:

$$E_{\text{kin}} = E_{\text{Core State}} - E_B - E'_C$$

where $E_{\text{Core State}} - E_B - E'_C$ are respectively the core level, first outer shell, and second outer shell electron energies, measured from the vacuum level. The apostrophe (tic) denotes a slight modification to the binding energy of the outer shell electrons due to the ionized nature of the atom; often however, this energy modification is ignored in order to ease calculations. Since orbital energies are unique to an atom of a specific element, analysis of the ejected electrons can yield information about the chemical composition of a surface. Figure 7.22 illustrates two schematic views of the Auger process.

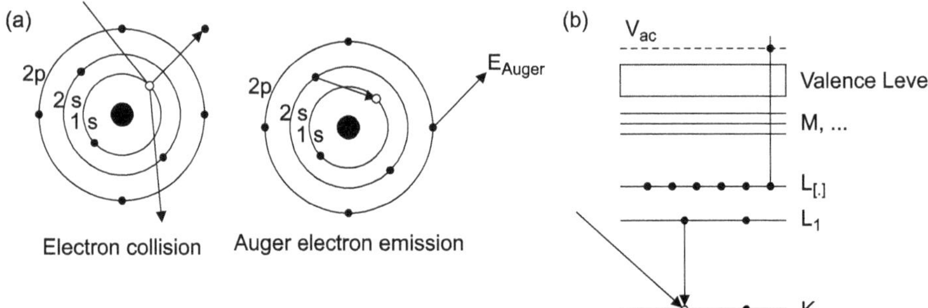

Figure 7.22: Two views of the Auger process. (a) illustrates sequentially the steps involved in Auger deexcitation. An incident electron creates a core hole in the 1s level. An electron from the 2s level fills in the 1s hole and the transition energy is imparted to a 2p electron that is emitted. The final atomic state thus has two holes, one in the 2s orbital and the other in the 2p orbital. (b) illustrates the same process using spectroscopic notation, $KL_1L_{2,3}$.

The types of state-to-state transitions available to electrons during an Auger event are dependent on several factors, ranging from initial excitation energy to relative interaction rates, yet are often dominated by a few characteristic transitions. Because of the interaction between an electron's spin and orbital angular momentum (spin-orbit coupling) and the concomitant energy level splitting for various shells in an atom, there are a variety of transition pathways for filling a core hole. Energy levels are labeled using a number of different schemes such as the j-j coupling method for heavy elements ($Z \geq 75$), the Russell-Saunders L-S method for lighter elements ($Z < 20$), and a combination of both for intermediate elements. The j-j coupling method, which is historically linked to X-ray notation, is almost always used to denote Auger transitions. Thus for a $KL_1L_{2,3}$ transition, K represents the core level hole, L_1 the relaxing electron's initial state, and $L_{2,3}$ the emitted electron's initial energy state. Figure 7.22(b) illustrates this transition with the corresponding spectroscopic notation. The energy level of the core hole will often determine which transition types will be favoured. For single energy levels, i.e. K, transitions can occur from the L levels, giving rise to strong KLL type peaks in an Auger spectrum. Higher level transitions can also occur, but are less probable. For multi-level shells, transitions are available from higher energy orbitals (different n, ℓ quantum numbers) or energy levels within the same shell (same$n$, different ℓ number). The results are transitions of the type LMM and KLL along with faster Coster–Kronig transitionssuch as LLM. While Coster–Kronig transitions are faster, they are also less energetic and thus harder to locate on an Auger spectrum. As the atomic number Z increases, so too does the number of potential Auger transitions. Fortunately, the strongest electron-electron interactions are between levels that are close together, giving rise to characteristic peaks in an Auger spectrum. KLL and LMM peaks are some of the most commonly identified transitions during surface analysis. Finally, valence band electrons can also fill core holes or be emitted during KVV-type transitions.

Several models, both phenomenological and analytical, have been developed to describe the energetics of Auger transitions. One of the most tractable descriptions, put forth by Jenkins and Chung, estimates the energy of Auger transition ABC as:

$$E_{ABC} = E_A(Z) - 0.5[E_B(Z) + E_B(Z+1)] - 0.5[E_C(Z) + E_C(Z+1)]\ E_i(Z)$$

are the binding energies of the ith level in element of atomic number Z and $E_i(Z+1)$ are the energies of the same levels in the next element up in the periodic table. While useful in practice, a more rigorous model accounting for effects such as screening and relaxation probabilities between energy levels gives the Auger energy as:

$$E_{ABC} = E_A - E_B - E_C - F(BC : x)] + R_{xin} + R_{xex}$$

where $F(BC : x)$ is the energy of interaction between the B and C level holes in a final atomic state x and the R's represent intra- and extra-atomic transition energies accounting for electronic screening. Auger electron energies can be calculated based on measured values of the various E_i and compared to peaks in the secondary electron spectrum in order to identify chemical species. This technique has been used to compile several reference databases used for analysis in current AES setups.

Experimental Setup and Quantification

Instrumentation

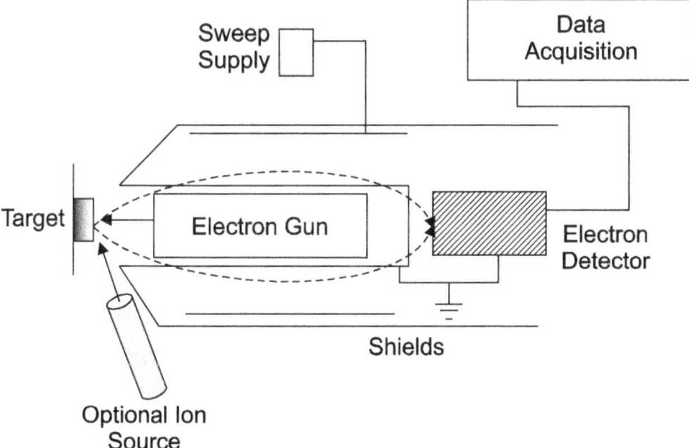

Figure 7.23: AES experimental setup using a cylindrical mirror analyzer (CMA). An electron beam is focused onto a specimen and emitted electrons are deflected around the electron gun and pass through an aperture towards the back of the CMA. These electrons are then directed into an electron multiplier for analysis. Varying voltage at the sweep supply allows derivative mode plotting of the Auger data. An optional ion gun can be integrated for depth profiling experiments.

Surface sensitivity in AES arises from the fact that emitted electrons usually have energies ranging from 50 eV to 3 keV and at these values, electrons have a short mean free path in a solid. The escape depth of electrons is therefore localized to within a few nanometers of the target surface, giving AES an extreme sensitivity to surface species. Because of the low energy of Auger electrons, most AES setups are run under ultra-high vacuum (UHV) conditions. Such measures prevent electron scattering off of residual gas atoms as well as the formation of a thin "gas (adsorbate) layer" on the surface of the specimen, which degrades analytical performance. A typical AES setup is shown schematically in figure 7.23. In this configuration, focused electrons are incident on a sample and emitted electrons are deflected into a cylindrical mirror analyzer (CMA). In the detection unit, Auger electrons are multiplied and the signal sent to data processing electronics. Collected Auger electrons are plotted as a function of energy against the broad secondary electron background spectrum.

Since the intensity of the Auger peaks may be small compared to the noise level of the background, AES is often run in a derivative mode that serves to highlight the peaks by modulating the electron collection current via a small applied AC voltage. Since this $\Delta V = k sin(\omega t)$, the collection current becomes $I(V + k\ sin(\omega t))$. Taylor expanding gives:

$$I(V + k\ \sin(wt)) \approx I_0 + I'(V + k\ \sin(\omega t)) + O(I'')$$

Using the setup in figure 7.23, detecting the signal at frequency ω will give a value

for I′ or $\frac{dN}{dE}$.

Plotting in derivative mode also emphasizes Auger fine structure, which appear as small secondary peaks surrounding the primary Auger peak. These secondary peaks, not to be confused with high energy satellites, which are discussed later, arise from the presence of the same element in multiple different chemical states on a surface (i.e. Adsorbate layers) or from relaxation transitions involving valence band electrons of the substrate. Figure 7.24 illustrates a derivative spectrum from a

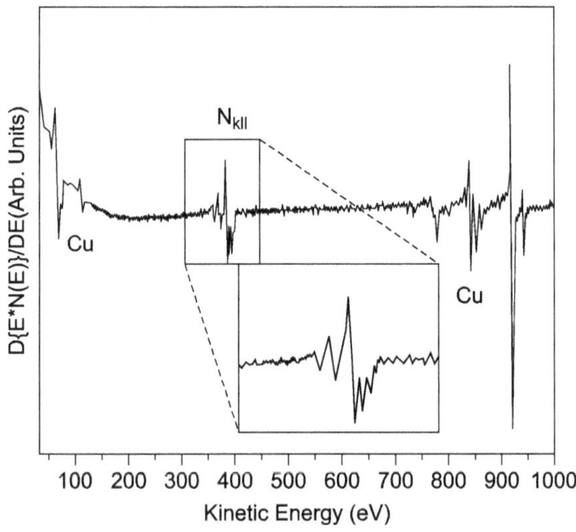

Figure 7.24: Auger spectrum of a copper nitride film in derivative mode plotted as a function of energy. Different peaks for Cu and N are apparent with the N KLL transition highlighted.

copper nitride film clearly showing the Auger peaks. The peak in derivative mode is not the true Auger peak, but rather the point of maximum slope of *N(E)*, but this concern is usually ignored.

Quantitative Analysis

Semi-quantitative compositional and element analysis of a sample using AES is dependent on measuring the yield of Auger electrons during a probing event. Electron yield, in turn, depends on several critical parameters such as electron-impact cross-section and fluorescence yield. Since the Auger effect is not the only mechanism available for atomic relaxation, there is a competition between radiative and non-radiative decay processes to be the primary de-excitation pathway. The total transition rate, ω, is a sum of the non-radiative (Auger) and radiative (photon emission) processes. The Auger yield, ω_A, is thus related to the fluorescence (x-ray) yield, ω_X, by the relation,

$$\omega_A = 1 - \omega_X = 1 - \frac{W_X}{W_X + W_A}$$

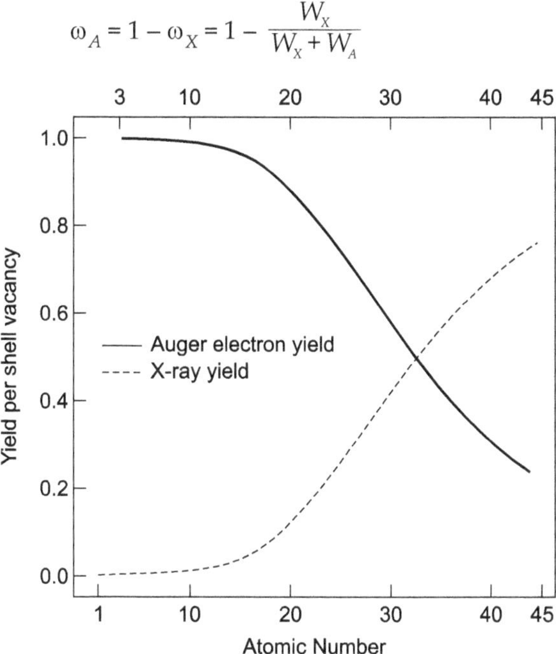

Figure 7.25: Fluorescence and Auger electron yields as a function of atomic number for K shell vacancies. Auger transitions (red curve) are more probable for lighter elements, while X-ray yield (dotted blue curve) becomes dominant at higher atomic numbers. Similar plots can be obtained for L and M shell transitions. Coster – Kronig (i.e. intra-shell) transitions are ignored in this analysis.

where W_X is the X-ray transition probability and W_A is the Auger transition probability. Attempts to relate the fluorescence and Auger yields to atomic number have resulted in plots similar to figure 7.25. A clear transition from electron to photon emission is evident in this chart for increasing atomic number. For heavier elements, x-ray yield becomes greater than Auger yield, indicating an increased difficulty in measuring the Auger peaks for large Z-values. Conversely, AES is sensitive to the lighter elements, and unlike X-ray fluorescence, Auger peaks can be detected for elements as light as lithium ($Z = 3$). Lithium represents the lower limit for AES sensitivity since the Auger effect is a "three state" event necessitating at least three electrons. Neither H nor He can be detected with this technique. For K-level based transitions, Auger effects are dominant for $Z < 15$ while for L- and M-level transitions, AES data can be measured for $Z \leq 50$. The yield limits effectively prescribe a cut off for AES sensitivity, but complex techniques can be utilized to identify heavier elements, such as uranium and americium, using the Auger effect.

Another critical quantity that determines yield of Auger electrons at a detector is the electron impact cross-section. Early approximations (in cm^2) of the cross-section were based on the work of Worthington and Tomlin,

$$\sigma_{az}(E) = 1.3 \times 10_{13} b \frac{C}{E_p}$$

with b acting as a scaling factor between 0.25 and 0.35, and C a function of the primary electron beam energy, E_P. While this value of σ_{ax} is calculated for an isolated atom, a simple modification can be made to account for matrix effects:

$$\sigma(E) = \sigma_{ax}[1 + r_m (E_p, \alpha)]$$

where α is the angle to the surface normal of the incident electron beam; r_m can be established empirically and encompasses electron interactions with the matrix such as ionization due to backscattered electrons. Thus the total yield can be written as:

$$Y(t) = N_x \times \delta t \times \sigma(E, t)[1 - w_X] \exp(-t\cos\frac{\theta}{\lambda}) \times \mathrm{I(t)} \times \mathrm{T} \times \frac{d(\Omega)}{4\pi}$$

Here N_x is the number of x atoms per volume, λ the electron escape depth, θ the analyzer angle, T the transmission of the analyzer, $I(t)$ the electron excitation flux at depth t, $d\Omega$ the solid angle, and δt is the thickness of the layer being probed. Encompassed in these terms, especially the Auger yield, which is related to the transition probability, is the quantum mechanical overlap of the initial and final state wave functions. Precise expressions for the transition probability, based on first-order perturbation Hamiltonians, can be found in Thompson and Baker. Often, all of these terms are not known, so most analyses compare measured yields with external standards of known composition. Ratios of the acquired data to standards can eliminate common terms, especially experimental setup characteristics and material parameters, and can be used to determine element composition. Comparison techniques work best for samples of homogeneous binary materials or uniform surface layers, while elemental identification is best obtained from comparison of pure samples.

Uses and Limitations

There are a number of electron microscopes that have been specifically designed for use in Auger spectroscopy; these are termed scanning Auger microscopes (SAM) and can produce high resolution, spatially resolved chemical images. SAM images are obtained by stepping a focused electron beam across a sample surface and measuring the intensity of the Auger peak above the background of scattered electrons. The intensity map is correlated to a gray scale on a monitor with whiter areas corresponding to higher element concentration. In addition, sputtering is sometimes used with Auger spectroscopy to perform depth profiling experiments. Sputtering removes thin outer layers of a surface so that AES can be used to determine the underlying composition. Depth profiles are shown as either Auger peak height vs. sputter time or atomic concentration vs. depth. Precise depth milling through sputtering has made profiling an invaluable technique for chemical analysis of nanostructured materials and thin films. AES is also used extensively as an evaluation tool on and off fab lines in the microelectronics industry, while the versatility and sensitivity of the Auger process makes it a standard analytical tool in research labs. Theoretically, Auger spectra can also be utilized to distinguish between protonation states. When a molecule is protonated or deprotonated, the geometry and electronic structure is changed, and AES spectra reflect this. In general, as a molecule becomes more protonated, the ionization potentials increase and the kinetic energy of the emitted outer shell electrons decreases.

Despite the advantages of high spatial resolution and precise chemical sensitivity attributed to AES, there are several factors that can limit the applicability of this technique, especially when evaluating solid specimens. One of the most common limitations encountered with Auger spectroscopy are charging effects in non-conducting samples. Charging results when the number of secondary electrons leaving the sample is different from the number of incident electrons, giving rise to a net positive or negative electric charge at the surface. Both positive and negative surface charges severely alter the yield of electrons emitted from the sample and hence distort the measured Auger peaks. To complicate matters, neutralization methods employed in other surface analysis techniques, such as secondary ion mass spectrometry (SIMS), are not applicable to AES, as these methods usually involve surface bombardment with either electrons or ions (i.e. flood gun). Several processes have been developed to combat the issue of charging, though none of them is ideal and still make quantification of AES data difficult. One such technique involves depositing conductive pads near the analysis area to minimize regional charging. However, this type of approach limits SAM applications as well as the amount of sample material available for probing. A related technique involves thinning or "dimpling" a non-conductive layer with Ar^+ ions and then mounting the sample to a conductive backing prior to AES. This method has been debated, with claims that the thinning process leaves elemental artifacts on a surface and/or creates damaged layers that distort bonding and promote chemical mixing in the sample. As a result, the compositional AES data is considered suspect. The most common setup to minimize charging effects includes use of a glancing angle (~10°) electron beam and a carefully tuned bombarding energy (between 1.5 keV and 3 keV). Control of both the angle and energy can subtly alter the number of emitted electrons vis-à-vis the incident electrons and thereby reduce or altogether eliminate sample charging.

In addition to charging effects, AES data can be obscured by the presence of characteristic energy losses in a sample and higher order atomic ionization events. Electrons ejected from a solid will generally undergo multiple scattering events and lose energy in the form of collective electron density oscillations called plasmons. If plasmon losses have energies near that of an Auger peak, the less intense Auger process may become dwarfed by the plasmon peak. As Auger spectra are normally weak and spread over many eV of energy, they are difficult to extract from the background and in the presence of plasmon losses; deconvolution of the two peaks becomes extremely difficult. For such spectra, additional analysis through chemical sensitive surface techniques like x-ray photoelectron spectroscopy (XPS) is often required to disentangle the peaks. Sometimes an Auger spectrum can also exhibit "satellite" peaks at well-defined off-set energies from the parent peak. Origin of the satellites is usually attributed to multiple ionization events in an atom or ionization cascades in which a series of electrons is emitted as relaxation occurs for core holes of multiple levels. The presence of satellites can distort the true Auger peak and/or small peak shift information due to chemical bonding at the surface. Several studies have been undertaken to further quantify satellite peaks.

Despite these sometimes substantial drawbacks, Auger electron spectroscopy is a widely used surface analysis technique that has been successfully applied to many diverse fields ranging from gas phase chemistry to nanostructure characterization. Very new class of high-resolving electrostatic energy analyzers recently developed – the face-field analyzers (FFA) can be used for remote electron spectroscopy of distant surfaces or surfaces with large roughness or even with deep dimples. These instruments are designed as if to be specifically used in combined scanning electron microscopes (SEMs). "FFA" in principle have no perceptible end-fields, which usually distort focusing in most of analysers known, for example, well known CMA.

Sensitivity, quantitative detail, and ease of use have brought AES from an obscure nuisance effect to a functional and practical characterization technique in just over fifty years. With applications both in the research laboratory and industrial settings, AES will continue to be a cornerstone of surface-sensitive electron-based spectroscopies.

3. SPECTROMETRY

Spectrometry May Refer to:

- Ion-mobility spectrometry, an analytical technique used to separate and identify ionized molecules in the gas phase based on their ion mobility in a carrier buffer gas
- Mass spectrometry, an analytical technique that measures the mass-to-charge ratio of charged particles
- Rutherford backscattering spectrometry, an analytical technique used to determine the structure and composition of materials by measuring the back-scattering of a beam of high energy ions impinging on a sample

- Neutron triple-axis spectrometry, a technique used in inelastic neutron scattering
- Optical spectrometry, a technique for measuring the distribution of light across the optical spectrum, from the UV spectral region to the visible and infrared
- Mass spectrometry (MS) is an analytical chemistry technique that helps identify the amount and type of chemicals present in a sample by measuring the mass-to-charge ratio and abundance of gas-phase ions
- A mass spectrum (plural *spectra*) is a plot of the ion signal as a function of the mass-to-charge ratio. The spectra are used to determine the elemental or isotopic signature of a sample, the masses of particles and of molecules, and to elucidate the chemical structures of molecules, such as peptides and other chemical compounds. Mass spectrometry works by ionizing chemical compounds to generate charged molecules or molecule fragments and measuring their mass-to-charge ratios
- In a typical MS procedure, a sample, which may be solid, liquid, or gas, is ionized, for example by bombarding it with electrons. This may cause some of the sample's molecules to break into charged fragments. These ions are then separated according to their mass-to-charge ratio, typically by accelerating them and subjecting them to an electric or magnetic field: ions of the same mass-to-charge ratio will undergo the same amount of deflection. The ions are detected by a mechanism capable of detecting charged particles, such as an electron multiplier. Results are displayed as spectra of the relative abundance of detected ions as a function of the mass-to-charge ratio. The atoms or molecules in the sample can be identified by correlating known masses to the identified masses or through a characteristic fragmentation pattern.

Creating Ions

The ion source is the part of the mass spectrometer that ionizes the material under analysis (the analyte). The ions are then transported by magnetic or electric fields to the mass analyzer.

Techniques for ionization have been key to determining what types of samples can be analyzed by mass spectrometry. Electron ionization and chemical ionization are used forgases and vapors. In chemical ionization sources, the analyte is ionized by chemical ion-molecule reactions during collisions in the source. Two techniques often used with liquidand solid biological samples include electrospray ionization (invented by John Fenn) and matrix-assisted laser desorption/ionization (MALDI, initially developed as a similar technique "Soft Laser Desorption (SLD)" by K. Tanaka for which a Nobel Prize was awarded and as MALDI by M. Karas and F. Hillenkamp.

Hard Ionization and Soft Ionization

In mass spectrometry (MS), ionization refers to the production of gas phase ions suitable for resolution in the mass analyser or mass filter. Ionization occurs in the instrument ion source. There are a plethora of ion sources available; each has advantages and disadvantages for particular applications. For example, electron ionization (EI) gives a high degree of fragmentation, yielding highly detailed mass spectra which when skilfully analysed can provide important information for structural elucidation/characterisation and facilitate identification of unknown compounds by comparison to mass spectral libraries obtained under identical operating conditions. However, EI is not suitable for coupling toHPLC, i.e. LC-MS, since at atmospheric pressure, the filaments used to generate electrons burn out rapidly. Thus EI is coupled predominantly with GC, i.e. GC-MS, where the entire system is under high vacuum.

Hard ionization techniques are processes which impart high quantities of residual energy in the subject molecule invoking large degrees of fragmentation (i.e. the systematic rupturing of bonds acts to remove the excess energy, restoring stability to the resulting ion). Resultant ions tend to have *m/z* lower than the molecular mass (other than in the case of proton transfer and not including isotope peaks). The most common example of hard ionization is electron ionization (EI).

Soft ionization refers to the processes which impart little residual energy onto the subject molecule and as such result in little fragmentation. Examples include fast atom bombardment (FAB), chemical ionization (CI), atmospheric-pressure chemical ionization (APCI), electrospray ionization (ESI), matrix-assisted laser desorption /ionization (MALDI).

Inductively Coupled Plasma

Inductively coupled plasma (ICP) sources are used primarily for cation analysis of a wide array of sample types. In this source, plasma that is electrically neutral overall, but that has had a substantial fraction of its atoms ionized by high temperature, is used to atomize introduced sample molecules and to further strip the outer electrons from those atoms. The plasma is usually generated from argon gas, since the first ionization energy of argon atoms is higher than the first of any other elements except He, O, F and Ne, but lower than the second ionization energy of all except the most electropositive metals. The heating is achieved by a radio-frequency current passed through a coil surrounding the plasma.

Other Ionization Techniques

Others include photoionization, glow discharge, field desorption (FD), fast atom bombardment (FAB), thermospray, desorption/ionization on silicon (DIOS), Direct Analysis in Real Time (DART), atmospheric pressure chemical ionization (APCI), secondary ion mass spectrometry (SIMS), spark ionization and thermal ionization (TIMS).

Mass Selection

Mass analyzers separate the ions according to their mass-to-charge ratio. The following two laws govern the dynamics of charged particles in electric and magnetic fields in vacuum:

$$F = Q(E + v \times B) \text{ (Lorentz force law);}$$

$$F = ma$$

(Newton's second law of motion in non-relativistic case, i.e. valid only at ion velocity much lower than the speed of light).

Here F is the force applied to the ion, m is the mass of the ion, a is the acceleration, Q is the ion charge, **E** is the electric field, and v × B is the vector cross product of the ion velocity and the magnetic field

Equating the above expressions for the force applied to the ion yields:

$$(m/Q)a = E + v \times B$$

This differential equation is the classic equation of motion for charged particles. Together with the particle's initial conditions, it completely determines the particle's motion in space and time in terms of m/Q. Thus mass spectrometers could be thought of as "mass-to-charge spectrometers". When presenting data, it is common to use the (officially)dimensionless m/z, where z is the number of elementary charges (e) on the ion (z=Q/e). This quantity, although it is informally called the mass-to-charge ratio, more accurately speaking represents the ratio of the mass number and the charge number, z.

There are many types of mass analyzers, using both static or dynamic fields, and magnetic or electric fields, but all operate according to the above differential equation. Each analyzer type has its strengths and weaknesses. Many mass spectrometers use two or more mass analyzers for tandem mass spectrometry (MS/MS). In addition to the more common mass analyzers listed below, there are others designed for special situations.

There are several important analyser characteristics. The mass resolving power is the measure of the ability to distinguish two peaks of slightly different m/z. The mass accuracy is the ratio of the m/z measurement error to the true m/z. Mass accuracy is usually measured in ppm or milli mass units. The mass range is the range of m/z amenable to analysis by a given analyzer. The linear dynamic range is the range over which ion signal is linear with analyte concentration. Speed refers to the time frame of the experiment and ultimately is used to determine the number of spectra per unit time that can be generated.

Sector Instruments

A sector field mass analyzer uses an electric and/or magnetic field to affect the path and/or velocity of the charged particles in some way. As shown above, sector instrumentsbend the trajectories of the ions as they pass through the mass analyzer, according to their mass-to-charge ratios, deflecting the more charged and faster-moving, lighter ions more. The analyzer can be used to select a narrow range of m/z or to scan through a range of m/z to catalog the ions present.

Time-of-Flight

The time-of-flight (TOF) analyzer uses an electric field to accelerate the ions through the same potential, and then measures the time they take to reach the detector. If the particles all have the same charge, the kinetic energies will be identical, and their velocities will depend only on their masses. Lighter ions will reach the detector first.

Quadrupole Mass Filter

Quadrupole mass analyzers use oscillating electrical fields to selectively stabilize or destabilize the paths of ions passing through a radio frequency (RF) quadrupole field created between 4 parallel rods. Only the ions in a certain range of mass/charge ratio are passed through the system at any time, but changes to the potentials on the rods allow a wide range of m/z values to be swept rapidly, either continuously or in a succession of discrete hops. A quadrupole mass analyzer acts as a mass-selective filter and is closely related to the quadrupole ion trap, particularly the linear quadrupole ion trap except that it is designed to pass the untrapped ions rather than collect the trapped ones, and is for that reason referred to as a transmission quadrupole. A common variation of the transmission quadrupole is the triple quadrupole mass spectrometer. The "triple quad" has three consecutive quadrupole stages, the first acting as a mass filter to transmit a particular incoming ion to the second quadrupole, a collision chamber, wherein that ion can be broken into fragments. The third quadrupole also acts as a mass filter, to transmit a particular fragment ion to the detector. If a quadrupole is made to rapidly and repetitively cycle through a range of mass filter settings, full spectra can be reported. Likewise, a triple quad can be made to perform various scan types characteristic of tandem mass spectrometry.

Ion Traps

Three-Dimensional Quadrupole ion Trap

The quadrupole ion trap works on the same physical principles as the quadrupole mass analyzer, but the ions are trapped and sequentially ejected. Ions are trapped in a mainly quadrupole RF field, in a space defined by a ring electrode (usually connected to the main RF potential) between two endcap electrodes (typically connected to DC or auxiliary AC potentials). The sample is ionized either internally (e.g. with an electron or laser beam), or externally, in which case the ions are often introduced through an aperture in an endcap electrode.

There are many mass/charge separation and isolation methods but the most commonly used is the mass instability mode in which the RF potential is ramped so that the orbit of ions with a mass $a > b$ are stable while ions with mass b become unstable and are ejected on the z-axis onto a detector. There are also non-destructive analysis methods.

Ions may also be ejected by the resonance excitation method, whereby a supplemental oscillatory excitation voltage is applied to the endcap electrodes, and the trapping voltage amplitude and/or excitation voltage frequency is varied to bring ions into a resonance condition in order of their mass/charge ratio. The cylindrical ion trap mass spectrometer is a derivative of the quadrupole ion trap mass spectrometer.

Linear Quadrupole ion Trap

A linear quadrupole ion trap is similar to a quadrupole ion trap, but it traps ions in a two dimensional quadrupole field, instead of a three-dimensional quadrupole field as in a 3D quadrupole ion trap. Thermo Fisher's LTQ ("linear trap quadrupole") is an example of the linear ion trap.

A toroidal ion trap can be visualized as a linear quadrupole curved around and connected at the ends or as a cross section of a 3D ion trap rotated on edge to form the toroid, donut shaped trap. The trap can store large volumes of ions by distributing them throughout the ring-like trap structure. This toroidal shaped trap is a configuration that allows the increased miniaturization of an ion trap mass analyzer. Additionally all ions are stored in the same trapping field and ejected together simplifying detection that can be complicated with array configurations due to variations in detector alignment and machining of the arrays.

Orbitrap

Orbitrap instruments are similar to Fourier transform ion cyclotron resonance mass spectrometers (see text below). Ions are electrostatically trapped in an orbit around a central, spindle shaped electrode. The electrode confines the ions so that they both orbit around the central electrode and oscillate back and forth along the central electrode's long axis. This oscillation generates an image current in the detector plates which is recorded by the instrument. The frequencies of these image currents depend on the mass to charge ratios of the ions. Mass spectra are obtained by Fourier transformation of the recorded image currents.

Orbitraps have a high mass accuracy, high sensitivity and a good dynamic range.

Fourier Transform ion Cyclotron Resonance

Fourier transform mass spectrometry (FTMS), or more precisely Fourier transform ion cyclotron resonance MS, measures mass by detecting the image current produced by ionscyclotroning in the presence of a magnetic field. Instead of measuring the deflection of ions with a detector such as an electron multiplier, the ions are injected into a Penning trap(a static electric/magnetic ion trap) where they effectively form part of a circuit. Detectors at fixed positions in space measure the electrical signal of ions which pass near them over time, producing a periodic signal. Since the frequency of an ion's cycling is determined by its mass to charge ratio, this can be deconvoluted by performing a Fourier transform on the signal. FTMS has the advantage of high sensitivity (since each ion is "counted" more than once) and much higher resolution and thus precision.

Ion cyclotron resonance (ICR) is an older mass analysis technique similar to FTMS except that ions are detected with a traditional detector. Ions trapped in a Penning trap are excited by an RF electric field until they impact the wall of the trap, where the detector is located. Ions of different mass are resolved according to impact time.

Detectors

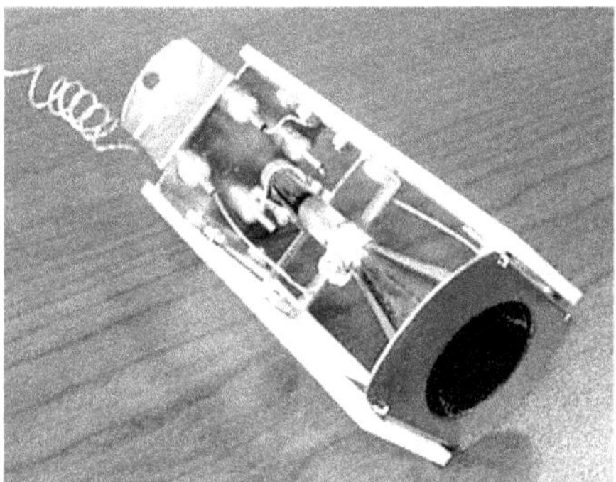

Figure 7.26: A continuous dynode particle multiplier detector.

The final element of the mass spectrometer is the detector. The detector records either the charge induced or the current produced when an ion passes by or hits a surface. In a scanning instrument, the signal produced in the detector during the course of the scan versus where the instrument is in the scan (at what m/Q) will produce a mass spectrum, a record of ions as a function of m/Q.

Typically, some type of electron multiplier is used, though other detectors including Faraday cups and ion-to-photon detectorsare also used. Because the number of ions leaving the mass analyzer at a particular instant is typically quite small, considerable amplification is often necessary to get a signal. Microchannel plate detectors are commonly used in modern commercial instruments. In FTMS and Orbitraps, the detector consists of a pair of metal surfaces within the mass analyzer/ion trap region which the ions only pass near as they oscillate. No direct current is produced, only a weak AC image current is produced in a circuit between the electrodes. Other inductive detectors have also been used.

Tandem Mass Spectrometry

A tandem mass spectrometer is one capable of multiple rounds of mass spectrometry, usually separated by some form of molecule fragmentation. For example, one mass analyzer can isolate one peptide from many entering a mass spectrometer. A second mass analyzer then stabilizes the peptide ions while they collide with a gas, causing them to fragment by collision-induced dissociation (CID). A third mass analyzer then sorts the fragments produced from the peptides. Tandem MS can also be done in a single mass analyzer over time, as in a quadrupole ion trap. There are various methods for fragmenting molecules for tandem MS, includingcollision-induced dissociation (CID), electron capture dissociation (ECD), electron transfer dissociation (ETD), infrared multiphoton dissociation (IRMPD), blackbody infrared radiative dissociation (BIRD), electron-detachment dissociation (EDD) and surface-induced dissociation (SID). An important application using tandem mass spectrometry is inprotein identification.

Tandem mass spectrometry enables a variety of experimental sequences. Many commercial mass spectrometers are designed to expedite the execution of such routine sequences as selected reaction monitoring (SRM) and precursor ion scanning. In SRM, the first analyzer allows only a single mass through and the second analyzer monitors for multiple user-defined fragment ions. SRM is most often used with scanning instruments where the second mass analysis event is duty cycle limited. These experiments are used to increase specificity of detection of known molecules, notably in pharmacokinetic studies. Precursor ion scanning refers to monitoring for a specific loss from the precursor ion. The first and second mass analyzers scan across the spectrum as partitioned by a user-defined *m/z* value. This experiment is used to detect specific motifs within unknown molecules.

Another type of tandem mass spectrometry used for radiocarbon dating is accelerator mass spectrometry (AMS), which uses very high voltages, usually in the mega-volt range, to accelerate negative ions into a type of tandem mass spectrometer.

Common Mass Spectrometer Configurations and Techniques

When a specific configuration of source, analyzer, and detector becomes conventional in practice, often a compound acronym arises to designate it, and the compound acronym may be better known among nonspectrometrists than the component acronyms. The epitome of this is MALDI-TOF, which simply refers to combining a matrix-assisted laser desorption/ionization source with a time-of-flight mass analyzer. The MALDI-TOF moniker is more widely recognized by the non-mass spectrometrists than MALDI or TOF individually. Other examples include inductively coupled plasma-mass spectrometry (ICP-MS), accelerator mass spectrometry (AMS), thermal ionization-mass spectrometry (TIMS) and spark source mass spectrometry (SSMS). Sometimes the use of the generic "MS" actually connotes a very specific mass analyzer and detection system, as is the case with AMS, which is always sector based.

Certain applications of mass spectrometry have developed monikers that although strictly speaking would seem to refer to a broad application, in practice have come instead to connote a specific or a limited number of instrument configurations. An example of this is isotope ratio mass spectrometry (IRMS), which refers in practice to the use of a limited number of sector based mass analyzers; this name is used to refer to both the application and the instrument used for the application.

Separation Techniques Combined with Mass Spectrometry

An important enhancement to the mass resolving and mass determining capabilities of mass spectrometry is using it in tandem with chromatographic and other separation techniques.

Gas Chromatography

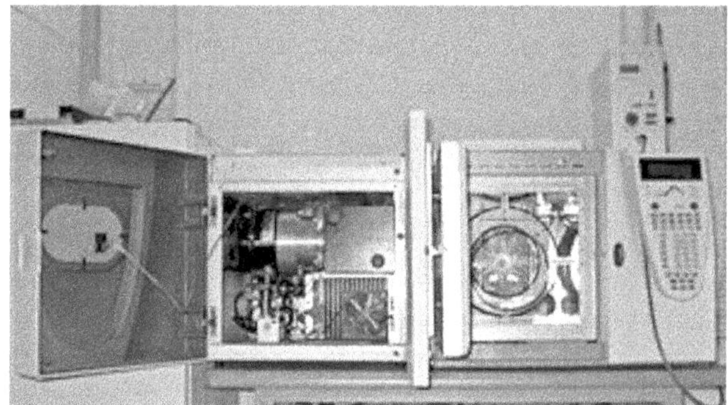

Figure 7.27: A gas chromatograph (right) directly coupled to a mass spectrometer (left)

A common combination is gas chromatography-mass spectrometry (GC/MS or GC-MS). In this technique, a gas chromatograph is used to separate different compounds. This stream of separated compounds is fed online into the ionsource, a metallic filament to which voltage is applied. This filament emits electrons which ionize the compounds. The ions can then further fragment, yielding predictable patterns. Intact ions and fragments pass into the mass spectrometer's analyzer and are eventually detected.

Liquid Chromatography

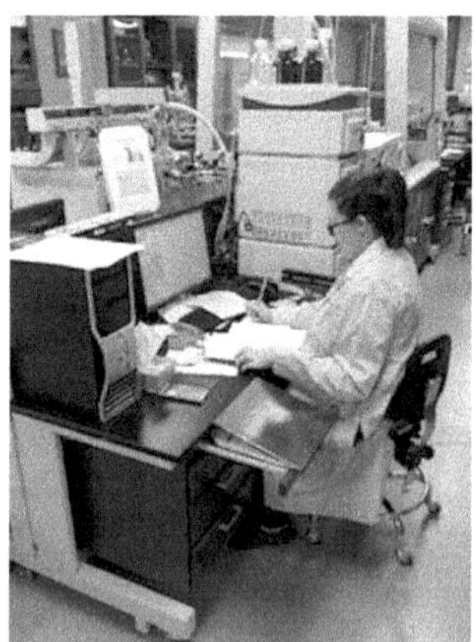

Figure 7.28: Indianapolis Museum of Art conservation scientist performing liquid chromatography mass spectrometry.

Similar to gas chromatography MS (GC/MS), liquid chromatography-mass spectrometry (LC/MS or LC-MS) separates compounds chromatographically before they are introduced to the ion source and mass spectrometer. It differs from GC/MS in that the mobile phase is liquid, usually a mixture of water and organic solvents, instead of gas. Most commonly, an electrospray ionization source is used in LC/MS. Other popular and commercially available LC/MS ion sources are atmospheric pressure chemical ionization and atmospheric pressure photoionization. There are also some newly developed ionization techniques like laser spray.

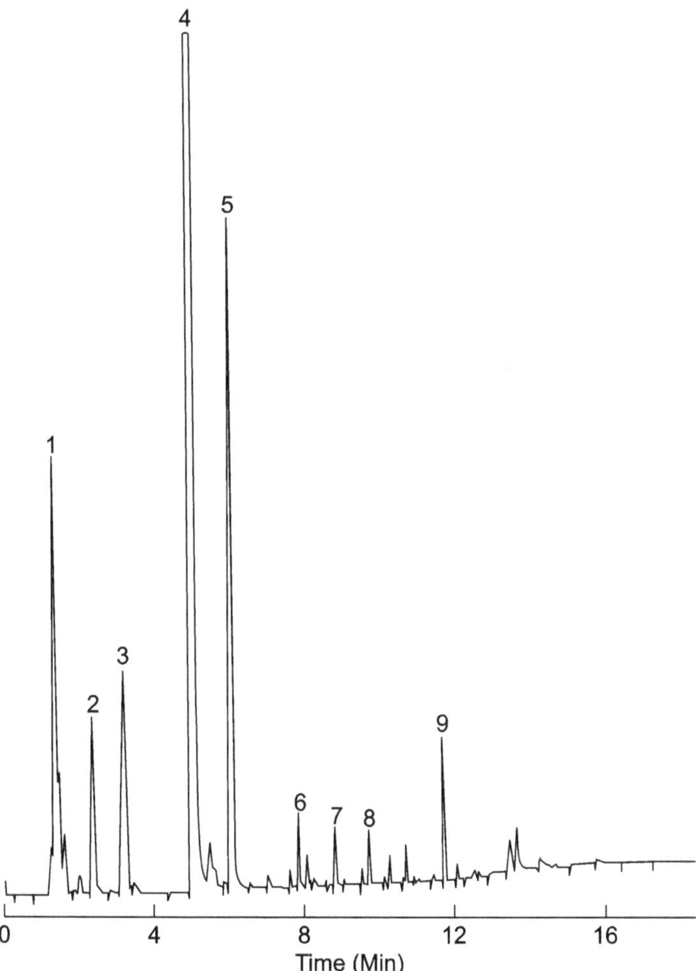

Figure 7.29: Gas chromatogram of the head space volatiles of beach pea seed meal, (1) acetaldehyde, (3) iso-butanol, (4) butanal, (6) hexanal, (8) trans-2-heptenal, (9) trans-2-octenal, (2, 5, 7) unknown.

Capillary Electrophoresis

Mass Spectrometry

Capillary electrophoresis mass spectrometry (CEMS) is a technique that combines the liquid separation process of capillary electrophoresis with mass spectrometry. CEMS is typically coupled to electrospray ionization.

Ion Mobility

Ion mobility spectrometry-mass spectrometry (IMS/MS or IMMS) is a technique where ions are first separated by drift time through some neutral gas under an applied electrical potential gradient before being introduced into a mass spectrometer. Drift time is a measure of the radius relative to the charge of the ion. The duty cycle of IMS (the time over which the experiment takes place) is longer than most mass spectrometric techniques, such that the mass spectrometer can sample along the course of the IMS separation. This produces data about the IMS separation and the mass-to-charge ratio of the ions in a manner similar to LC/MS. The duty cycle of IMS is short relative to liquid chromatography or gas chromatography separations and can thus be coupled to such techniques, producing triple modalities such as LC/IMS/MS.

Data and Analysis

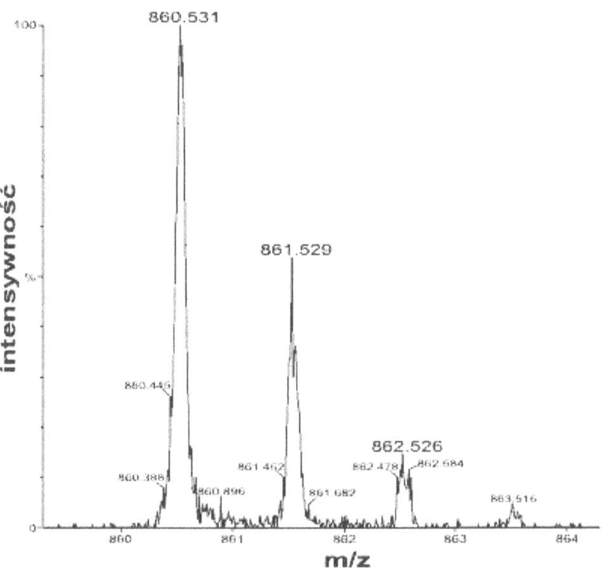

Figure 7.30: Mass spectrum of a peptide showing the isotopic distribution

Data Representations

1. Mass spectrometry produces various types of data. The most common data representation is the mass spectrum.

2. Certain types of mass spectrometry data are best represented as a mass chromatogram. Types of chromatograms include selected ion monitoring (SIM), total ion current (TIC), and selected reaction monitoring (SRM), among many others.
3. Other types of mass spectrometry data are well represented as a three-dimensional contour map. In this form, the mass-to-charge, m/z is on the x-axis, intensity the y-axis, and an additional experimental parameter, such as time, is recorded on the z-axis.

Data Analysis

1. Mass spectrometry data analysis is specific to the type of experiment producing the data. General subdivisions of data are fundamental to understanding any data.
2. Many mass spectrometers work in either negative ion mode or positive ion mode. It is very important to know whether the observed ions are negatively or positively charged. This is often important in determining the neutral mass but it also indicates something about the nature of the molecules.
3. Different types of ion source result in different arrays of fragments produced from the original molecules. An electron ionization source produces many fragments and mostly single-charged (1-) radicals (odd number of electrons), whereas an electrospray source usually produces non-radical quasimolecular ions that are frequently multiply charged. Tandem mass spectrometry purposely produces fragment ions post-source and can drastically change the sort of data achieved by an experiment.
4. Knowledge of the origin of a sample can provide insight into the component molecules of the sample and their fragmentations. A sample from a synthesis/manufacturing process will probably contain impurities chemically related to the target component. A crudely prepared biological sample will probably contain a certain amount of salt, which may form adduct with the analyte molecules in certain analyses.
5. Results can also depend heavily on sample preparation and how it was run/introduced. An important example is the issue of which matrix is used for MALDI spotting, since much of the energetics of the desorption/ionization event is controlled by the matrix rather than the laser power. Sometimes samples are spiked with sodium or another ion-carrying species to produce adducts rather than a protonated species.
6. Mass spectrometry can measure molar mass, molecular structure, and sample purity. Each of these questions requires a different experimental procedure; therefore, adequate definition of the experimental goal is a prerequisite for collecting the proper data and successfully interpreting it.

Interpretation of Mass Spectra

Since the precise structure or peptide sequence of a molecule is deciphered through the set of fragment masses, the interpretation of mass spectra requires combined use of various techniques. Usually the first strategy for identifying an unknown compound is to compare its experimental mass spectrum against a library of mass spectra. If no matches result from the search, then manual interpretation or software assisted interpretation of mass spectra must be performed. Computer simulation of ionization and fragmentation processes occurring in mass spectrometer is the primary tool for assigning structure or peptide sequence to a molecule. An *a priori* structural information is fragmented *in silico*and the resulting pattern is compared with observed spectrum. Such simulation is often supported by a fragmentation library that contains published patterns of known decomposition reactions. Software taking advantage of this idea has been developed for both small molecules and proteins.

Analysis of mass spectra can also be spectra with accurate mass. A mass-to-charge ratio value (*m*/*z*) with only integer precision can represent an immense number of theoretically possible ion structures; however, more precise mass figures significantly reduce the number of candidate molecular formulas. A computer algorithm called formula generator calculates all molecular formulas that theoretically fit a given mass with specified tolerance.

A recent technique for structure elucidation in mass spectrometry, called precursor ion fingerprinting, identifies individual pieces of structural information by conducting a search of the tandem spectra of the molecule under investigation against a library of the product-ion spectra of structurally characterized precursor ions.

Applications

Mass spectrometry has both qualitative and quantitative uses. These include identifying unknown compounds, determining the isotopic composition of elements in a molecule, and determining the structure of a compound by observing its fragmentation. Other uses include quantifying the amount of a compound in a sample or studying the fundamentals of gas phase ion chemistry (the chemistry of ions and neutrals in a vacuum). MS is now in very common use in analytical laboratories that study physical, chemical, or biological properties of a great variety of compounds.

As an analytical technique it possesses distinct advantages such as: Increased sensitivity over most other analytical techniques because the analyzer, as a mass-charge filter, reduces background interference, Excellent specificity from characteristic fragmentation patterns to identify unknowns or confirm the presence of suspected compounds, Information about molecular weight, Information about the isotopic abundance of elements, Temporally resolved chemical data.

A few of the disadvantages of the method is that often fails to distinguish between optical and geometrical isomers and the positions of substituent in *o*-, *m*- and *p*- positions in an aromatic ring. Also, its scope is limited in identifying hydrocarbons that produce similar fragmented ions.

Isotope Ratio MS: Isotope Dating and Tracing

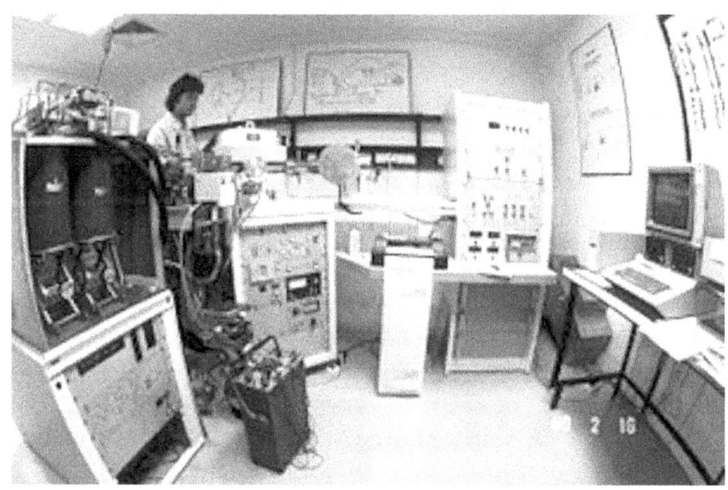

Mass spectrometer to determine the $^{16}O/^{18}O$ and $^{12}C/^{13}C$ isotope ratio on biogenous carbonate

Mass spectrometry is also used to determine the isotopic composition of elements within a sample. Differences in mass among isotopes of an element are very small, and the less abundant isotopes of an element are typically very rare, so a very sensitive instrument is required. These instruments, sometimes referred to as isotope ratio mass spectrometers (IR-MS), usually use a single magnet to bend a beam of ionized particles towards a series of Faraday cups which convert particle impacts to electric current. A fast on-line analysis of deuterium content of water can be done using Flowing afterglow mass spectrometry, FA-MS. Probably the most sensitive and accurate mass spectrometer for this purpose is the accelerator mass spectrometer (AMS). This is because it provides ultimate sensitivity, capable of measuring individual atoms and measuring nuclides with a dynamic range of $\sim10^{15}$ relative to the major stable isotope. Isotope ratios are important markers of a variety of processes. Some isotope ratios are used to determine the age of materials for example as in carbon dating. Labeling with stable isotopes is also used for protein quantification.

Trace Gas Analysis

Several techniques use ions created in a dedicated ion source injected into a flow tube or a drift tube: selected ion flow tube (SIFT-MS), and proton transfer reaction (PTR-MS), are variants of chemical ionization dedicated for trace gas analysis of air, breath or liquid headspace using well defined reaction time allowing calculations of analyte concentrations from the known reaction kinetics without the need for internal standard or calibration.

Atom Probe

An atom probe is an instrument that combines time-of-flight mass spectrometry and field ion microscopy (FIM) to map the location of individual atoms.

Pharmacokinetics

Pharmacokinetics is often studied using mass spectrometry because of the complex nature of the matrix (often blood or urine) and the need for high sensitivity to observe low dose and long-time point data. The most common instrumentation used in this application is LC-MS with a triple quadrupole mass spectrometer. Tandem mass spectrometry is usually employed for added specificity. Standard curves and internal standards are used for quantitation of usually a single pharmaceutical in the samples. The samples represent different time points as a pharmaceutical is administered and then metabolized or cleared from the body. Blank or t=0 samples taken before administration are important in determining background and ensuring data integrity with such complex sample matrices. Much attention is paid to the linearity of the standard curve; however it is not uncommon to use curve fitting with more complex functions such as quadratics since the response of most mass spectrometers is less than linear across large concentration ranges. There is currently considerable interest in the use of very high sensitivity mass spectrometry for microdosing studies, which are seen as a promising alternative to animal experimentation.

Protein Characterization

Mass spectrometry is an important method for the characterization and sequencing of proteins. The two primary methods for ionization of whole proteins are electrospray ionization (ESI) and matrix-assisted laser desorption/ ionization (MALDI). In keeping with the performance and mass range of available mass spectrometers, two approaches are used for characterizing proteins. In the first, intact proteins are ionized by either of the two techniques described above, and then introduced to a mass analyzer. This approach is referred to as "top-down" strategy of protein analysis. In the second, proteins are enzymatically digested into smaller peptides using proteases such as trypsin or pepsin, either insolution or in gel after electrophoretic separation. Other proteolytic agents are also used. The collection of peptide products are then introduced to the mass analyzer. When the characteristic pattern of peptides is used for the identification of the protein the method is called peptide mass fingerprinting (PMF), if the identification is performed using the sequence data determined in tandem MS analysis it is called de novo peptide sequencing. These procedures of protein analysis are also referred to as the "bottom-up" approach.

Glycan Analysis

Mass spectrometry (MS), with its low sample requirement and high sensitivity, has been predominantly used in glycobiology for characterization and elucidation of glycan structures. Mass spectrometry provides a complementary method to HPLC for the analysis of glycans. Intact glycans may be detected directly as singly charged ions bymatrix-assisted laser desorption/ionization mass spectrometry (MALDI-MS) or, following permethylation or peracetylation, by fast atom bombardment mass spectrometry (FAB-MS). Electrospray ionization mass spectrometry (ESI-MS) also gives good signals for the smaller glycans. Various free and commercial software are now available which interpret MS data and aid in Glycan structure characterization.

Space Exploration

As a standard method for analysis, mass spectrometers have reached other planets and moons. Two were taken to Mars by the Viking program. In early 2005 the Cassini–Huygens mission delivered a specialized GC-MS instrument aboard the Huygens probe through the atmosphere of Titan, the largest moon of the planet Saturn. This instrument analyzed atmospheric samples along its descent trajectory and was able to vaporize and analyze samples of Titan's frozen, hydrocarbon covered surface once the probe had landed. These measurements compare the abundance of isotope(s) of each particle comparatively to earth's natural abundance. Also on board the Cassini–Huygensspacecraft is an ion and neutral mass spectrometer which has been taking measurements of Titan's atmospheric composition as well as the composition of Enceladus' plumes. AThermal and Evolved Gas Analyzer mass spectrometer was carried by the Mars Phoenix Lander launched in 2007. Mass spectrometers are also widely used in space missions to measure the composition of plasmas. For example, the Cassini spacecraft carries the Cassini Plasma Spectrometer (CAPS), which measures the mass of ions in Saturn's magnetosphere.

Respired Gas Monitor

Mass spectrometers were used in hospitals for respiratory gas analysis beginning around 1975 through the end of the century. Some are probably still in use but none are currently being manufactured. Found mostly in the operating room, they were a part of a complex system, in which respired gas samples from patients undergoing anesthesia were drawn into the instrument through a valve mechanism designed to sequentially connect up to 32 rooms to the mass spectrometer. A computer directed all operations of the system. The data collected from the mass spectrometer was delivered to the individual rooms for the anesthesiologist to use.

The uniqueness of this magnetic sector mass spectrometer may have been the fact that a plane of detectors, each purposely positioned to collect all of the ion species expected to be in the samples, allowed the instrument to simultaneously report all of the gases respired by the patient. Although the mass range was limited to slightly over 120 u, fragmentation of some of the heavier molecules negated the need for a higher detection limit.

Preparative Mass Spectrometry

The primary function of mass spectrometry is as a tool for chemical analyses based on detection and quantification of ions according to their mass-to-charge ratio. However, mass spectrometry also shows promise for material synthesis. Ion soft landing is characterized by deposition of intact species on surfaces at low kinetic energies which precludes the fragmentation of the incident species. The soft landing technique was first reported in 1977 for the reaction of low energy sulfur containing ions on a lead surface.

Nuclear Magnetic Resonance Spectroscopy (NMR)

Nuclear magnetic resonance spectroscopy, most commonly known as NMR spectroscopy, is a research technique that exploits the magnetic properties of certain atomic nuclei. It determines the physical and chemical properties of atoms or the molecules in which they are contained. It relies on the phenomenon of nuclear magnetic resonance and can provide detailed information about the structure, dynamics, reaction state, and chemical environment of molecules. The intramolecular magnetic field around an atom in a molecule changes the resonance frequency, thus giving access to details of the electronic structure of a molecule.

Most frequently, NMR spectroscopy is used by chemists and biochemists to investigate the properties of organic molecules, although it is applicable to any kind of sample that contains nuclei possessing spin. Suitable samples range from small compounds analyzed with 1-dimensional proton or carbon-13 NMR spectroscopy to large proteins or nucleic acids using 3 or 4-dimensional techniques. The impact of NMR spectroscopy on the sciences has been substantial because of the range of information and the diversity of samples, including solutions and solids.

NMR spectra are unique, well-resolved, analytically tractable and often highly predictable for small molecules. Thus, in organic chemistry practice, NMR analysis is used to confirm the identity of a substance. Different functional groups are obviously distinguishable, and identical functional groups with differing neighbouring substituents still give distinguishable signals. NMR has largely replaced traditional wet chemistry tests such as colour reagents for identification. A disadvantage is that a relatively large amount, 2–50 mg, of a purified substance is required, although it may be recovered. Preferably, the sample should be dissolved in a solvent, because NMR analysis of solids requires a dedicated MAS machine and may not give equally well-resolved spectra. The timescale of NMR is relatively long, and thus it is not suitable for observing fast phenomena, producing only an averaged spectrum. Although large amounts of impurities do show on an NMR spectrum, better methods exist for detecting impurities, as NMR is inherently not very sensitive.

NMR spectrometers are relatively expensive; universities usually have them, but they are less common in private companies. Modern NMR spectrometers have a very strong, large and expensive liquid helium-cooled superconducting magnet, because resolution directly depends on magnetic field strength. Less expensive machines using permanent magnets and lower resolution are also available, which still give sufficient performance for certain application such as reaction monitoring and quick checking of samples. There are even bench top NMR spectrometers.

History

The Purcell group at Harvard University and the Bloch group at Stanford University independently developed NMR spectroscopy in the late 1940s and early 1950s. Dr. Edward Mills Purcell and Dr. Felix Bloch shared the 1952 Nobel Prize in Physics for their discoveries.

Basic NMR Techniques

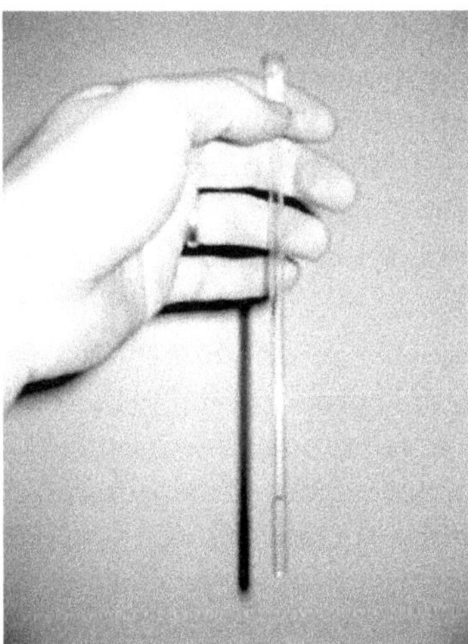

Figure 7.31: The NMR sample is prepared in a thin-walled glass tube - an NMR tube.

When placed in a magnetic field, NMR active nuclei (such as ^{1}H or ^{13}C) absorb electromagnetic radiation at a frequency characteristic of theisotope. The resonant frequency, energy of the absorption, and the intensity of the signal are proportional to the strength of the magnetic field. For example, in a 21 Tesla magnetic field, protons resonate at 900 MHz. It is common to refer to a 21 T magnet as a 900 MHz magnet, although different nuclei resonate at a different frequency at this field strength in proportion to their nuclear magnetic moments.

Acquisition of Spectra

Upon excitation of the sample with radio frequency pulse, a nuclear magnetic resonance response - a free induction decay (FID) - is obtained. It is a very weak signal, and requires sensitive radio receivers to pick up. A Fourier transform is done to extract the frequency-domain spectrum from the raw time-domain FID. A spectrum from a single FID has a low signal-to-noise ratio, but fortunately it improves readily with averaging of repeated acquisitions. Good ^{1}H NMR spectra can be acquired with 16 repeats, which takes only minutes. However, for heavier elements than hydrogen, the relaxation time is rather long, e.g. around 8 seconds for ^{13}C. Thus, acquisition of quantitative heavy-element spectra can be time-consuming, taking tens of minutes to hours. If the second excitation pulse is sent prematurely before the relaxation is complete, the average magnetization vector still points in a nonparallel direction, giving suboptimal absorption and emission of the pulse. In practice, the peak areas are then not proportional to the stoichiometry; only the presence, but not the amount of functional groups is possible to discern.

Chemical Shift

A spinning charge generates a magnetic field that results in a magnetic moment proportional to the spin. In the presence of an external magnetic field, two spin states exist (for a spin 1/2 nucleus): one spin up and one spin down, where one aligns with the magnetic field and the other oppose it. The difference in energy (ΔE) between the two spin states increases as the strength of the field increases, but this difference is usually very small, leading to the requirement for strong NMR magnets (1-20 T for modern NMR instruments). Irradiation of the sample with energy corresponding to the exact spin state separation of a specific set of nuclei will cause excitation of those set of nuclei in the lower energy state to the higher energy state.

For spin 1/2 nuclei, the energy difference between the two spin states at a given magnetic field strength is proportional to their magnetic moment. However, even if all protons have the same magnetic moments, they do not give resonant signals at the same frequency values. This difference arises from the differing electronic environments of the nucleus of interest. Upon application of an external magnetic field, these electrons move in response to the field and generate local magnetic fields that oppose the much stronger applied field. This local field thus "shields" the proton from the applied magnetic field, which must therefore be increased in order to achieve resonance (absorption of rf energy). Such increments are very small, usually in parts per million (ppm). For instance, the proton peak from an aldehyde is shifted ca. 10 ppm compared to a hydrocarbon peak, since as an electron-withdrawing group, the carbonyl deshields the proton by reducing the local electron density. The difference between 2.3487 T and 2.3488 T is therefore about 42 ppm. However a frequency scale is commonly used to designate the NMR signals, even though the spectrometer may operate by sweeping the magnetic field, and thus the 42 ppm is 4200 Hz for a 100 MHz reference frequency (rf).

However given that the location of different NMR signals is dependent on the external magnetic field strength and the reference frequency, the signals are usually reported relative to a reference signal, usually that of TMS (tetramethylsilane). Additionally, since the distribution of NMR signals is field dependent, these frequencies are divided by the spectrometer frequency. However since we are dividing Hz by MHz, the resulting number would be too small, and thus it is multiplied by a million. This operation therefore gives a locator number called the "chemical shift" with units of parts per million.[3] To detect such small frequency differences the applied magnetic field must be constant throughout the sample volume. High resolution NMR spectrometers use shims to adjust the homogeneity of the magnetic field to parts per billion (ppb) in a volume of a few cubic centimeters. In general, chemical shifts for protons are highly predictable since the shifts are primarily determined by simpler shielding effects (electron density), but the chemical shifts for many heavier nuclei are more strongly influenced by other factors including excited states ("paramagnetic" contribution to shielding tensor).

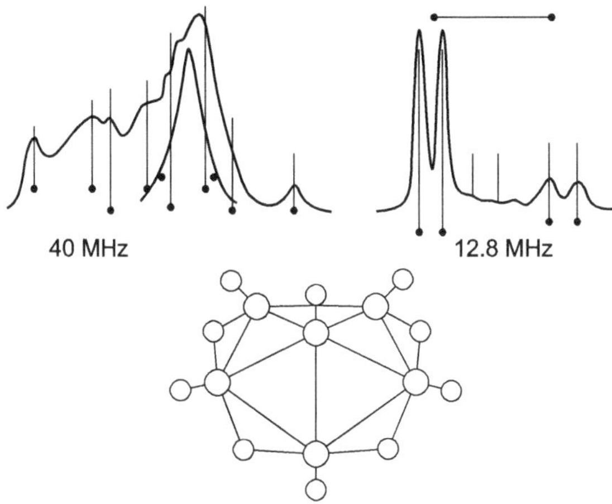

Example of the chemical shift: NMR spectrum of hexaborane B_6H_{10}showing peaks shifted in frequency, which give clues as to the molecular structure.

The chemical shift provides information about the structure of the molecule. The conversion of the raw data to this information is called assigning the spectrum. For example, for the ^{1}H-NMR spectrum for ethanol (CH_3CH_2OH), one would expect signals at each of three specific chemical shifts: one for the CH_3 group, one for the CH_2 group and one for the *OH* group. A typical CH_3 group has a shift around 1 ppm, a CH_2 attached to an OH has a shift of around 4 ppm and an OH has a shift anywhere from 2–6 ppm depending on the solvent used and the amount of hydrogen bonding. While the O atom does draw electron density away from the attached H through their mutual sigma bond, the electron lone pairs on the O bathe the H in their shielding effect.

In Paramagnetic NMR spectroscopy, measurements are conducted on paramagnetic samples. The paramagnetism gives rise to very diverse chemical shifts. In 1H NMR spectroscopy, the chemical shift range can span 500 ppm.

Because of molecular motion at room temperature, the three methyl protons *average out* during the NMR experiment (which typically requires a few ms). These protons become degenerate and form a peak at the same chemical shift.

The shape and area of peaks are indicators of chemical structure too. In the example above the proton spectrum of ethanol—the CH_3peak has three times the area as the OH peak. Similarly the CH_2 peak would be twice the area of the OH peak but only 2/3 the area of the CH_3 peak.

Software allows analysis of signal intensity of peaks, which under conditions of optimal relaxation, correlate with the number of protons of that type. Analysis of signal intensity is done by integration the mathematical process that calculates the area under a curve. The analyst must integrate the peak and not measure its height because the peaks also have width—and thus its size is dependent on its area not its height. However, it should be mentioned that the number of protons, or any other observed nucleus, is only proportional to the intensity, or the integral, of the NMR signal in the very simplest one-dimensional NMR experiments. In more elaborate experiments, for instance, experiments typically used to obtain carbon-13 NMR spectra; the integral of the signals depends on the relaxation rate of the nucleus, and its scalar and dipolar coupling constants. Very often these factors are poorly known - therefore, the integral of the NMR signal is very difficult to interpret in more complicated NMR experiments.

J-Coupling

Multiplicity	**Intensity Ratio**
Singlet (s)	1
Doublet (d)	1:1
Triplet (t)	1:2:1
Quartet (q)	1:3:3:1
Quintet	1:4:6:4:1
Sextet	1:5:10:10:5:1
Septet	1:6:15:20:15:6:1

Ethanol

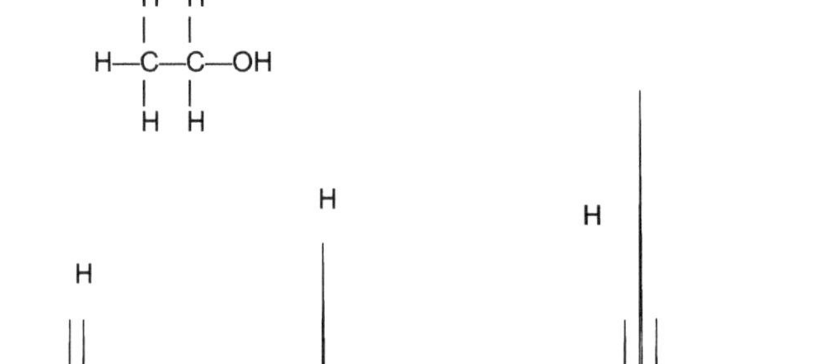

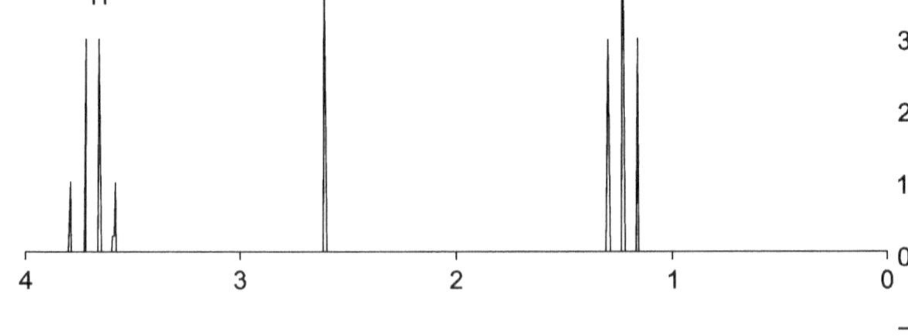

Example ^{1}H NMR spectrum (1-dimensional) of ethanol plotted as signal intensity vs. chemical shift. There are three different types of H atoms in ethanol regarding NMR. The hydrogen (H) on the -OH group is not coupling with the other H atoms and appears as a singlet, but the CH_3- and the -CH_2- hydrogens are coupling with each other, resulting in a triplet and quartet respectively.

Some of the most useful information for structure determination in a one-dimensional NMR spectrum comes from J-coupling or scalar coupling (a special case of spin-spin coupling) between NMR active nuclei. This coupling arises from the interaction of different spin states through the chemical bonds of a molecule and results in the splitting of NMR signals. These splitting patterns can be complex or simple and, likewise, can be straightforwardly interpretable or deceptive. This coupling provides detailed insight into the connectivity of atoms in a molecule.

Coupling to n equivalent (spin ½) nuclei splits the signal into a n+1 multiplet with intensity ratios following Pascal's triangle as described on the right. Coupling to additional spins will lead to further splittings of each component of the multiplet e.g. coupling to two different spin ½ nuclei with significantly different coupling constants will lead to a doublet of doublets (abbreviation: dd). Note that coupling between nuclei that are chemically equivalent (that is, have the same chemical shift) has no effect on the NMR spectra and couplings between nuclei that are distant (usually more than 3 bonds apart for protons in flexible molecules) are usually too small to cause observable splittings. Long-range couplings over more than three bonds can often be observed in cyclic and aromatic compounds, leading to more complex splitting patterns.

For example, in the proton spectrum for ethanol described above, the CH_3 group is split into a triplet with an intensity ratio of 1:2:1 by the two neighboring CH_2 protons. Similarly, the CH_2 is split into aquartet with an intensity ratio of 1:3:3:1 by the three neighboring CH_3 protons. In principle, the two CH_2 protons would also be split again into a doublet to form a doublet of quartets by the hydroxyl proton, but intermolecular exchange of the acidic hydroxyl proton often results in a loss of coupling information.

Coupling to any spin ½ nuclei such as phosphorus-31 or fluorine-19 works in this fashion (although the magnitudes of the coupling constants may be very different). But the splitting patterns differ from those described above for nuclei with spin greater than ½ because the spin quantum number has more than two possible values. For instance, coupling to deuterium (a spin 1 nucleus) splits the signal into a 1:1:1 triplet because the spin 1 has three spin states. Similarly, a spin 3/2 nucleus splits a signal into a 1:1:1:1 quartet and so on.

Coupling combined with the chemical shift (and the integration for protons) tells us not only about the chemical environment of the nuclei, but also the number of *neighboring* NMR active nuclei within the molecule. In more complex spectra with multiple peaks at similar chemical shifts or in spectra of nuclei other than hydrogen, coupling is often the only way to distinguish different nuclei.

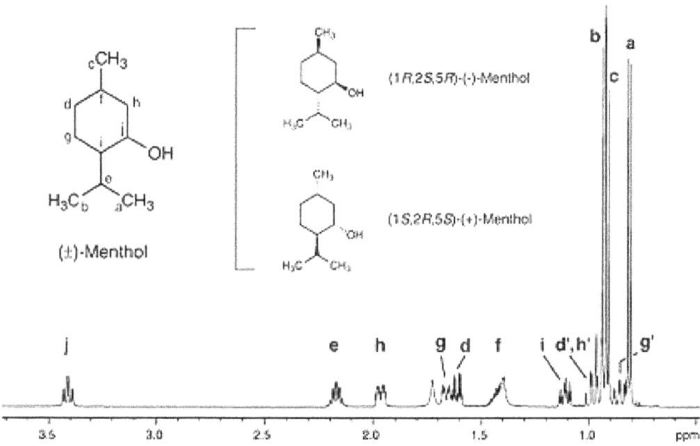

^{1}H NMR spectrum of menthol with chemical shift in ppm on the horizontal axis. Each magnetically inequivalent proton has a characteristic shift, and couplings to other protons appear as splitting of the peaks into multiplets: e.g. peak *a*, due to the three magnetically equivalent protons in methyl group *a*, couple to one adjacent proton (*e*) and thus appears as a doublet.

Second-Order (Or Strong) Coupling

The above description assumes that the coupling constant is small in comparison with the difference in NMR frequencies between the inequivalent spins. If the shift separation decreases (or the coupling strength increases), the multiplet intensity patterns are first distorted, and then become more complex and less easily analyzed (especially if more than two spins are involved). Intensification of some peaks in a multiplet is achieved at the expense of the remainder, which sometimes almost disappear in the background noise, although the integrated area under the peaks remains constant. In most high-field NMR, however, the distortions are usually modest and the characteristic distortions (roofing) can in fact help to identify related peaks.

Some of these patterns can be analyzed with the method published by John Pople, though it has limited scope.

Second-order effects decrease as the frequency difference between multiplets increases, so that high-field (i.e. high-frequency) NMR spectra display less distortion than lower frequency spectra. Early spectra at 60 MHz were more prone to distortion than spectra from later machines typically operating at frequencies at 200 MHz or above.

Magnetic Inequivalence

More subtle effects can occur if chemically equivalent spins (i.e., nuclei related by symmetry and so having the same NMR frequency) have different coupling relationships to external spins. Spins that are chemically equivalent but are not indistinguishable (based on their coupling relationships) are termed magnetically inequivalent. For example, the 4 H sites of 1,2-dichlorobenzene divide into two chemically equivalent pairs by symmetry, but an individual member of one of the pairs has different couplings to the spins making up the other pair. Magnetic inequivalence can lead to highly complex spectra which can only be analyzed by computational modeling. Such effects are more common in NMR spectra of aromatic and other non-flexible systems, while conformational averaging about C-C bonds in flexible molecules tends to equalize the couplings between protons on adjacent carbons, reducing problems with magnetic inequivalence.

Deuterated Solvents

The vast majority of nuclei in a solution would belong to the solvent, and most regular solvents are hydrocarbons and would contain NMR-reactive protons. Thus, deuterium (hydrogen-2) is substituted (99+%). The most used deuterated solvent is deuterochloroform ($CDCl_3$), although deuterium oxide (D_2O) and deuterated DMSO (DMSO-d_6) are used for hydrophilic analytes. NMR spectra are often calibrated against the known solvent residual proton peak instead of added tetramethylsilane.

Correlation Spectroscopy

Correlation spectroscopy is one of several types of two-dimensional nuclear magnetic resonance (NMR) spectroscopy or 2D-NMR. This type of NMR experiment is best known by its acronym, COSY. Other types of two-dimensional NMR include J-spectroscopy, exchange spectroscopy (EXSY), Nuclear Overhauser effect spectroscopy (NOESY), total correlation spectroscopy (TOCSY) and heteronuclear correlation experiments, such as HSQC, HMQC, and HMBC. Two-dimensional NMR spectra provide more information about a molecule than one-dimensional NMR spectra and are especially useful in determining the structure of a molecule, particularly for molecules that are too complicated to work with using one-dimensional NMR. The first two-dimensional experiment, COSY, was proposed by Jean Jeener, a professor at Université Libre de Bruxelles, in 1971. This experiment was later implemented by Walter P. Aue, Enrico Bartholdi and Richard R. Ernst, who published their work in 1976.

Solid-State Nuclear Magnetic Resonance

A variety of physical circumstances do not allow molecules to be studied in solution, and at the same time not by other spectroscopic techniques to an atomic level, either. In solid-phase media, such as crystals, microcrystalline powders, gels, anisotropic solutions, etc., it is in particular the dipolar coupling and chemical shift anisotropy that become dominant to the behaviour of the nuclear spin systems. In conventional solution-state NMR spectroscopy, these additional interactions would lead to a significant broadening of spectral lines. A variety of techniques allows establishing high-resolution conditions, that can, at least for ^{13}C spectra, be comparable to solution-state NMR spectra.

Two important concepts for high-resolution solid-state NMR spectroscopy are the limitation of possible molecular orientation by sample orientation, and the reduction of anisotropic nuclear magnetic interactions by sample spinning. Of the latter approach, fast spinning around the magic angle is a very prominent method, when the system comprises spin 1/2 nuclei. A number of intermediate techniques, with samples of partial alignment or reduced mobility, are currently being used in NMR spectroscopy.

Applications in which solid-state NMR effects occur are often related to structure investigations on membrane proteins, protein fibrils or all kinds of polymers, and chemical analysis in inorganic chemistry, but also include "exotic" applications like the plant leaves and fuel cells.

Bimolecular NMR Spectroscopy

Proteins

Much of the innovation within NMR spectroscopy has been within the field of protein NMR spectroscopy, an important technique in structural biology. A common goal of these investigations is to obtain high resolution 3-dimensional structures of the protein, similar to what can be achieved by X-ray crystallography. In contrast to X-ray crystallography, NMR spectroscopy is usually limited to proteins smaller than 35 kDa, although larger structures have been solved. NMR spectroscopy is often the only way to obtain high resolution information on partially or wholly intrinsically unstructured proteins. It is now a common tool for the determination of Conformation Activity Relationships where the structure before and after interaction with, for example, a drug candidate is compared to its known biochemical activity. Proteins are orders of magnitude larger than the small organic molecules discussed earlier in this article, but the basic NMR techniques and some NMR theory also applies. Because of the much higher number of atoms present in a protein molecule in comparison with a small organic compound, the basic 1D spectra become crowded with overlapping signals to an extent where direct spectra analysis becomes untenable. Therefore, multidimensional (2, 3 or 4D) experiments have been devised to deal with this problem. To facilitate these experiments, it is desirable toisotopically label the protein with ^{13}C and ^{15}N because the predominant naturally occurring isotope ^{12}C is not NMR-active, whereas the nuclear quadrupole moment of the predominant naturally occurring ^{14}N isotope prevents high resolution information to be obtained from this nitrogen isotope. The most important method used for structure determination of proteins utilizes NOE experiments to measure distances between pairs of atoms within the molecule. Subsequently, the obtained distances are used to generate a 3D structure of the molecule by solving a distance geometry problem. NMR can also be used to obtain information on the dynamics and conformational flexibility of different regions of a protein.

Nucleic Acids

"Nucleic acid NMR" is the use of NMR spectroscopy to obtain information about the structure and dynamics of polynucleic acids, such as DNA or RNA. As of 2003, nearly half of all known RNA structures had been determined by NMR spectroscopy.

Nucleic acid and protein NMR spectroscopy are similar but differences exist. Nucleic acids have a smaller percentage of hydrogen atoms, which are the atoms usually observed in NMR spectroscopy, and because nucleic acid double helices are stiff and roughly linear, they do not fold back on themselves to give "long-range" correlations. The types of NMR usually done with nucleic acids are ^{1}H or proton NMR, ^{13}C NMR, ^{15}N NMR, and ^{31}P NMR. Two-dimensional NMR methods are almost always used, such as correlation spectroscopy (COSY) and total coherence transfer spectroscopy (TOCSY) to detect through-bond nuclear couplings, and nuclear Overhauser effect spectroscopy (NOESY) to detect couplings between nuclei that are close to each other in space.

Parameters taken from the spectrum, mainly NOESY cross-peaks and coupling constants, can be used to determine local structural features such as glycosidic bond angles, dihedral angles (using the Karplus equation), and sugar pucker conformations. For large-scale structure, these local parameters must be supplemented with other structural assumptions or models, because errors add up as the double helix is traversed, and unlike with proteins, the double helix does not have a compact interior and does not fold back upon itself. NMR is also useful for investigating nonstandard geometries such as bent helices, non-Watson–Crick base pairing, and coaxial stacking. It has been especially useful in probing the structure of natural RNA oligonucleotides, which tend to adopt complex conformations such as stem-loops and pseudo knots. NMR is also useful for probing the binding of nucleic acid molecules to other molecules, such as proteins or drugs, by seeing which resonances are shifted upon binding of the other molecule.

Carbohydrates

Carbohydrate NMR spectroscopy addresses questions on the structure and conformation of carbohydrates.

CHAPTER 8

Chromatography

1. CHROMATOGRAPHY

Principles and Applications

Chromatography is the collective term for a set of laboratory techniques for the separation of mixtures. The mixture is dissolved in a fluid called the *mobile* phase, which carries it through a structure holding another material called the stationary phase. The various constituents of the mixture travel at different speeds, causing them to separate. The separation is based on differential partitioning between the mobile and stationary phases. Subtle differences in a compound's partition coefficient result in differential retention on the stationary phase and thus changing the separation.

Chromatography may be preparative or analytical. The purpose of preparative chromatography is to separate the components of a mixture for more advanced use (and is thus a form of purification). Analytical chromatography is done normally with smaller amounts of material and is for measuring the relative proportions of analytes in a mixture. The two are not mutually exclusive.

History

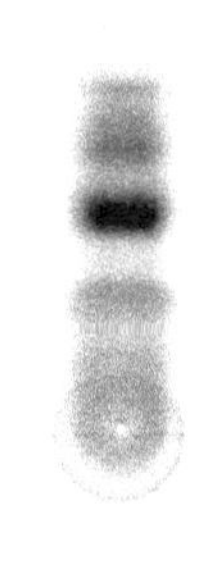

Thin layer chromatography is used to separate components of a plant extract, illustrating the experiment with plant pigments that gave chromatography its name.

Chromatography was first employed in Russia by the Italian-born scientist Mikhail Tsvet in 1900. He continued to work with chromatography in the first decade of the 20th century, primarily for the separation of plant pigments such as chlorophyll, carotenes, and xanthophylls. Since these components have different colours (green, orange, and yellow, respectively) they gave the technique its name. New types of chromatography developed during the 1930s and 1940s made the technique useful for many separation processes.

Chromatography technique developed substantially as a result of the work of Archer John Porter Martin and Richard Laurence Millington Synge during the 1940s and 1950s. They established the principles and basic techniques of partition chromatography, and their work encouraged the rapid development of several chromatographic methods: paper chromatography, gas chromatography, and what would become known as high performance liquid chromatography. Since then, the technology has advanced rapidly. Researchers found that the main principles of Tsvet's chromatography could be applied in many different ways, resulting in the different varieties of chromatography described below. Advances are continually improving the technical performance of chromatography, allowing the separation of increasingly similar molecules.

Chromatography Terms

- The analyte is the substance to be separated during chromatography. It is also normally what is needed from the mixture.
- Analytical chromatography is used to determine the existence and possibly also the concentration of analyte(s) in a sample.
- A bonded phase is a stationary phase that is covalently bonded to the support particles or to the inside wall of the column tubing.
- A chromatogram is the visual output of the chromatograph. In the case of an optimal separation, different peaks or patterns on the chromatogram correspond to different components of the separated mixture.

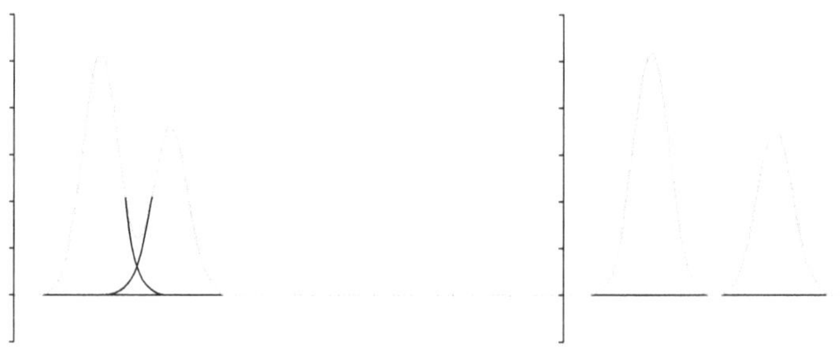

Plotted on the x-axis is the retention time and plotted on the y-axis a signal (for example obtained by a spectrophotometer, mass spectrometer or a variety of other detectors) corresponding to the response created by the analytes exiting the system. In the case of an optimal system the signal is proportional to the concentration of the specific analyte separated.

- A chromatograph is equipment that enables a sophisticated separation, e.g. gas chromatographic or liquid chromatographic separation.
- Chromatography is a physical method of separation that distributes components to separate between two phases, one stationary (stationary phase), the other (the mobile phase) moving in a definite direction.
- The eluate is the mobile phase leaving the column.
- The eluent is the solvent that carries the analyte.
- An eluotropic series is a list of solvents ranked according to their eluting power.
- An immobilized phase is a stationary phase that is immobilized on the support particles, or on the inner wall of the column tubing.

- The mobile phase is the phase that moves in a definite direction. It may be a liquid (LC and Capillary Electrochromatography (CEC)), a gas (GC), or a supercritical fluid (supercritical-fluid chromatography, SFC). The mobile phase consists of the sample being separated/analyzed and the solvent that moves the sample through the column. In the case of HPLC the mobile phase consists of a non-polar solvent(s) such as hexane in normal phase or polar solvents in reverse phase chromatography and the sample being separated. The mobile phase moves through the chromatography column (the stationary phase) where the sample interacts with the stationary phase and is separated.
- Preparative chromatography is used to purify sufficient quantities of a substance for further use, rather than analysis.
- The retention time is the characteristic time it takes for a particular analyte to pass through the system (from the column inlet to the detector) under set conditions.
- The sample is the matter analyzed in chromatography. It may consist of a single component or it may be a mixture of components. When the sample is treated in the course of an analysis, the phase or the phases containing the analytes of interest is/are referred to as the sample whereas everything out of interest separated from the sample before or in the course of the analysis is referred to as waste.
- The solute refers to the sample components in partition chromatography.
- The solvent refers to any substance capable of solubilizing another substance, and especially the liquid mobile phase in liquid chromatography.
- The stationary phase is the substance fixed in place for the chromatography procedure. Examples include the silica layer in thin layer chromatography
- The detector refers to the instrument used for qualitative and quantitative detection of analytes after separation.

Chromatography is based on the concept of partition coefficient. Any solute partitions between two immiscible solvents. When we make one solvent immobile (by adsorption on a solid support matrix) and another mobile it results in most common applications of chromatography. If matrix support is polar (e.g. paper, silica etc.) it is forward phase chromatography, and if it is non-polar (C-18) it is reverse phase.

Techniques by Chromatographic Bed Shape

Column Chromatography

Column chromatography is a separation technique in which the stationary bed is within a tube. The particles of the solid stationary phase or the support coated with a liquid stationary phase may fill the whole inside volume of the tube (packed column) or be concentrated on or along the inside tube wall leaving an open, unrestricted path for the mobile phase in the middle part of the tube (open tubular column). Differences in rates of movement through the medium are calculated to different retention times of the sample.

In 1978, W. Clark Still introduced a modified version of column chromatography called flash column chromatography (flash). The technique is very similar to the traditional column chromatography, except for that the solvent is driven through the column by applying positive pressure. This allowed most separations to be performed in less than 20 minutes, with improved separations compared to the old method. Modern flash chromatography systems are sold as pre-packed plastic cartridges, and the solvent is pumped through the cartridge. Systems may also be linked with detectors and fraction collectors providing automation. The introduction of gradient pumps resulted in quicker separations and less solvent usage.

In expanded bed adsorption, a fluidized bed is used, rather than a solid phase made by a packed bed. This allows omission of initial clearing steps such as centrifugation and filtration, for culture broths or slurries of broken cells.

Phosphocellulose chromatography utilizes the binding affinity of many DNA-binding proteins for phosphocellulose. The stronger a protein's interaction with DNA, the higher the salt concentration needed to elute that protein.

Use of Adsorption Chromatography for Separation of Pigments

- Separation of compounds by column chromatography must be one of the most widely used techniques in biochemical work.
- Separation of compounds/substances is based on the differences in adsorption coefficients. A mixture of compounds can be separated by distribution between two phases one of which is stationary and other is mobile, the first ma)' be solid or liquid and the second may be liquid or gas.
- The substances to be separated are distributed between the stationary phase and the mobile phase. Different substances are distributed differently and are thereby separated from one another.
- The principal application of chromatography is in the separation of mixtures of compounds for analytical or preparative purposes. This process can also serve in the identification, isolation, purification and quantitation of individual compounds.
- This technique may be used for determination of homogeneity of the chemical substances, determination of molecular structure, determination of reaction products, enzyme substrate specificity's and monitoring of chemical and biochemical products and processes.

Following compounds separated from the mixture of compounds by chromatography techniques.

• Anthocyanins	• Lycopene
• Flavonoids	• Neoxanthin
• Proanthocyanidins	• Zeaxanthin
• Tannins	• Capsanthin
• Betalains	• Begin
• Quinones	• Asthaxanthin
• Xanthones	• Croqueting
	• Carotenoids
	• Fucoxanthin
• Chlorophyll	• Lutein
	• Violaxanthin
	• β-Carotene

Adsorbents and Solvents Used in Chromatography

Adsorbent	Solvent
• Fullers earth (Aluminium silicate)	• Petroleum ether (30-50° C)
• Charcoal	• Petroleum ether (50-70°C)
• Activated alumina	• Petroleum ether (50-100°C)
• Magnesium silicate (Florisil)	• Carbon tetrachloride
• Silica gel	• Cyclohexane
• Calcium oxide	• Carbon disulphite
• Magnesium oxide	• Ether
• Calcium carbonate	• Acetone
• Calcium phosphate	• Benzene
• Potassium carbonate	• Toluene
• Sodium carbonate	• Ester of organic acids
•Talc	• 1,2-dichloromcthane • Dichloromethane
• Inulin	• Alcohol, chloroform
• Starch	• Water (var. pH & salt conc.)
• Powdered sugar	• Pyridine, Organic acids

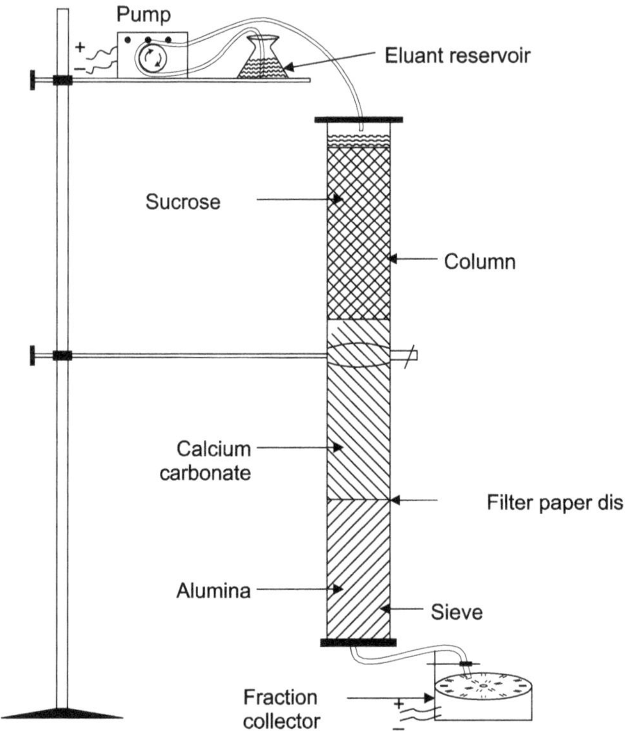

Figure 8.1: Column chromatography.

Estimation of β-Carotene

- The tissue pigments can be extracted from the material using acetone-hexane as solvent The carotene's are then separate from other pigments on magnesium oxide supercel adsorption column and measure at 436 nm on colorimeter/spectronic-20.

Preparation of Column and Separation of β-carotene

- Prepare column chromatography with activated magnesium oxide and supercel at 1:1 mixture upto 10 cm in length and apply enough vacuum to pack the column. Place 1 cm of Na_2SO_4 over the top of the column. With vacuum continuously apply to flask, transfer 50 n11 of acetone-hexane extract of pigment into column and apply the eluting solvent with vacuum during entire operation.
- Carotene's pass rapidly through the column. Bands of Xanthophylls, carotene oxidation products and chlorophyll's remain absorbed on the column. Collect the elute, concentrate under reduced pressure upto 50 ml with 9% acetone in hexane and measure the colour intensity at 436 nm using 9% acetone in hexane as blank.

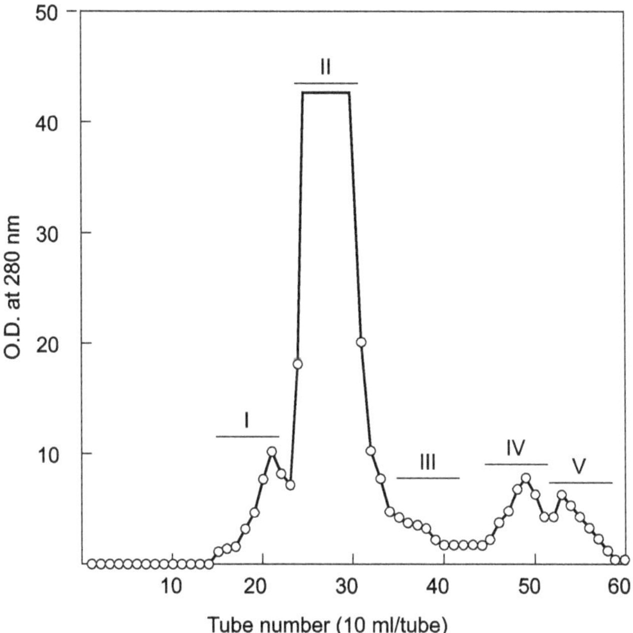

Figure 8.2: Separation of phenolic fractions of beach pea extracts by Sephadex LH-20 column chromatography.

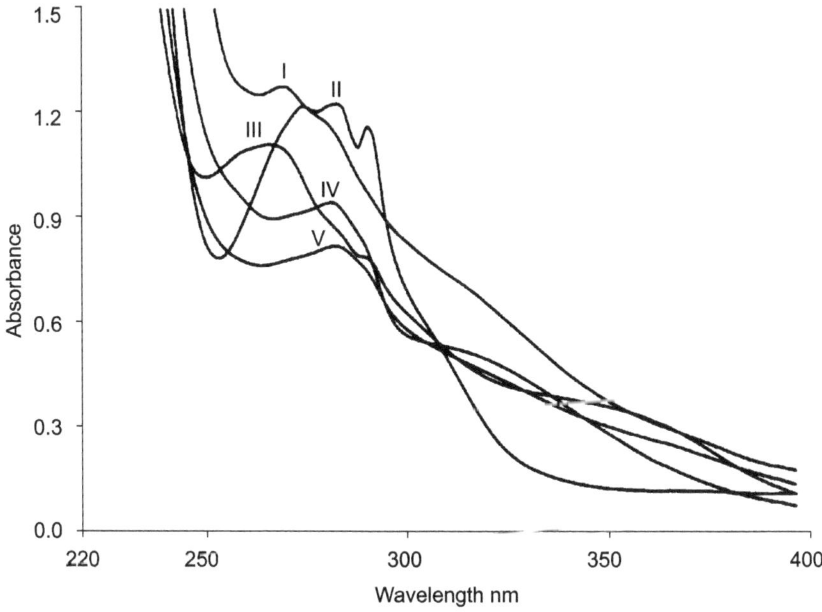

Figure 8.3: UV spectra of individual fractions of beach pea extracts separated from Spehadex LH-20 column.

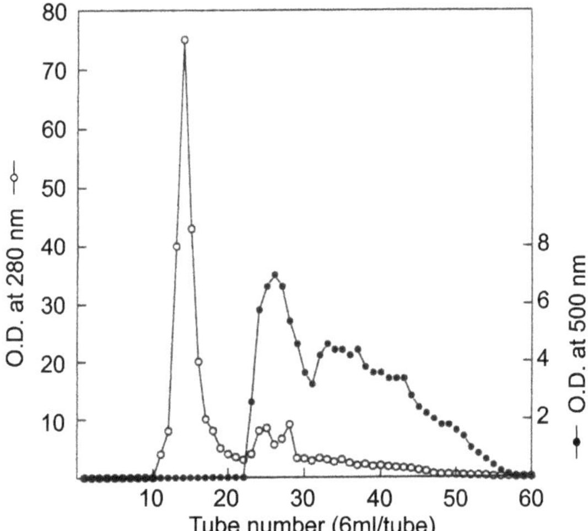

Figure 8.4: Eluates following Sephadex LH-20 column chromatography: UV absorbance of phenolics at 280 nm and condensed tannins after colour development at 500 nm.

PLANAR CHROMATOGRAPHY

Planar chromatography is a separation technique in which the stationary phase is present as or on a plane. The plane can be a paper, serving as such or impregnated by a substance as the stationary bed (paper chromatography) or a layer of solid particles spread on a support such as a glass plate (thin layer chromatography). Different compoundsin the sample mixture travel different distances according to how strongly they interact with the stationary phase as compared to the mobile phase. The specific Retention factor (R_f) of each chemical can be used to aid in the identification of an unknown substance.

PAPER CHROMATOGRAPHY

Paper chromatography is a technique that involves placing a small dot or line of sample solution onto a strip of chromatography paper. The paper is placed in a container with a shallow layer of solvent and sealed. As the solvent rises through the paper, it meets the sample mixture, which starts to travel up the paper with the solvent. This paper is made ofcellulose, a polar substance, and the compounds within the mixture travel farther if they are non-polar. More polar substances bond with the cellulose paper more quickly, and therefore do not travel as far.

THIN LAYER CHROMATOGRAPHY

Thin layer chromatography (TLC) is a widely employed laboratory technique and is similar to paper chromatography. However, instead of using a stationary phase of paper, it involves a stationary phase of a thin layer of adsorbent like silica gel, alumina, or cellulose on a flat, inert substrate. Compared to paper, it has the advantage of faster runs, better separations, and the choice between different adsorbents. For even better resolution and to allow for quantification, high-performance TLC can be used. An older popular use had been to differentiate chromosomes by observing distance in gel.

Thin-Layer Chromatography

- Thin layer chromatography (TLC), the subject of this experiment is a solid-liquid technique based on both absorptivity and solubility. The stationary phase is a finely divided polar material, usually silica gel G (Silicic acid, H_2SIO_3) or alumina (Al_2O_3)
- The interactions that can occur between organic molecules and silica gel/ alumina are of several types
- Non-polar molecules are attracted to silica gel by Van der Waals forces
- Dipole-dipole interactions occur with polar molecules
- Co-ordination with a Lewis base, hydrogen bonding with hydroxylic compounds
- Salt formation with a base Salt formation > Co-ordination > Hydrogen bonding, dipole- dipole > van der Waal's.

TLC Visualizing Methods

1. An iodine chamber → Yellow or brown spots
2. Viewing under UV lamp → Bright, Dark spots
3. Spraying the plate with → Blue, black or brown spots suitable reagent/ solvents.

Where We Can Use TLC

1. Establishing that two compounds are identical.
2. Determining the numbers of compounds in a mixture.
3. Verifying the purity of a compound.

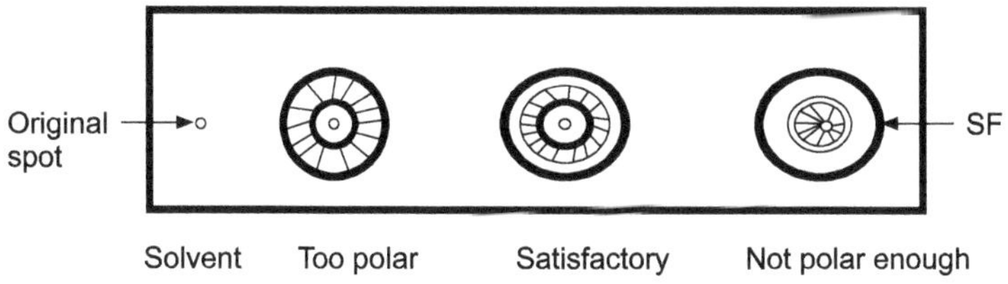

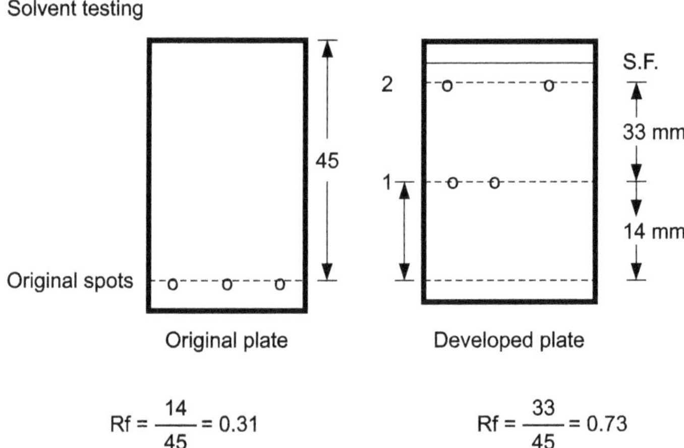

Figure 8.5: TLC development system and calculation of Rf values.

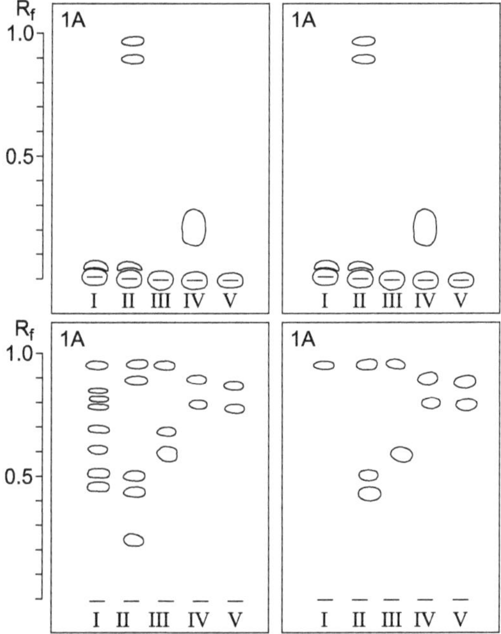

Figure 8.6: TLC chromatograms of phenolic fractions separated from beach pea extracts; chromatograms were developed using (1) B: diethyl ether-petroleum ether-acetic acid (80:20:1) and (2) n-butanol-acetic acid-water (3:1:1); plates were sprayed with a solutions of ferric chloride (A) to give spots of phenolic compounds and (B) β–Carotene-linoleate in order to evaluate antioxidant activity of spots of fractions I-V.

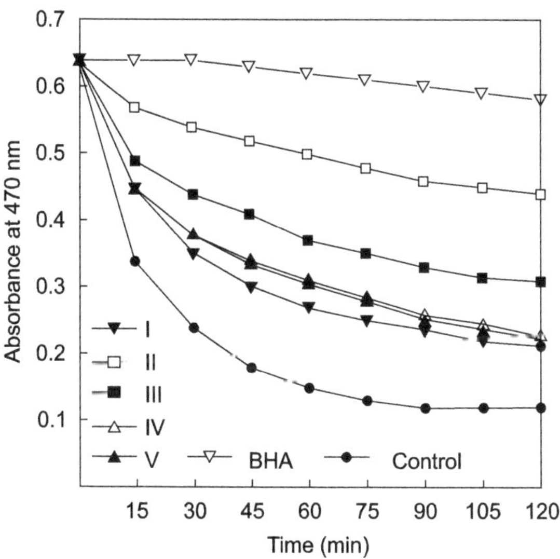

Figure 8.7: Inhibition of bleaching of β–Carotene in model system containing individual fractions of beach pea extracts separated on Sephadex LH-20 column.

Displacement Chromatography

The basic principle of displacement chromatography is: A molecule with a high affinity for the chromatography matrix (the displacer) competes effectively for binding sites, and thus displaces all molecules with lesser affinities. There are distinct differences between displacement and elution chromatography. In elution mode, substances typically emerge from a column in narrow, Gaussian peaks. Wide separation of peaks, preferably to baseline, is desired for maximum purification. The speed at which any component of a mixture travels down the column in elution mode depends on many factors. But for two substances to travel at different speeds, and thereby be resolved, there must be substantial differences in some interaction between the biomolecules and the chromatography matrix. Operating parameters are adjusted to maximize the effect of this difference. In many cases, baseline separation of the peaks can be achieved only with gradient elution and low column loadings. Thus, two drawbacks to elution mode chromatography, especially at the preparative scale, are operational complexity, due to gradient solvent pumping, and low throughput, due to low column loadings. Displacement chromatography has advantages over elution chromatography in that components are resolved into consecutive zones of pure substances rather than "peaks". Because the process takes advantage of the nonlinearity of the isotherms, a larger column feed can be separated on a given column with the purified components recovered at significantly higher concentrations.

Techniques by Physical State of Mobile Phase

Gas Chromatography

Gas chromatography (GC), also sometimes known as gas-liquid chromatography, (GLC), is a separation technique in which the mobile phase is a gas. Gas chromatographic separation is always carried out in a column, which is typically "packed" or "capillary". Packed columns are the routine work horses of gas chromatography, being cheaper and easier to use and often giving adequate performance. Capillary columns generally give far superior resolution and although more expensive are becoming widely used, especially for complex mixtures. Both types of column are made from non-adsorbent and chemically inert materials. Stainless steel and glass are the usual materials for packed columns and quartz or fused silica for capillary columns.

Gas chromatography is based on partition equilibrium of analyte between a solid or viscous liquid stationary phase (often a liquid silicone-based material) and a mobile gas (most often helium). The stationary phase is adhered to the inside of a small-diameter (commonly 0.53 – 0.18mm inside diameter) glass or fused-silica tube (a capillary column) or a solid matrix inside a larger metal tube (a packed column). It is widely used in analytical chemistry; though the high temperatures used in GC make it unsuitable for high molecular weight biopolymers or proteins (heat denatures them), frequently encountered in biochemistry, it is well suited for use in the petrochemical, environmental monitoringand remediation, and industrial chemical fields. It is also used extensively in chemistry research.

Liquid Chromatography

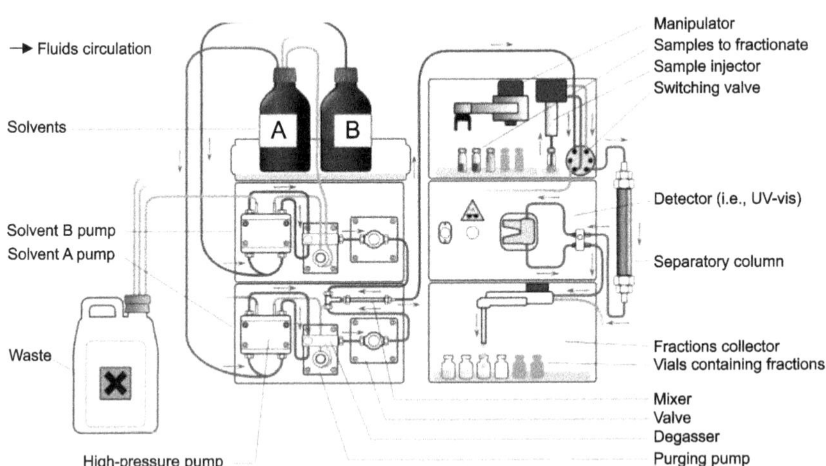

Figure 8.8: Preparative HPLC apparatus

Liquid chromatography (LC) is a separation technique in which the mobile phase is a liquid. It can be carried out either in a column or a plane. Present day liquid chromatography that generally utilizes very small packing particles and a relatively high pressure is referred to as high performance liquid chromatography (HPLC).

In HPLC the sample is forced by a liquid at high pressure (the mobile phase) through a column that is packed with a stationary phase composed of irregularly or spherically shaped particles, a porous monolithic layer, or a porous membrane. HPLC is historically divided into two different sub-classes based on the polarity of the mobile and stationary phases. Methods in which the stationary phase is more polar than the mobile phase (e.g., toluene as the mobile phase, silica as the stationary phase) are termed normal phase liquid chromatography (NPLC) and the opposite (e.g., water-methanol mixture as the mobile phase and C18 = octadecylsilyl as the stationary phase) is termed reversed phase liquid chromatography (RPLC).

Specific Techniques under this Broad Heading are Listed Below.

Affinity Chromatography

Affinity chromatography is based on selective non-covalent interaction between an analyte and specific molecules. It is very specific, but not very robust. It is often used in biochemistry in the purification of proteins bound to tags. These fusion proteins are labeled with compounds such as His-tags, biotin or antigens, which bind to the stationary phase specifically. After purification, some of these tags are usually removed and the pure protein is obtained.

Affinity chromatography often utilizes a biomolecule's affinity for a metal (Zn, Cu, Fe, *etc.*). Columns are often manually prepared. Traditional affinity columns are used as a preparative step to flush out unwanted biomolecules.

However, HPLC techniques exist that do utilize affinity chromatogaphy properties. Immobilized Metal Affinity Chromatography (IMAC) is useful to separate aforementioned molecules based on the relative affinity for the metal (i.e. Dionex IMAC). Often these columns can be loaded with different metals to create a column with a targeted affinity.

Supercritical Fluid Chromatography

Supercritical fluid chromatography is a separation technique in which the mobile phase is a fluid above and relatively close to its critical temperature and pressure.

Techniques by Separation Mechanism

Ion Exchange Chromatography

Ion exchange chromatography (usually referred to as ion chromatography) uses an ion exchange mechanism to separate analytes based on their respective charges. It is usually performed in columns but can also be useful in planar mode. Ion exchange chromatography uses a charged stationary phase to separate charged compounds including anions, cations, amino acids, peptides, and proteins. In conventional methods the stationary phase is an ion exchange resin that carries charged functional groups that interact with oppositely charged groups of the compound to retain. Ion exchange chromatography is commonly used to purify proteins using FPLC.

Size-Exclusion Chromatography

Size-exclusion chromatography (SEC) is also known as gel permeation chromatography (GPC) or gel filtration chromatography and separates molecules according to their size (or more accurately according to their hydrodynamic diameter or hydrodynamic volume). Smaller molecules are able to enter the pores of the media and, therefore, molecules are trapped and removed from the flow of the mobile phase. The average residence time in the pores depends upon the effective size of the analyte molecules. However, molecules that are larger than the average pore size of the packing are excluded and thus suffer essentially no retention; such species are the first to be eluted. It is generally a low-resolution chromatography technique and thus it is often reserved for the final, "polishing" step of purification. It is also useful for determining the tertiary structure and quaternary structure of purified proteins, especially since it can be carried out under native solution conditions.

Expanded Bed Adsorption (EBA) Chromatographic Separation

Expanded Bed Adsorption (EBA) Chromatographic Separation captures a target protein from a crude feed stream when it passes through a chromatography column system containing adsorbent beads. With this technique the crude feedstock can be treated directly in the chromatographic column, avoiding the traditional clarification and pre-treatment steps. EBA Chromatographic Separation is highly scalable, from laboratory-based 1 cm diameter columns to large production columns up to 2 meter in diameter. These columns can typically handle feed stock throughput of more than 1,000,000 liter per day with a production capacity of 1000 MT protein per year.

Special Techniques

Reversed-Phase Chromatography

Reversed-phase chromatography (RPC) is any liquid chromatography procedure in which the mobile phase is significantly more polar than the stationary phase. It is so named because in normal-phase liquid chromatography, the mobile phase is significantly less polar than the stationary phase. Hydrophobic molecules in the mobile phase tend to adsorb to the relatively hydrophobic stationary phase. Hydrophilic molecules in the mobile phase will tend to elute first. Separating columns typically comprise a C8 or C18 carbon-chain bonded to a silica particle substrate.

Hydrophobic interactions between proteins and the chromatographic matrix can be exploited to purify the proteins. In hydrophobic interaction chromatography, the matrix material is lightly substituted with octyl or phenyl groups. At high salt concentrations, nonpolar groups on the surface on proteins "interact" with the hydrophobic groups; that is, both types of groups are excluded by the polar solvent (hydrophobic effects are augmented by increased ionic strength). The eluant is typically an aqueous buffer with decreasing salt concentrations, increasing concentrations of detergent (which disrupts hydrophobic interactions), or changes in pH.

Two-Dimensional Chromatography

In some cases, the chemistry within a given column can be insufficient to separate some analytes. It is possible to direct a series of unresolved peaks onto a second column with different physico-chemical (Chemical classification) properties. Since the mechanism of retention on this new solid support is different from the first dimensional separation, it can be possible to separate compounds that are indistinguishable by one-dimensional chromatography. The sample is spotted at one corner of a square plate,developed, air-dried, then rotated by 90° and usually redeveloped in a second solvent system.

Simulated Moving-Bed Chromatography

The simulated moving bed (SMB) technique is a variant of high performance liquid chromatography; it is used to separate particles and/or chemical compounds that would be difficult or impossible to resolve otherwise. This increased separation is brought about by a valve-and-column arrangement that is used to lengthen the stationary phase indefinitely. In the moving bed technique of preparative chromatography the feed entry and the analyte recovery are simultaneous and continuous, but because of practical difficulties with a continuously moving bed, simulated moving bed technique was proposed. In the simulated moving bed technique instead of moving the bed, the sample inlet and the analyte exit positions are moved continuously, giving the impression of a moving bed. True moving bed chromatography (TMBC) is only a theoretical concept. Its simulation, SMBC is achieved by the use of a multiplicity of columns in series and a complex valve arrangement, which provides for sample and solvent feed, and also analyte and waste takeoff at appropriate locations of any column, whereby it allows switching at regular intervals the sample entry in one direction, the solvent entry in the opposite direction, whilst changing the analyte and waste takeoff positions appropriately as well.

Pyrolysis Gas Chromatography

Pyrolysis gas chromatography mass spectrometry is a method of chemical analysis in which the sample is heated to decomposition to produce smaller molecules that are separated by gas chromatography and detected using mass spectrometry.

Pyrolysis is the thermal decomposition of materials in an inert atmosphere or a vacuum. The sample is put into direct contact with a platinum wire, or placed in a quartz sample tube, and rapidly heated to 600–1000 °C. Depending on the application even higher temperatures are used. Three different heating techniques are used in actual pyrolyzers: Isothermal furnace, inductive heating (Curie Point filament), and resistive heating using platinum filaments. Large molecules cleave at their weakest points and produce smaller, more volatile fragments. These fragments can be separated by gas chromatography. Pyrolysis GC chromatograms are typically complex because a wide range of different decomposition products is formed. The data can either be used as fingerprint to prove material identity or the GC/MS data is used to identify individual fragments to obtain structural information. To increase the volatility of polar fragments, various methylating reagents can be added to a sample before pyrolysis.

Besides the usage of dedicated pyrolyzers, pyrolysis GC of solid and liquid samples can be performed directly inside Programmable Temperature Vaporizer (PTV) injectors that provide quick heating (up to 30 °C/s) and high maximum temperatures of 600–650 °C. This is sufficient for some pyrolysis applications. The main advantage is that no dedicated instrument has to be purchased and pyrolysis can be performed as part of routine GC analysis. In this case quartz GC inlet liners have to be used. Quantitative data can be acquired, and good results of derivatization inside the PTV injector are published as well.

Fast Protein Liquid Chromatography

Fast protein liquid chromatography (FPLC), is a form of liquid chromatography that is often used to analyze or purify mixtures of proteins. As in other forms of chromatography, separation is possible because the different components of a mixture have different affinities for two materials, a moving fluid (the "mobile phase") and a porous solid (the stationary phase). In FPLC the mobile phase is an aqueous solution, or "buffer". The buffer flow rate is controlled by a positive-displacement pump and is normally kept constant, while the composition of the buffer can be varied by drawing fluids in different proportions from two or more external reservoirs. The stationary phase is a resin composed of beads, usually of cross-linked agarose, packed into a cylindrical glass or plastic column. FPLC resins are available in a wide range of bead sizes and surface ligands depending on the application.

Counter Current Chromatography

Counter current chromatography (CCC) is a type of liquid-liquid chromatography, where both the stationary and mobile phases are liquids. The operating principle of CCC equipment requires a column consisting of an open tube coiled around a bobbin. The bobbin is rotated in a double-axis gyratory motion (a cardioid), which causes a variable gravity (G)

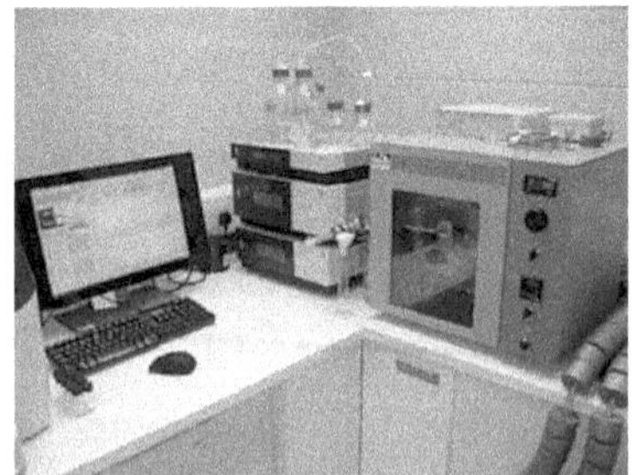

Figure 8.9: An example of a HPCCC system

field to act on the column during each rotation. This motion causes the column to see one partitioning step per revolution and components of the sample separate in the column due to their partitioning coefficient between the two immiscible liquid phases used. There are many types of CCC available today. These include HSCCC (High Speed CCC) and HPCCC (High Performance CCC). HPCCC is the latest and best performing version of the instrumentation available currently.

Chiral Chromatography

Chiral chromatography involves the separation of stereoisomers. In the case of enantiomers, these have no chemical or physical differences apart from being three-dimensional mirror images. Conventional chromatography or other separation processes are incapable of separating them. To enable chiral separations to take place, either the mobile phase or the stationary phase must themselves be made chiral, giving differing affinities between the analytes. Chiral chromatography HPLC columns (with a chiral stationary phase) in both normal and reversed phase are commercially available.

2. GAS CHROMATOGRAPHY–MASS SPECTROMETRY

Gas chromatography–mass spectrometry (GC-MS) is an analytical method that combines the features of gas-chromatography and mass spectrometry to identify different substances within a test sample. Applications of GC-MS include drug detection, fire investigation, environmental analysis, explosives investigation, and identification of unknown samples. GC-MS can also be used in airport security to detect substances in luggage or on human beings. Additionally, it can identify trace elements in materials that were previously thought to have disintegrated beyond identification.

GC-MS has been widely heralded as a "gold standard" for forensic substance identification because it is used to perform a specific test. A specific test positively identifies the actual presence of a particular substance in a given sample. A non-specific test merely indicates that a substance falls into a category of substances. Although a non-specific test could statistically suggest the identity of the substance, this could lead to false positive identification.

History

The use of a mass spectrometer as the detector in gas chromatography was developed during the 1950s after being originated by James and Martin in 1952. These comparatively sensitive devices were originally limited to laboratory settings.

The development of affordable and miniaturized computers has helped in the simplification of the use of this instrument, as well as allowed great improvements in the amount of time it takes to analyze a sample. In 1964, Electronic Associates, Inc. (EAI), a leading U.S. supplier of analog computers, began development of a computer controlledquadrupole mass spectrometer under the direction of Robert

E. Finnigan. By 1966 Finnigan and collaborator Mike Uthe's EAI division had sold over 500 quadrupole residual gas-analyzer instruments. In 1967, Finnigan left EAI to form the Finnigan Instrument Corporation along with Roger Sant, T. Z. Chou, Michael Story, and William Fies. In early 1968, they delivered the first prototype quadrupole GC/MS instruments to Stanford and Purdue University. When Finnigan Instrument Corporation was acquired by Thermo Instrument Systems (later Thermo Fisher Scientific) in 1990, it was considered "the world's leading manufacturer of mass spectrometers".

In 1996 the top-of-the-line high-speed GC-MS units completed analysis of fire accelerants in less than 90 seconds, whereas first-generation GC-MS would have required at least 16 minutes.[7] By the 2000s computerized GC/MS instruments using quadrupole technology had become both essential to chemical research and one of the foremost instruments used for organic analysis. Today computerized GC/MS instruments are widely used in environmental monitoring of water, air, and soil; in the regulation of agriculture and food safety; and in the discovery and production of medicine.

Instrumentation

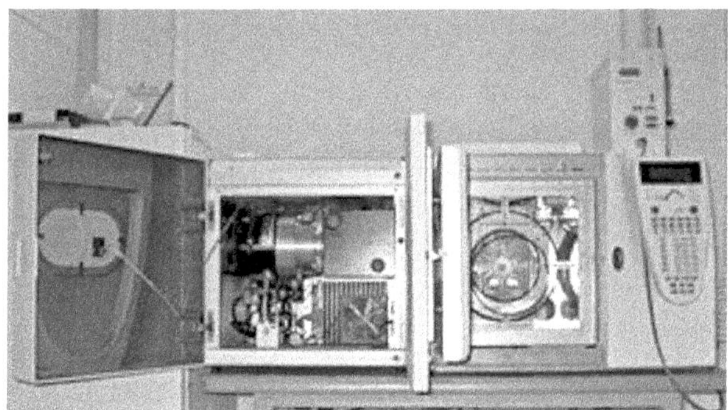

Figure 8.10: The insides of the GC-MS, with the column of the gas chromatograph in the oven on the right.

The GC-MS is composed of two major building blocks: the gas chromatograph and the mass spectrometer. The gas chromatograph utilizes a capillary column which depends on the column's dimensions (length, diameter, film thickness) as well as the phase properties (e.g. 5% phenyl polysiloxane). The difference in the chemical properties between different molecules in a mixture and their relative affinity for the stationary phase of the column will promote separation of the molecules as the sample travels the length of the column. The molecules are retained by the column and then elute (come off) from the column at different times (called the retention time), and this allows the mass spectrometer downstream to capture, ionize, accelerate, deflect, and detect the ionized molecules separately. The mass spectrometer does this by breaking each molecule into ionized fragments and detecting these fragments using their mass-to-charge ratio.

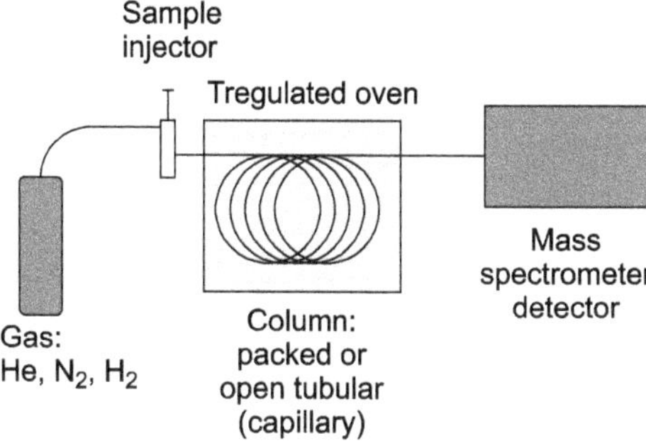

Figure 8.11: GC-MS schematic.

These two components, used together, allow a much finer degree of substance identification than either unit used separately. It is not possible to make an accurate identification of a particular molecule by gas chromatography or mass spectrometry alone. The mass spectrometry process normally requires a very pure sample while gas chromatography using a traditional detector (e.g. Flame ionization detector) cannot differentiate between multiple molecules that happen to take the same amount of time to travel through the column (*i.e.* have the same retention time), which results in two or more molecules that co-elute. Sometimes two different molecules can also have a similar pattern of ionized fragments in a mass spectrometer (mass spectrum). Combining the two processes reduces the possibility of error, as it is extremely unlikely that two different molecules will behave in the same way in both a gas chromatograph and a mass spectrometer. Therefore, when an identifying mass spectrum appears at a characteristic retention time in a GC-MS analysis, it typically increases certainty that the analyte of interest is in the sample.

Purge and Trap GC-MS

For the analysis of volatile compounds, a purge and trap (P&T) concentrator system may be used to introduce samples. The target analytes are extracted and mixed with water and introduced into an airtight chamber. An inert gas such as Nitrogen (N_2) is bubbled through the water; this is known as purging. The volatile compounds move into the headspace above the water and are drawn along a pressure gradient (caused by the introduction of the purge gas) out of the chamber. The volatile compounds are drawn along a heated line onto a 'trap'. The trap is a column of adsorbent material at ambient temperature that holds the compounds by returning them to the liquid phase. The trap is then heated and the sample compounds are introduced to the GC-MS column via a volatiles interface, which is a split inlet system. P&T GC-MS is particularly suited to volatile organic compounds (VOCs) and BTEX compounds (aromatic compounds associated with petroleum).

Types of Mass Spectrometer Detectors

The most common type of mass spectrometer (MS) associated with a gas chromatograph (GC) is the quadrupole mass spectrometer, sometimes referred to by the Hewlett-Packard (now Agilent) trade name "Mass Selective Detector" (MSD). Another relatively common detector is the ion trap mass spectrometer. Additionally one may find a magnetic sector mass spectrometer, however these particular instruments are expensive and bulky and not typically found in high-throughput service laboratories. Other detectors may be encountered such as time of flight (TOF), tandem quadrupoles (MS-MS) (see below), or in the case of an ion trap MS where n indicates the number mass spectrometry stages.

GC-tandem MS

When a second phase of mass fragmentation is added, for example using a second quadrupole in a quadrupole instrument, it is called tandem MS (MS/MS). MS/MS can sometimes be used to quantitate low levels of target compounds in the presence of a high sample matrix background.

The first quadrupole (Q1) is connected with a collision cell (Q2) and another quadrupole (Q3). Both quadrupoles can be used in scanning or static mode, depending on the type of MS/MS analysis being performed. Types of analysis include product ion scan, precursor ion scan, selected reaction monitoring (SRM) (sometimes referred to as multiple reaction monitoring (MRM)) and neutral loss scan. For example: When Q1 is in static mode (looking at one mass only as in SIM), and Q3 is in scanning mode, one obtains a so-called product ion spectrum (also called "daughter spectrum"). From this spectrum, one can select a prominent product ion which can be the product ion for the chosen precursor ion. The pair is called a "transition" and forms the basis for SRM. SRM is highly specific and virtually eliminates matrix background.

Ionization

After the molecules travel the length of the column, pass through the transfer line and enter into the mass spectrometer they are ionized by various methods with typically only one method being used at any given time. Once the sample is fragmented it will then be detected, usually by an electron multiplier diode, which essentially turns the ionized mass fragment into an electrical signal that is then detected. The ionization technique chosen is independent of using full scan or SIM.

Electron Ionization

By far the most common and perhaps standard form of ionization is electron ionization (EI). The molecules enter into the MS (the source is a quadrupole or the ion trap itself in an ion trap MS) where they are bombarded with free electrons emitted from a filament, not unlike the filament one would find in a standard light bulb. The electrons bombard the molecules, causing the molecule to fragment in a characteristic and reproducible way. This "hard ionization" technique results in the creation of more fragments of low mass to charge ratio (m/z) and few, if any, molecules approaching the molecular mass unit. Hard ionization is considered by mass spectrometrists as the employ of molecular electron bombardment, whereas "soft ionization" is charge by molecular collision with an introduced gas. The molecular fragmentation pattern is dependent upon the electron energy applied to the system, typically 70 eV (electron Volts). The use of 70 eV facilitates comparison of generated spectra with library spectra using manufacturer-supplied software or software developed by the National Institute of Standards (NIST-USA). Spectral library searches employ matching algorithms such as Probability Based Matching and dot product matching that is used with methods of analysis written by many method standardization agencies. Sources of libraries include NIST, Wiley, the AAFS, and instrument manufacturers.

Cold Electron Ionization

The "hard ionization" process of electron ionization can be softened by the cooling of the molecules before their ionization, resulting in mass spectra that are richer in information. In this method named cold electron ionization (Cold-EI) the molecules exit the GC column, mixed with added helium make up gas and expand into vacuum through a specially designed supersonic nozzle, forming a supersonic molecular beam (SMB). Collisions with the makeup gas at the expanding supersonic jet reduce the internal vibrational (and rotational) energy of the analyte molecules, hence reducing the degree of fragmentation caused by the electrons during the ionization process. Cold-EI mass spectra are characterized by an abundant molecular ion while the usual fragmentation pattern is retained, thus making Cold-EI mass spectra compatible with library search identification techniques. The enhanced molecular ions increase the identification probabilities of both known and unknown compounds, amplify isomer mass spectral effects and enable the use of isotope abundance analysis for the elucidation of elemental formulae.

Chemical Ionization

In chemical ionization a reagent gas, typically methane or ammonia is introduced into the mass spectrometer. Depending on the technique (positive CI or negative CI) chosen, this reagent gas will interact with the electrons and analyte and cause a 'soft' ionization of the molecule of interest. A softer ionization fragments the molecule to a lower degree than the hard ionization of EI. One of the main benefits of using chemical ionization is that a mass fragment closely corresponding to the molecular weight of the analyte of interest is produced.

In positive chemical ionization (PCI) the reagent gas interacts with the target molecule, most often with a proton exchange. This produces the species in relatively high amounts.

In negative chemical ionization (NCI) the reagent gas decreases the impact of the free electrons on the target analyte. This decreased energy typically leaves the fragment in great supply.

Analysis

A mass spectrometer is typically utilized in one of two ways: full scan or selected ion monitoring (SIM). The typical GC-MS instrument is capable of performing both functions either individually or concomitantly, depending on the setup of the particular instrument.

The primary goal of instrument analysis is to quantify an amount of substance. This is done by comparing the relative concentrations among the atomic masses in the generated spectrum. Two kinds of analysis are possible, comparative and original. Comparative analysis essentially compares the given spectrum to a spectrum library to see if its characteristics are present for some sample in the library. This is best performed by a computer because there are a myriad of visual distortions that can take place due to variations in scale. Computers can also simultaneously correlate more data (such as the retention times identified by GC), to more accurately relate certain data.

Another method of analysis measures the peaks in relation to one another. In this method, the tallest peak is assigned 100% of the value, and the other peaks being assigned proportionate values. All values above 3% are assigned. The total mass of the unknown compound is normally indicated by the parent peak. The value of this parent peak can be used to fit with a chemical formula containing the various elements which are believed to be in the compound. The isotope pattern in the spectrum, which is unique for elements that have many isotopes, can also be used to identify the various elements present. Once a chemical formula has been matched to the spectrum, the molecular structure and bonding can be identified, and must be consistent with the characteristics recorded by GC-MS. Typically, this identification done automatically by programs which come with the instrument, given a list of the elements which could be present in the sample.

A "full spectrum" analysis considers all the "peaks" within a spectrum. Conversely, selective ion monitoring (SIM) only monitors selected ions associated with a specific substance. This is done on the assumption that at a given retention time, a set of ions is characteristic of a certain compound. This is a fast and efficient analysis, especially if the analyst has previous information about a sample or is only looking for a few specific substances. When the amount of information collected about the ions in a given gas chromatographic peak decreases, the sensitivity of the analysis increases. So, SIM analysis allows for a smaller quantity of a compound to be detected and measured, but the degree of certainty about the identity of that compound is reduced.

Full Scan MS

When collecting data in the full scan mode, a target range of mass fragments is determined and put into the instrument's method. An example of a typical broad range of mass fragments to monitor would be *m/z* 50 to *m/z* 400. The determination of what range to use is largely dictated by what one anticipates being in the sample while being cognizant of the solvent and other possible interferences. A MS should not be set to look for mass fragments too low or else one may detect air (found as *m/z* 28 due to nitrogen), carbon dioxide (*m/z* 44) or other possible interferences. Additionally if one is to use a large scan range then sensitivity of the instrument is decreased due to performing fewer scans per second since each scan will have to detect a wide range of mass fragments.

Full scan is useful in determining unknown compounds in a sample. It provides more information than SIM when it comes to confirming or resolving compounds in a sample. During instrument method development it may be common to first analyze test solutions in full scan mode to determine the retention time and the mass fragment fingerprint before moving to a SIM instrument method.

Selected Ion Monitoring

In selected ion monitoring (SIM) certain ion fragments are entered into the instrument method and only those mass fragments are detected by the mass spectrometer. The advantages of SIM are that the detection limit is lower since the instrument is only looking at a small number of fragments (e.g. three fragments) during each scan. More scans can take place each second. Since only a few mass fragments of interest are being monitored, matrix interferences are typically lower. To additionally confirm the likelihood of a potentially positive result, it is relatively important to be sure that the ion ratios of the various mass fragments are comparable to a known reference standard.

Applications

Environmental Monitoring and Cleanup

GC-MS is becoming the tool of choice for tracking organic pollutants in the environment. The cost of GC-MS equipment has decreased significantly, and the reliability has increased at the same time, which has contributed to its increased adoption in environmental studies. There are some compounds for which GC-MS is not sufficiently sensitive, including certain pesticides and herbicides, but for most organic analysis of environmental samples, including many major classes of pesticides, it is very sensitive and effective.

Criminal Forensics

GC-MS can analyze the particles from a human body in order to help link a criminal to a crime. The analysis of fire debris using GC-MS is well established, and there is even an established American Society for Testing and Materials (ASTM) standard for fire debris analysis. GCMS/MS is especially useful here as samples often contain very complex matrices and results, used in court, need to be highly accurate.

Law Enforcement

GC-MS is increasingly used for detection of illegal narcotics, and may eventually supplant drug-sniffing dogs.] It is also commonly used in forensic toxicology to find drugs and/or poisons in biological specimens of suspects, victims, or the deceased.

Sports Anti-Doping Analysis

GC-MS is the main tool used in sports anti-doping laboratories to test athletes' urine samples for prohibited performance-enhancing drugs, for example anabolic steroids.

Security

A post–September 11 development, explosive detection systems have become a part of all US airports. These systems run on a host of technologies, many of them based on GC-MS. There are only three manufacturers certified by the FAA to provide these systems, one of which is Thermo Detection (formerly Thermedics), which produces the EGIS, a GC-MS-based line of explosives detectors. The other two manufacturers are Barringer Technologies, now owned by Smith's Detection Systems, and Ion Track Instruments, part of General Electric Infrastructure Security Systems.

Chemical Warfare Agent Detection

As part of the post-September 11 drive towards increased capability in homeland security and public health preparedness, traditional GC-MS units with transmission quadrupole mass spectrometers, as well as those with cylindrical ion trap (CIT-MS) and toroidal ion trap (T-ITMS) mass spectrometers have been modified for field portability and near real-time detection of chemical warfare agents (CWA) such as sarin, soman, and VX. These complex and large GC-MS systems have been modified and configured with resistively heated low thermal mass (LTM) gas chromatographs that reduce analysis time to less than ten percent of the time required in traditional laboratory systems. Additionally, the systems are smaller, and more mobile, including units that are mounted in mobile analytical laboratories (MAL), such as those used by the United States Marine Corps Chemical and Biological Incident Response Force MAL and other similar laboratories, and systems that are hand-carried by two-person teams or individuals, much ado to the smaller mass detectors. Depending on the system, the analytes can be introduced via liquid injection, desorbed from sorbent tubes through a thermal desorption process, or with solid-phase micro extraction (SPME).

Food, Beverage and Perfume Analysis

Foods and beverages contain numerous aromatic compounds, some naturally present in the raw materials and some forming during processing. GC-MS is extensively used for the analysis of these compounds which include esters, fatty acids, alcohols, aldehydes, terpenes etc. It is also used to detect and measure contaminants from spoilage or adulteration which may be harmful and which is often controlled by governmental agencies, for example pesticides.

Astrochemistry

Several GC-MS have left earth. Two were brought to Mars by the Viking program. Venera 11 and 12 and Pioneer Venus analysed the atmosphere of Venus with GC-MS. The Huygens probe of the Cassini-Huygens mission landed one GC-MS on Saturn's largest moon, Titan. The material in the comet 67P/ Churyumov-Gerasimenko will be analysed by the Rosetta mission with a chiral GC-MS in 2014.

Medicine

Dozens of congenital metabolic diseases also known as Inborn error of metabolism are now detectable by newborn screening tests, especially the testing using gas chromatography–mass spectrometry. GC-MS can determine compounds in urine even in minor concentration. These compounds are normally not present but appear in individuals suffering with metabolic disorders. This is increasingly becoming a common way to diagnose IEM for earlier diagnosis and institution of treatment eventually leading to a better outcome. It is now possible to test a newborn for over 100 genetic metabolic disorders by a urine test at birth based on GC-MS.

In combination with isotopic labelling of metabolic compounds, the GC-MS is used for determining metabolic activity. Most applications are based on the use of ^{13}C as the labelling and the measurement of ^{13}C-^{12}C ratios with an isotope ratio mass spectrometer (IRMS); an MS with a detector designed to measure a few select ions and return values as ratios.

3. HIGH PERFORMANCE THIN LAYER CHROMATOGRAPHY (HPLC)

High performance thin layer chromatography (HPTLC) is an enhanced form of thin layer chromatography (TLC). A number of enhancements can be made to the basic method of thin layer chromatography to automate the different steps, to increase the resolution achieved and to allow more accurate quantitative measurements.

Automation is useful to overcome the uncertainty in droplet size and position when the sample is applied to the TLC plate by hand. One recent approach to automation has been the use of piezoelectric devices and inkjet printers for applying the sample.

The spot capacity (analogous to peak capacity in HPLC) can be increased by developing the plate with two different solvents, using two-dimensional chromatography. The procedure begins with development of sample loaded plate with first solvent. After removing it, the plate is rotated 90° and developed with a second solvent.

Commonly used HPLC column packing material

Material	Typical application	Code
Octadecylsilyl-bonded silica	General purpose RPLC	ODS
Octylsilyl-bonded silica	Solutes strongly retained on ODS	OSD
Phenyl-bonded silica	Fatty acids, peptides	PBS
Cyanopropyl-bonded silica	General-purpose NPLC/ RPLC	CPB
Diol-bonded silica	Organic acids and aqueous SEC	DBS
Aminopropyl-bonded silica	Carbohydrates, ion-exchange	APS
Controlled-pore glass	Aqueous SEC	CPG
Microparticulate silica	General purpose	SIL
Cross-linked polystyrene	Organic SEC, RPLC	CPS
Silica-based cation exchanger	Nucleic acids, metals, amines, nitrogenous bases	SCX
Polystyrene-based cation exchanger	Amino acids, carbohydrate analysis	PCX
Silica-based anion exchanger	Proteins, nucleic acids, phophorylated nucleotides	SAX
Polystyrene-based anion exchanger	Nucleotides, organic acids, purines & carbohydrates	PAX

Instrumentation

Widely used instrument for HPTLC is from CAMAG, Switzerland. It provides automated sample application (loading), plate development, detection and documentation.

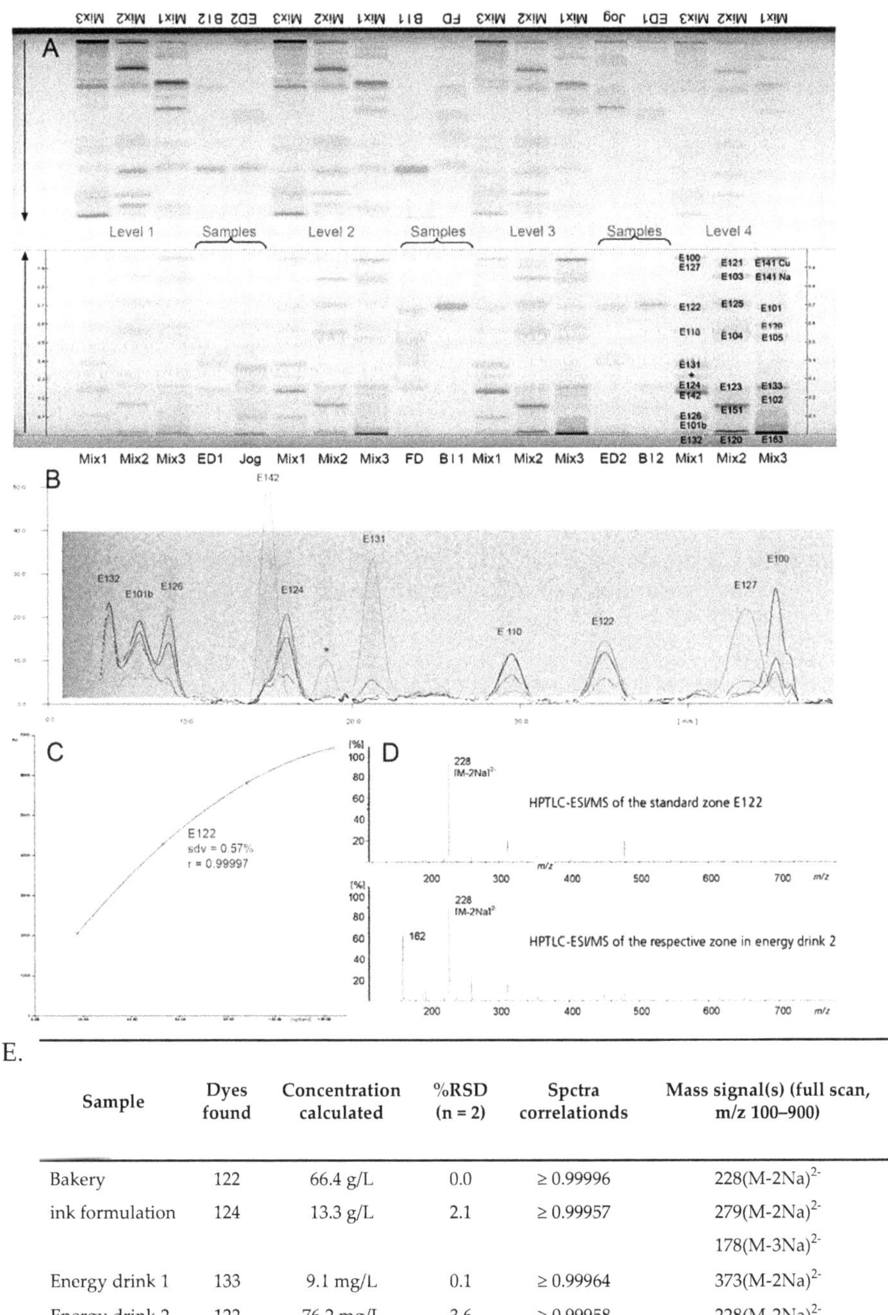

E.

Sample	Dyes found	Concentration calculated	%RSD (n = 2)	Spctra correlationds	Mass signal(s) (full scan, m/z 100–900)
Bakery	122	66.4 g/L	0.0	≥ 0.99996	$228(M\text{-}2Na)^{2-}$
ink formulation	124	13.3 g/L	2.1	≥ 0.99957	$279(M\text{-}2Na)^{2-}$
					$178(M\text{-}3Na)^{2-}$
Energy drink 1	133	9.1 mg/L	0.1	≥ 0.99964	$373(M\text{-}2Na)^{2-}$
Energy drink 2	122	76.2 mg/L	3.6	≥ 0.99958	$228(M\text{-}2Na)^{2-}$

Figure 8.12: Analysis of food-dyes: (A) photo of HPTLC plate (developed from both sides), (B) multi-wavelength scan of mix 1, (C) calibration function, (D) mass spectra of selected zones, (E) results.

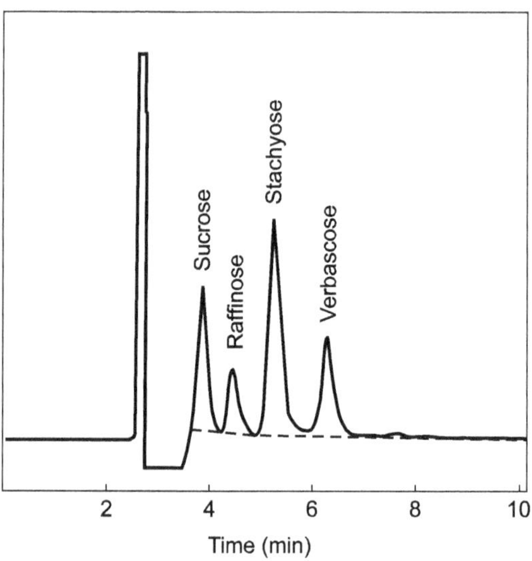

Figure 8.13: Chromatogram of the analytically separated sucrose, raffinose, stacyose and verbascose from beach pea meal by semi-preparative HPLC.

4. POLYMERASE CHAIN REACTION (PCR)

The polymerase chain reaction (PCR) is a technology in molecular biology used to amplify a single copy or a few copies of a piece of DNA across several orders of magnitude, generating thousands to millions of copies of a particular DNA sequence.

Developed in 1983 by Kary Mullis, PCR is now a common and often indispensable technique used in medical and biological research labs for a variety of applications. These include DNA cloning for sequencing, DNA-based phylogeny, or functional analysis of genes; the diagnosis of hereditary diseases; the identification of genetic fingerprints (used in forensic sciences and paternity testing); and the detection and diagnosis of infectious diseases. In 1993, Mullis was awarded the Nobel Prize in Chemistry along with Michael Smith for his work on PCR.

The method relies on thermal cycling, consisting of cycles of repeated heating and cooling of the reaction for DNA melting and enzymatic replication of the DNA. Primers (short DNA fragments) containing sequences complementary to the target region along with a DNA polymerase, which the method is named after, are key components to enable selective and repeated amplification. As PCR progresses, the DNA generated is itself used as a template for replication, setting in motion a chain reaction in which the DNA template is exponentially amplified. PCR can be extensively modified to perform a wide array of genetic manipulations.

Almost all PCR applications employ a heat-stable DNA polymerase, such as Taq polymerase (an enzyme originally isolated from the bacterium *Thermus aquaticus*). This DNA polymerase enzymatically assembles a new DNA strand from DNA building-blocks, the nucleotides, by using single-stranded DNA as a template and DNA oligonucleotides (also called DNA primers), which are required for initiation of DNA synthesis. The vast majority of PCR methods use thermal cycling, i.e., alternately heating and cooling the PCR sample through a defined series of temperature steps.

In the first step, the two strands of the DNA double helix are physically separated at a high temperature in a process called DNA melting. In the second step, the temperature is lowered and the two DNA strands become templates for DNA polymerase to selectively amplify the target DNA. The selectivity of PCR results from the use of primers that are complementary to the DNA region targeted for amplification under specific thermal cycling conditions.

Principles and Procedure

PCR amplifies a specific region of a DNA strand (the DNA target). Most PCR methods typically amplify DNA fragments of between 0.1 and 10kilo base pairs (kbp), although some techniques allow for amplification of fragments up to 40 kbp in size. The amount of amplified product is determined by the available substrates in the reaction, which become limiting as the reaction progresses.

A basic PCR set up requires several components and reagents. These components include:

- *DNA* template that contains the DNA region (target) to amplify
- Two primers that are complementary to the 3′ (three prime) ends of each of the sense and anti-sense strand of the DNA target
- Taq polymerase or another DNA polymerase with a temperature optimum at around 70 °C
- Deoxynucleoside triphosphates (dNTPs, sometimes called "deoxynucleotide triphosphates"; nucleotides containing triphosphate groups), the building-blocks from which the DNA polymerase synthesizes a new DNA strand
- Buffer solution, providing a suitable chemical environment for optimum activity and stability of the DNA polymerase
- Bivalent cations, magnesium or manganese ions; generally Mg^{2+} is used, but Mn^{2+} can be used for PCR-mediated DNA mutagenesis, as higher Mn^{2+} concentration increases the error rate during DNA synthesis
- Monovalent cation potassium ions

The PCR is commonly carried out in a reaction volume of 10–200 μl in small reaction tubes (0.2–0.5 ml volumes) in a thermal cycler. The thermal cycler heats and cools the reaction tubes to achieve the temperatures required at each step of the reaction (see below). Many modern thermal cyclers make use of the Peltier effect, which permits both heating and cooling of the block holding the PCR tubes simply by reversing the electric current. Thin-walled reaction tubes permit favorable thermal conductivity to allow for rapid thermal equilibration. Most thermal cyclers have heated lids to prevent condensation at the top of the reaction tube. Older thermocyclers lacking a heated lid require a layer of oil on top of the reaction mixture or a ball of wax inside the tube.

Procedure

Typically, PCR consists of a series of 20–40 repeated temperature changes, called cycles, with each cycle commonly consisting of 2–3 discrete temperature steps, usually three (Figure below). The cycling is often preceded by a single temperature step at a high temperature (>90 °C), and followed by one hold at the end for final product extension or brief storage. The temperatures used and the length of time they are applied in each cycle depend on a variety of parameters. These include the enzyme used for DNA synthesis, the concentration of divalent ions and dNTPs in the reaction, and the melting temperature (Tm) of the primers.

- *Initialization step*: (Only required for DNA polymerases that require heat activation by hot-start PCR.): This step consists of heating the reaction to a temperature of 94–96 °C (or 98 °C if extremely thermostable polymerases are used), which is held for 1–9 minutes.
- *Denaturation step*: This step is the first regular cycling event and consists of heating the reaction to 94–98 °C for 20–30 seconds. It causes DNA melting of the DNA template by disrupting the hydrogen bonds between complementary bases, yielding single-stranded DNA molecules.
- *Annealing step*: The reaction temperature is lowered to 50–65 °C for 20–40 seconds allowing annealing of the primers to the single-stranded DNA template. This temperature must be low enough to allow for hybridization of the primer to the strand, but high enough for the hybridization to be specific, i.e., the primer should only bind to a perfectly complementary part of the template. If the temperature is too low, the primer could bind imperfectly. If it is too high, the primer might not bind. Typically the annealing temperature is about 3–5 °C below the Tm of the primers used. Stable DNA–DNA hydrogen bonds are only formed when the primer sequence very closely matches the template sequence. The polymerase binds to the primer-template hybrid and begins DNA formation.
- *Extension/elongation step*: The temperature at this step depends on the DNA polymerase used; Taq polymerase has its optimum activity temperature at 75–80 °C, and commonly a temperature of 72 °C is used with this enzyme. At this step the DNA polymerase synthesizes a new DNA strand complementary to the DNA template strand by adding dNTPs that are complementary to the template in 5′ to 3′ direction, condensing the 5′-phosphate group of the dNTPs with the 3′-hydroxyl group at the end of the nascent (extending) DNA strand. The extension time depends both on the DNA polymerase used and on the length of the DNA fragment to amplify. As a rule-of-thumb, at its optimum temperature, the DNA polymerase polymerizes a thousand bases per minute. Under optimum conditions, i.e., if there are no limitations due to limiting substrates or reagents, at each extension step,

the amount of DNA target is doubled, leading to exponential (geometric) amplification of the specific DNA fragment.

- *Final elongation*: This single step is occasionally performed at a temperature of 70–74 °C (this is the temperature needed for optimal activity for most polymerases used in PCR) for 5–15 minutes after the last PCR cycle to ensure that any remaining single-stranded DNA is fully extended.
- *Final hold*: This step at 4–15 °C for an indefinite time may be employed for short-term storage of the reaction.

Polymerase Chain Reaction – PCR

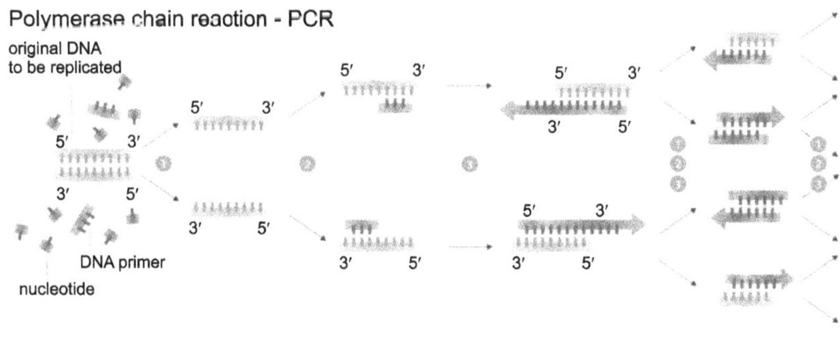

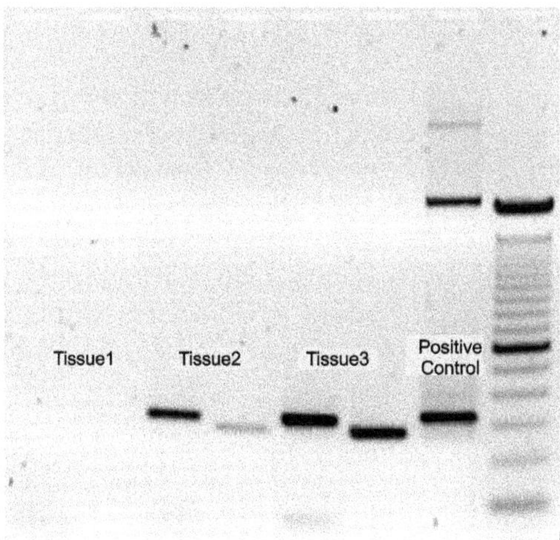

Figure 8.14: Ethidium bromide-stained PCR products after gel electrophoresis. Two sets of primers were used to amplify a target sequence from three different tissue samples. No amplification is present in sample #1; DNA bands in sample #2 and #3 indicate successful amplification of the target sequence. The gel also shows a positive control, and a DNA ladder containing DNA fragments of defined length for sizing the bands in the experimental PCRs.

To check whether the PCR generated the anticipated DNA fragment (also sometimes referred to as the amplimer oramplicon), agarose gel electrophoresis is employed for size separation of the PCR products. The size(s) of PCR products is determined by comparison with a DNA ladder (a molecular weight marker), which contains DNA fragments of known size, run on the gel alongside the PCR products.

Stages

The PCR process can be divided into three stages:

Exponential amplification: At every cycle, the amount of product is doubled (assuming 100% reaction efficiency). The reaction is very sensitive: only minute quantities of DNA must be present.

Leveling off stage: The reaction slows as the DNA polymerase loses activity and as consumption of reagents such as dNTPs and primers causes them to become limiting.

Plateau: No more products accumulate due to exhaustion of reagents and enzyme.

Optimization

In practice, PCR can fail for various reasons, in part due to its sensitivity to contamination causing amplification of spurious DNA products. Because of this, a number of techniques and procedures have been developed for optimizing PCR conditions. Contamination with extraneous DNA is addressed with lab protocols and procedures that separate pre-PCR mixtures from potential DNA contaminants. This usually involves spatial separation of PCR-setup areas from areas for analysis or purification of PCR products, use of disposable plastic ware, and thoroughly cleaning the work surface between reaction setups. Primer-design techniques are important in improving PCR product yield and in avoiding the formation of spurious products, and the usage of alternate buffer components or polymerase enzymes can help with amplification of long or otherwise problematic regions of DNA. Addition of reagents, such as formamide, in buffer systems may increase the specificity and yield of PCR. Computer simulations of theoretical PCR results (Electronic PCR) may be performed to assist in primer design.

Applications

Selective DNA Isolation

PCR allows isolation of DNA fragments from genomic DNA by selective amplification of a specific region of DNA. This use of PCR augments many methods, such as generating hybridization probes for Southern or northern hybridization and DNA cloning, which require larger amounts of DNA, representing a specific DNA region. PCR supplies these techniques with high amounts of pure DNA, enabling analysis of DNA samples even from very small amounts of starting material.

Other applications of PCR include DNA sequencing to determine unknown PCR-amplified sequences in which one of the amplification primers may be used in Sanger sequencing, isolation of a DNA sequence to expedite recombinant DNA technologies involving the insertion of a DNA sequence into a plasmid, phage, or cosmid (depending on size) or the genetic material of another organism. Bacterial colonies (such as *E. coli*) can be rapidly screened by PCR for correct DNA vector constructs. PCR may also be used for genetic fingerprinting; a forensic technique used to identify a person or organism by comparing experimental DNAs through different PCR-based methods.

Some PCR 'fingerprints' methods have high discriminative power and can be used to identify genetic relationships between individuals, such as parent-child or between siblings, and are used in paternity testing (Fig. 4). This technique may also be used to determine evolutionary relationships among organisms when certain molecular clocks are used (*i.e.*, the 16S rRNA and recA genes of microorganisms).

Amplification and Quantification of DNA

Because PCR amplifies the regions of DNA that it targets, PCR can be used to analyze extremely small amounts of sample. This is often critical for forensic analysis, when only a trace amount of DNA is available as evidence. PCR may also be used in the analysis of ancient DNAthat is tens of thousands of years old. These PCR-based techniques have been successfully used on animals, such as a forty-thousand-year-old mammoth, and also on human DNA, in applications ranging from the analysis of Egyptian mummies to the identification of a Russian tsarand the body of English king Richard III.

Quantitative PCR methods allow the estimation of the amount of a given sequence present in a sample a technique often applied to quantitatively determine levels of gene expression. Quantitative PCR is an established tool for DNA quantification that measures the accumulation of DNA product after each round of PCR amplification.

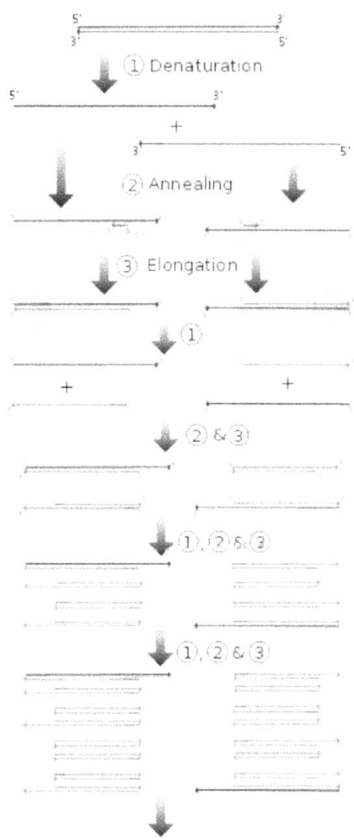

Disease Diagnosis

PCR permits early diagnosis of malignant diseases such as leukemia and lymphomas, which is currently the highest-developed in cancer research and is already being used routinely. PCR assays can be performed directly on genomic DNA samples to detect translocation-specific malignant cells at a sensitivity that is at least 10,000 fold higher than that of other methods.

PCR allows for rapid and highly specific diagnosis of infectious diseases, including those caused by bacteria or viruses. PCR also permits identification of non-cultivatable or slow-growing microorganisms such as mycobacteria, anaerobic bacteria, or viruses from tissue culture assays and animal models. The basis for PCR diagnostic applications in microbiology is the detection of infectious agents and the discrimination of non-pathogenic from pathogenic strains by virtue of specific genes.

Viral DNA can likewise be detected by PCR. The primers used must be specific to the targeted sequences in the DNA of a virus, and the PCR can be used for diagnostic analyses or DNA sequencing of the viral genome. The high sensitivity of PCR permits virus detection soon after infection and even before the onset of disease. Such early detection may give physicians a significant lead time in treatment. The amount of virus ("viral load") in a patient can also be quantified by PCR-based DNA quantitation techniques.

Limitations

DNA polymerase is prone to error, which in turn causes mutations in the PCR fragments that are made. Additionally, the specificity of the PCR fragments can mutate to the template DNA, due to nonspecific binding of primers. Furthermore prior information on the sequence is necessary in order to generate the primers.

Variations

- *Allele-specific PCR*: a diagnostic or cloning technique based on single-nucleotide variations (SNVs not to be confused with SNPs) (single-base differences in a patient). It requires prior knowledge of a DNA sequence, including differences between alleles, and uses primers whose 3′ ends encompass the SNV (base pair buffer around SNV usually incorporated). PCR amplification under stringent conditions is much less efficient in the presence of a mismatch between template and primer, so successful amplification with an SNP-specific primer signals presence of the specific SNP in a sequence. See SNP genotyping for more information.
- *Assembly PCR* or *Polymerase Cycling Assembly (PCA)*: artificial synthesis of long DNA sequences by performing PCR on a pool of long oligonucleotides with short overlapping segments. The oligonucleotides alternate between sense and antisense directions, and the overlapping segments determine the order of the PCR fragments, thereby selectively producing the final long DNA product.

- *Asymmetric PCR*: preferentially amplifies one DNA strand in a double-stranded DNA template. It is used in sequencing and hybridization probing where amplification of only one of the two complementary strands is required. PCR is carried out as usual, but with a great excess of the primer for the strand targeted for amplification. Because of the slow (arithmetic) amplification later in the reaction after the limiting primer has been used up, extra cycles of PCR are required. A recent modification on this process, known as Linear-After-The-Exponential-PCR (LATE-PCR), uses a limiting primer with a higher melting temperature (Tm) than the excess primer to maintain reaction efficiency as the limiting primer concentration decreases mid-reaction.
- *Dial out PCR*: a highly parallel method for retrieving accurate DNA molecules for gene synthesis. A complex library of DNA molecules is modified with unique flanking tags before massively parallel sequencing. Tag-directed primers then enable the retrieval of molecules with desired sequences by PCR.
- *Digital PCR (dPCR)*: used to measure the quantity of a target DNA sequence in a DNA sample. The DNA sample is highly diluted so that after running many PCRs in parallel, some of them do not receive a single molecule of the target DNA. The target DNA concentration is calculated using the proportion of negative outcomes. Hence the name 'digital PCR'.
- *Helicase-dependent amplification*: similar to traditional PCR, but uses a constant temperature rather than cycling through denaturation and annealing/extension cycles. DNA helicase, an enzyme that unwinds DNA, is used in place of thermal denaturation.
- *Hot start PCR*: a technique that reduces non-specific amplification during the initial set up stages of the PCR. It may be performed manually by heating the reaction components to the denaturation temperature (e.g., 95 °C) before adding the polymerase. Specialized enzyme systems have been developed that inhibit the polymerase's activity at ambient temperature, either by the binding of an antibody or by the presence of covalently bound inhibitors that dissociate only after a high-temperature activation step. Hot-start/cold-finish PCR is achieved with new hybrid polymerases that are inactive at ambient temperature and are instantly activated at elongation temperature.
- *In silico PCR* (digital PCR, virtual PCR, electronic PCR, e-PCR): refers to computational tools used to calculate theoretical polymerase chain reaction results using a given set of primers (probes) to amplify DNA sequences from a sequenced genome or transcriptome. In silico PCR was proposed as an educational tool for molecular biology.
- *Intersequence-specific PCR* (ISSR): a PCR method for DNA fingerprinting that amplifies regions between simple sequence repeats to produce a unique fingerprint of amplified fragment lengths.

- *Inverse PCR*: is commonly used to identify the flanking sequences around genomic inserts. It involves a series of DNA digestions and self-ligation, resulting in known sequences at either end of the unknown sequence.
- *Ligation-mediated PCR*: uses small DNA linkers ligated to the DNA of interest and multiple primers annealing to the DNA linkers; it has been used for DNA sequencing, genome walking, and DNA foot printing.
- *Methylation-specific PCR* (MSP): developed by Stephen Baylin and Jim Herman at the Johns Hopkins School of Medicine, and is used to detect methylation of CpG islands in genomic DNA. DNA is first treated with sodium bisulfite, which converts unmethylated cytosine bases to uracil, which is recognized by PCR primers as thymine. Two PCRs are then carried out on the modified DNA, using primer sets identical except at any CpG islands within the primer sequences. At these points, one primer set recognizes DNA with cytosines to amplify methylated DNA, and one set recognizes DNA with uracil or thymine to amplify unmethylated DNA. MSP using qPCR can also be performed to obtain quantitative rather than qualitative information about methylation.
- *Miniprimer PCR*: uses a thermostable polymerase (S-Tbr) that can extend from short primers ("smalligos") as short as 9 or 10 nucleotides. This method permits PCR targeting to smaller primer binding regions, and is used to amplify conserved DNA sequences, such as the 16S (or eukaryotic 18S) rRNA gene.
- *Multiplex Ligation-dependent Probe Amplification* (*MLPA*): permits amplifying multiple targets with a single primer pair, thus avoiding the resolution limitations of multiplex PCR (see below).
- *Multiplex-PCR*: consists of multiple primer sets within a single PCR mixture to produce amplicons of varying sizes that are specific to different DNA sequences. By targeting multiple genes at once, additional information may be gained from a single test-run that otherwise would require several times the reagents and more time to perform. Annealing temperatures for each of the primer sets must be optimized to work correctly within a single reaction, and amplicon sizes. That is, their base pair length should be different enough to form distinct bands when visualized by gel electrophoresis.
- *Nanoparticle-Assisted PCR (nanoPCR)*: In recent years, it has been reported that some nanoparticles (NPs) can enhance the efficiency of PCR (thus being called nano–PCR), and some even perform better than the original PCR enhancers. It was also found that quantum dots (QDs) can improve PCR specificity and efficiency. Single-walled carbon nanotubes (SWCNTs) and multi-walled carbon nanotubes (MWCNTs) are efficient in enhancing the amplification of long PCR. Carbon nanopowder (CNP) was reported be able to improve the efficiency of repeated PCR and long PCR. ZnO, TiO_2, and Ag NPs were also found to increase PCR yield. Importantly, already

known data has indicated that non-metallic NPs retained acceptable amplification fidelity. Given that many NPs are capable of enhancing PCR efficiency, it is clear that there is likely to be great potential for nanoPCR technology improvements and product development.

- *Nested PCR*: increases the specificity of DNA amplification, by reducing background due to non-specific amplification of DNA. Two sets of primers are used in two successive PCRs. In the first reaction, one pair of primers is used to generate DNA products, which besides the intended target, may still consist of non-specifically amplified DNA fragments. The product(s) are then used in a second PCR with a set of primers whose binding sites are completely or partially different from and located 3′ of each of the primers used in the first reaction. Nested PCR is often more successful in specifically amplifying long DNA fragments than conventional PCR, but it requires more detailed knowledge of the target sequences.
- *Overlap-extension PCR* or *Splicing by overlap extension (SOEing)*: a genetic engineering technique that is used to splice together two or more DNA fragments that contain complementary sequences. It is used to join DNA pieces containing genes, regulatory sequences, or mutations; the technique enables creation of specific and long DNA constructs. It can also introduce deletions, insertions or point mutations into a DNA sequence.
- *PAN-AC*: uses isothermal conditions for amplification, and may be used in living cells.
- *quantitative PCR* (qPCR): used to measure the quantity of a target sequence (commonly in real-time). It quantitatively measures starting amounts of DNA, cDNA, or RNA. Quantitative PCR is commonly used to determine whether a DNA sequence is present in a sample and the number of its copies in the sample. *Quantitative PCR* has a very high degree of precision. Quantitative PCR methods use fluorescent dyes, such as Sybr Green, EvaGreen or fluorophore-containing DNA probes, such as TaqMan, to measure the amount of amplified product in real time. It is also sometimes abbreviated to RT-PCR (*real-time* PCR) but this abbreviation should be used only for reverse transcription PCR. qPCR is the appropriate contractions for quantitative PCR (real-time PCR).
- *Reverse Transcription PCR (RT-PCR)*: for amplifying DNA from RNA. Reverse transcriptase reverse transcribes RNA into cDNA, which is then amplified by PCR. RT-PCR is widely used in expression profiling, to determine the expression of a gene or to identify the sequence of an RNA transcript, including transcription start and termination sites. If the genomic DNA sequence of a gene is known, RT-PCR can be used to map the location of exons and introns in the gene. The 5′ end of a gene (corresponding to the transcription start site) is typically identified by RACE-PCR (*Rapid Amplification of cDNA Ends*).

- *Solid Phase PCR*: encompasses multiple meanings, including Polony Amplification (where PCR colonies are derived in a gel matrix, for example), Bridge PCR (primers are covalently linked to a solid-support surface), conventional Solid Phase PCR (where Asymmetric PCR is applied in the presence of solid support bearing primer with sequence matching one of the aqueous primers) and Enhanced Solid Phase PCR (where conventional Solid Phase PCR can be improved by employing high Tm and nested solid support primer with optional application of a thermal 'step' to favour solid support priming).
- *Suicide PCR*: typically used in paleogenetics or other studies where avoiding false positives and ensuring the specificity of the amplified fragment is the highest priority. It was originally described in a study to verify the presence of the microbe Yersinia pestis in dental samples obtained from 14th Century graves of people supposedly killed by plague during the medieval Black Death epidemic. The method prescribes the use of any primer combination only once in a PCR (hence the term "suicide"), which should never have been used in any positive control PCR reaction, and the primers should always target a genomic region never amplified before in the lab using this or any other set of primers. This ensures that no contaminating DNA from previous PCR reactions is present in the lab, which could otherwise generate false positives.
- *Thermal asymmetric interlaced PCR (TAIL-PCR)*: for isolation of an unknown sequence flanking a known sequence. Within the known sequence, TAIL-PCR uses a nested pair of primers with differing annealing temperatures; a degenerate primer is used to amplify in the other direction from the unknown sequence.
- *Touchdown PCR* (*Step-down PCR*): a variant of PCR that aims to reduce nonspecific background by gradually lowering the annealing temperature as PCR cycling progresses. The annealing temperature at the initial cycles is usually a few degrees (3–5 °C) above the T_m of the primers used, while at the later cycles, it is a few degrees (3–5 °C) below the primer T_m. The higher temperatures give greater specificity for primer binding, and the lower temperatures permit more efficient amplification from the specific products formed during the initial cycles.
- *Universal Fast Walking*: for genome walking and genetic fingerprinting using a more specific 'two-sided' PCR than conventional 'one-sided' approaches (using only one gene-specific primer and one general primerwhich can lead to artefactual 'noise') by virtue of a mechanism involving lariat structure formation. Streamlined derivatives of UFW are LaNe RAGE (lariat-dependent nested PCR for rapid amplification of genomic DNA ends), 5'RACE LaNe and 3'RACE LaNe.

History

A 1971 paper in the Journal of Molecular Biology by Kjell Kleppe and co-workers in the laboratory of H. Gobind Khorana first described a method using an enzymatic assay to replicate a short DNA template with primers *in vitro*. However, this early manifestation of the basic PCR principle did not receive much attention at the time, and the invention of the polymerase chain reaction in 1983 is generally credited to Kary Mullis.

When Mullis developed the PCR in 1983, he was working in Emeryville, California for Cetus Corporation, one of the first biotechnologycompanies. There, he was responsible for synthesizing short chains of DNA. Mullis has written that he conceived of PCR while cruising along the Pacific Coast Highway one night in his car. He was playing in his mind with a new way of analyzing changes (mutations) in DNA when he realized that he had instead invented a method of amplifying any DNA region through repeated cycles of duplication driven by DNA polymerase. In *Scientific American*, Mullis summarized the procedure: "Beginning with a single molecule of the genetic material DNA, the PCR can generate 100 billion similar molecules in an afternoon. The reaction is easy to execute. It requires no more than a test tube, a few simple reagents, and a source of heat." He was awarded the Nobel Prize in Chemistry in 1993 for his invention, seven years after he and his colleagues at Cetus first put his proposal to practice. However, some controversies have remained about the intellectual and practical contributions of other scientists to Mullis' work, and whether he had been the sole inventor of the PCR principle.

At the core of the PCR method is the use of a suitable DNA polymerase able to withstand the high temperatures of >90 °C (194 °F) required for separation of the two DNA strands in the DNA double helix after each replication cycle. The DNA polymerases initially employed for in vitro experiments presaging PCR were unable to withstand these high temperatures. So the early procedures for DNA replication were very inefficient and time consuming, and required large amounts of DNA polymerase and continuous handling throughout the process.

The discovery in 1976 of Taq polymerase a DNA polymerase purified from the thermophilic bacterium, *Thermus aquaticus,* which naturally lives in hot (50 to 80 °C (122 to 176 °F)) environments such as hot springs paved the way for dramatic improvements of the PCR method. The DNA polymerase isolated from *T. aquaticus* is stable at high temperatures remaining active even after DNA denaturation, thus obviating the need to add new DNA polymerase after each cycle. This allowed an automated thermocycler-based process for DNA amplification.

Patent Disputes

The PCR technique was patented by Kary Mullis and assigned to Cetus Corporation, where Mullis worked when he invented the technique in 1983. The *Taq* polymerase enzyme was also covered by patents. There have been several high-profile lawsuits related to the technique, including an unsuccessful lawsuit brought by DuPont. The pharmaceutical company Hoffmann-La Roche purchased the rights to the patents in 1992 and currently holds those that are still protected.

A related patent battle over the Taq polymerase enzyme is still ongoing in several jurisdictions around the world between Roche and Promega. The legal arguments have extended beyond the lives of the original PCR and Taq polymerase patents.

5. ELECTRON MICROSCOPY (EM)

An electron microscope is a microscope that uses a beam of accelerated electrons as a source of illumination. Because the wavelength of an electron can be up to 100,000 times shorter than that of visible light photons, the electron microscope has a higher resolving power than a light microscope and can reveal the structure of smaller objects. A transmission electron microscope can achieve better than 50 pm resolution and magnifications of up to about 10,000,000x whereas most light microscopes are limited by diffraction to about 200 nm resolution and useful magnifications below 2000x.

The transmission electron microscope uses electrostatic and electromagnetic lenses to control the electron beam and focus it to form an image. These electron optical lenses are analogous to the glass lenses of an optical light microscope.

Electron microscopes are used to investigate the ultrastructure of a wide range of biological and inorganic specimens including microorganisms, cells, large molecules, biopsy samples, metals, and crystals. Industrially, the electron microscope is often used for quality control and failure analysis. Modern electron microscopes produce electron micrographs using specialized digital cameras and frame grabbers to capture the image.

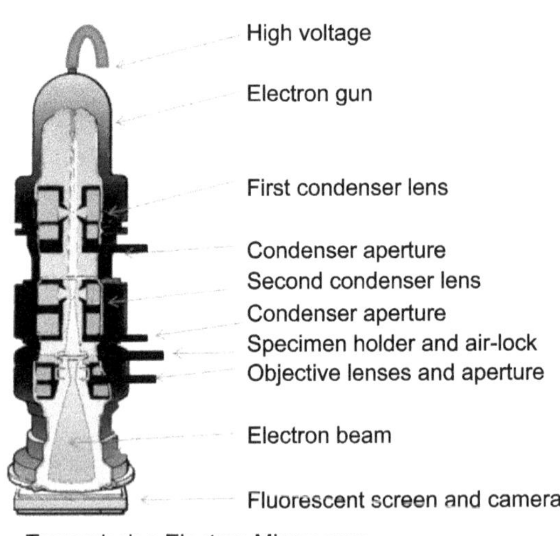

Figure 8.15: Transmission electron microscope

History

According to Dennis Gabor, the physicist Leó Szilárd tried in 1928 to convince Busch to build an electron microscope, for which he had filed a patent.

German physicist Ernst Ruska and the electrical engineer Max Knoll constructed the prototype electron microscope in 1931, capable of four-hundred-power magnification; the apparatus was the first demonstration of the principles of electron microscopy. Two years later, in 1933, Ruska built an electron microscope that exceeded the resolution attainable with an optical (light) microscope. Moreover, Reinhold Rudenberg, the scientific director of Siemens-Schuckertwerke, obtained the patent for the electron microscope in May 1931.

In 1932, Ernst Lubcke of Siemens & Halske built and obtained images from a prototype electron microscope, applying concepts described in the Rudenberg patent applications. Five years later (1937), the firm financed the work of Ernst Ruska and Bodo von Borries, and employed Helmut Ruska (Ernst's brother) to develop applications for the microscope, especially with biological specimens. Also in 1937, Manfred von Ardenne pioneered the scanning electron microscope. The first *practical* electron microscope was constructed in 1938, at the University of Toronto, by Eli Franklin Burton and students Cecil Hall, James Hillier, and Albert Prebus; and Siemens produced the first commercial transmission electron microscope (TEM) in 1939. Although contemporary electron microscopes are capable of two million-power magnification, as scientific instruments, they remain based upon Ruska's prototype.

Types

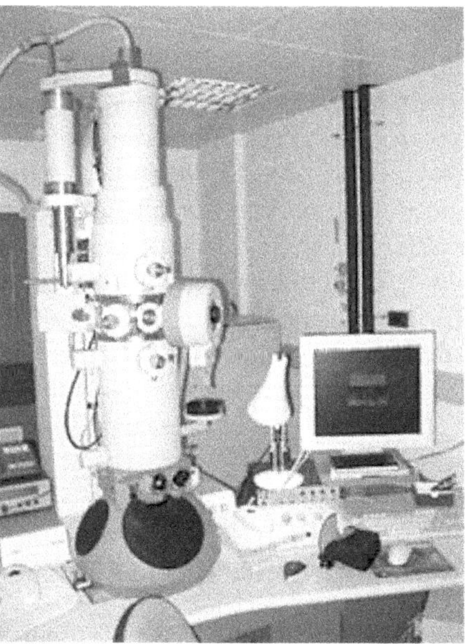

Figure 8.16: A modern transmission electron microscope

TRANSMISSION ELECTRON MICROSCOPE (TEM)

The original form of electron microscope, the transmission electron microscope (TEM) uses a high voltage electron beam to create an image. The electron beam is produced by an electron gun, commonly fitted with a tungsten filament cathode as the electron source. The electron beam is accelerated by an anode typically at +100 keV (40 to 400 keV) with respect to the cathode, focused by electrostatic andelectromagnetic lenses, and transmitted through the specimen that is in part transparent to electrons and in part scatters them out of the beam. When it emerges from the specimen, the electron beam carries information about the structure of the specimen that is magnified by the objective lens system of the microscope. The spatial variation in this information (the "image") may be viewed by projecting the magnified electron image onto a fluorescent viewing screen coated with a phosphor or scintillator material such as zinc sulfide. Alternatively, the image can be photographically recorded by exposing a photographic film or plate directly to the electron beam, or a high-resolution phosphor may be coupled by means of a lens optical system or a fibre optic light-guide to the sensor of a CCD (charge-coupled device) camera. The image detected by the CCD may be displayed on a monitor or computer.

Resolution of the TEM is limited primarily by spherical aberration, but a new generation of aberration correctors have been able to partially overcome spherical aberration to increase resolution. Hardware correction of spherical aberration for the high-resolution transmission electron microscopy (HRTEM) has allowed the production of images with resolution below 0.5 angstrom (50 picometres) and magnifications above 50 million times. The ability to determine the positions of atoms within materials has made the HRTEM an important tool for nano-technologies research and development.

An important mode of TEM utilization is electron diffraction. The advantages of electron diffraction over X-ray crystallography are that the specimen need not be a single crystal or even a polycrystalline powder, and also that the Fourier transform reconstruction of the object's magnified structure occurs physically and thus avoids the need for solving the phase problem faced by the X-ray crystallographers after obtaining their X-ray diffraction patterns of a single crystal or polycrystalline powder. The major disadvantage of the transmission electron microscope is the need for extremely thin sections of the specimens, typically about 100 nanometers. Biological specimens are typically required to be chemically fixed, dehydrated and embedded in a polymer resin to stabilize them sufficiently to allow ultrathin sectioning. Sections of biological specimens, organic polymers and similar materials may require special treatment with heavy atom labels in order to achieve the required image contrast.

SCANNING ELECTRON MICROSCOPE (SEM)

The SEM produces images by probing the specimen with a focused electron beam that is scanned across a rectangular area of the specimen (raster scanning). When the electron beam interacts with the specimen, it loses energy by a variety of mechanisms. The lost energy is converted into alternative forms such as heat, emission of low-energy secondary electrons and high-energy backscattered electrons, light emission (cathodoluminescence) or X-ray emission, all of which provide signals carrying information about the properties of the specimen surface, such as its topography and composition. The image displayed by an SEM maps the varying intensity of any of these signals into the image in a position corresponding to the position of the beam on the specimen when the signal was generated. In the SEM image of an ant shown at right, the image was constructed from signals produced by a secondary electron detector, the normal or conventional imaging mode in most SEMs.

Generally, the image resolution of an SEM is at least an order of magnitude poorer than that of a TEM. However, because the SEM image relies on surface processes rather than transmission, it is able to image bulk samples up to many centimetres in size and (depending on instrument design and settings) has a great depth of field, and so can produce images that are good representations of the three-dimensional shape of the sample. Another advantage of SEM is its variety called environmental scanning electron microscope (ESEM) can produce images of sufficient quality and resolution with the samples being wet or contained in low vacuum or gas. This greatly facilitates imaging biological samples that are unstable in the high vacuum of conventional electron microscopes.

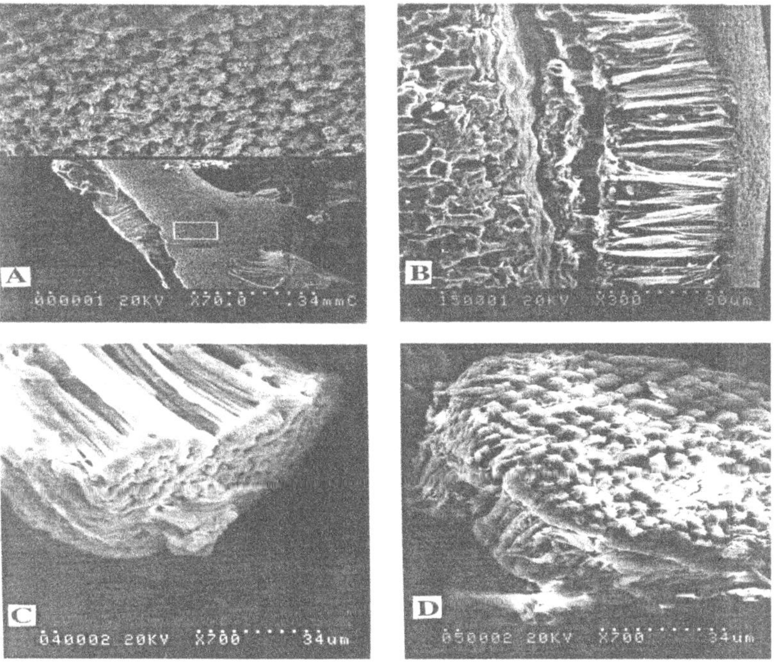

Figure 8.17: Scanning electron micrographs of beach pea seed coat structure (A: Seed coat structure; B: cross section of seed coat; C: after soaking 30 min in H_2SO_4 and then 12 h in distilled water and D: heat processing for 30 min).

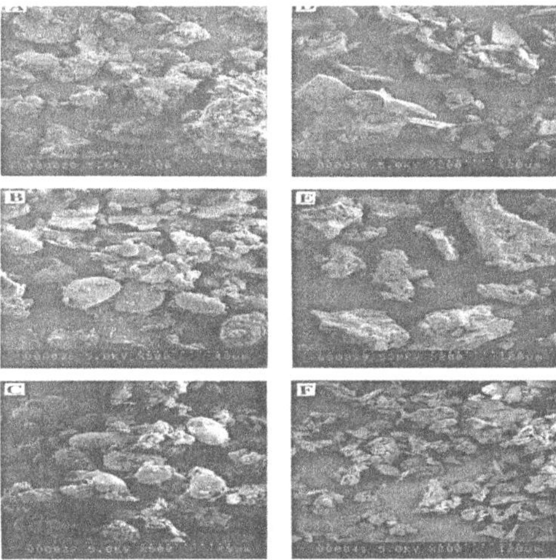

Figure 8.18: Scanning electron micrographs of beach pea flours and protein isolates (NaOH-extracted): A, beach pea flour; B, green pea flour; C, Canadian grass pea flour; D, beach pea protein isolates; E, green pea protein isolates and F, Canadian grass pea protein isolate.

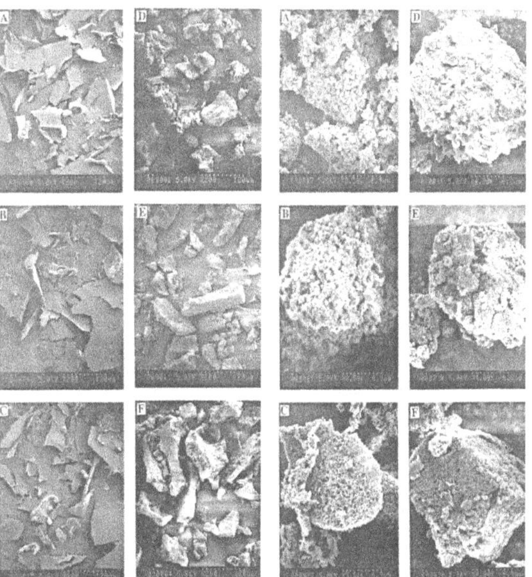

Figure 8.19: Scanning electron micrographs of beach pea protein fractions [**First plate**] (A, beach pea albumin; B, grass pea albumin; C, Canadian grass pea albumin; D, beach pea globulin: E, grass pea globulin and F, Canadian grass pea globulin).

[**Second plate**] (A, beach pea prolamine; B, grass pea prolamine; C, Canadian grass pea prolamine; D, beach pea glutelin: E, grass pea glutelin and F, Canadian grass pea glutelin).

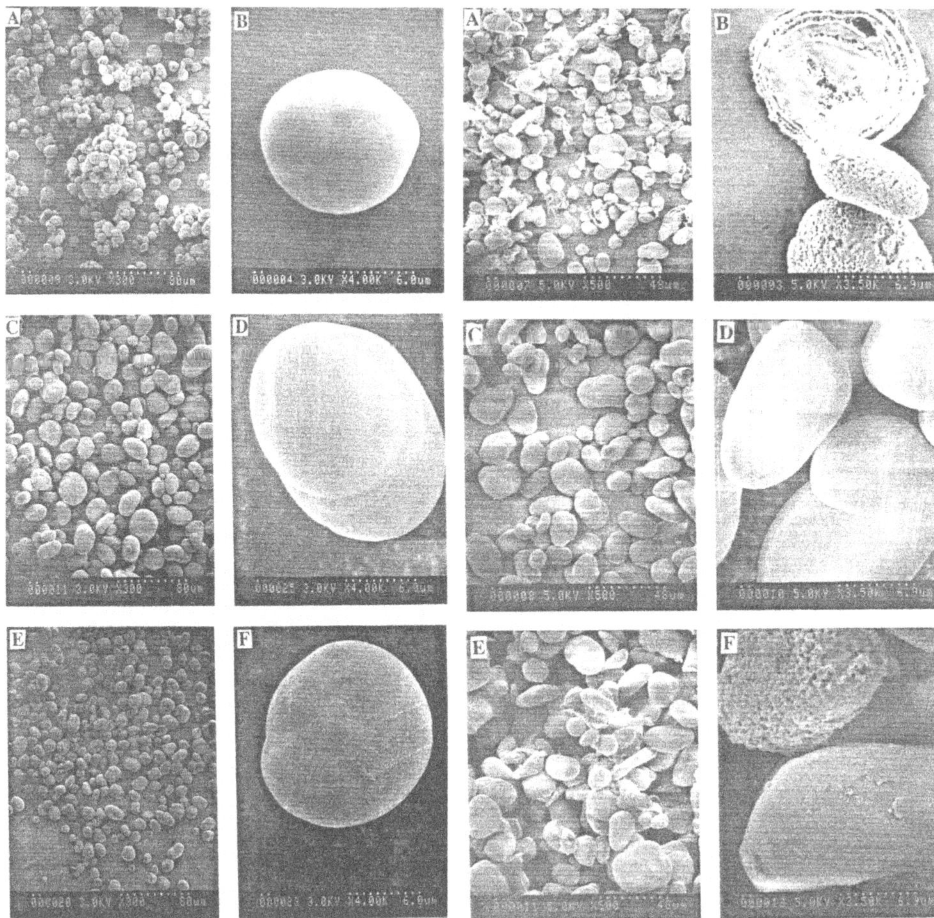

Figure 8.20: Scanning electron micrographs of legume starches: [**First plate**] (A) and (B) beach pea; (C) and (D) green pea and (E) and (F) Canadian grass pea.

[**Second plate**] Scanning electron micrographs of native and digested starches after 24 h attack by porcine pancreatic α-amylase: (A) and (B) beach pea; (C) and (D) green pea and (E) and (F) Canadian grass pea.

Colour

In their most common configurations, electron microscopes produce images with a single brightness value per pixel, with the results usually rendered in grayscale. However, often these images are then colourized through the use of feature-detection software, or simply by hand-editing using a graphics editor. This is usually for aesthetic effect or for clarifying structure, and generally does not add information about the specimen.

In some configurations more information about specimen properties is gathered per pixel, usually by the use of multiple detectors. In SEM, the attributes of topography and material contrast can be obtained by a pair of backscattered electron detectors and such attributes can be superimposed in a single colour image by assigning a different primary colour to each attribute. Similarly, a combination of backscattered and secondary electron signals can be assigned to different colours and superimposed on a single colour micrograph displaying simultaneously the properties of the specimen.

Some types of detectors used in SEM have analytical capabilities, and can provide several items of data at each pixel. Examples are the Energy-dispersive X-ray spectroscopy(EDS) detectors used in elemental analysis and Cathodoluminescence microscope (CL) systems that analyse the intensity and spectrum of electron-induced luminescence in (for example) geological specimens. In SEM systems using these detectors it is common to colour code the signals and superimpose them in a single colour image, so that differences in the distribution of the various components of the specimen can be seen clearly and compared. Optionally, the standard secondary electron image can be merged with the one or more compositional channels, so that the specimen's structure and composition can be compared. Such images can be made while maintaining the full integrity of the original signal, which is not modified in any way.

REFLECTION ELECTRON MICROSCOPE (REM)

In the reflection electron microscope (REM) as in the TEM, an electron beam is incident on a surface but instead of using the transmission (TEM) or secondary electrons (SEM), the reflected beam of elastically scattered electrons is detected. This technique is typically coupled with reflection high energy electron diffraction (RHEED) and reflection high-energy loss spectroscopy (RHELS). Another variation is spin-polarized low-energy electron microscopy (SPLEEM), which is used for looking at the microstructure ofmagnetic domains.

SCANNING TRANSMISSION ELECTRON MICROSCOPE (STEM)

The STEM rasters a focused incident probe across a specimen that (as with the TEM) has been thinned to facilitate detection of electrons scattered *through* the specimen. The high resolution of the TEM is thus possible in STEM. The focusing actions (and aberrations) occur before the electrons hit the specimen in the STEM, but afterward in the TEM. The STEMs use of SEM-like beam rastering simplifies annular dark-field imaging, and other analytical techniques, but also means that image data is acquired in serial rather than in parallel fashion. Often TEM can be equipped with the scanning option and then it can function both as TEM and STEM.

Sample Preparation

Materials to be viewed under an electron microscope may require processing to produce a suitable sample. The technique required varies depending on the specimen and the analysis required:

- *Chemical fixation:* For biological specimens aims to stabilize the specimen's mobile macromolecular structure by chemical crosslinking of proteins with aldehydes such as formaldehyde and glutaraldehyde, and lipids with osmium tetroxide.
- *Negative stain:* Suspensions containing nanoparticles or fine biological material (such as viruses and bacteria) are briefly mixed with a dilute solution of an electron-opaque solution such as ammonium molybdate, uranyl acetate (or formate), or phosphotungstic acid. This mixture is applied to a suitably coated EM grid, blotted, then allowed to dry. Viewing of this preparation in the TEM should be carried out without delay for best results. The method is important in microbiology for fast but crude morphological identification, but can also be used as the basis for high resolution 3D reconstruction using EM tomography methodology when carbon films are used for support. Negative staining is also used for observation of nanoparticles.
- *Cryofixation:* Freezing a specimen so rapidly, in liquid ethane, and maintained at liquid nitrogen or even liquid helium temperatures, so that the water forms vitreous (non-crystalline) ice. This preserves the specimen in a snapshot of its solution state. An entire field calledcryo-electron microscopy has branched from this technique. With the development of cryo-electron microscopy of vitreous sections(CEMOVIS), it is now possible to observe samples from virtually any biological specimen close to its native state.
- *Dehydration:* Or replacement of water with organic solvents such as ethanol or acetone, followed by critical point drying or infiltration with embedding resins. Also freeze drying.
- *Embedding, biological specimens:* After dehydration, tissue for observation in the transmission electron microscope is embedded so it can be sectioned ready for viewing. To do this the tissue is passed through a 'transition solvent' such as Propylene oxide (epoxypropane) and then infiltrated with an epoxy resin such as Araldite, Epon, orDurcupan; tissues may also be embedded directly in water-miscible acrylic resin. After the resin has been polymerized (hardened) the sample is thin sectioned (ultrathin sections) and stained – it is then ready for viewing.
- *Embedding, materials:* After embedding in resin, the specimen is usually ground and polished to a mirror-like finish using ultra-fine abrasives. The polishing process must be performed carefully to minimize scratches and other polishing artifacts that reduce image quality.

- *Metal shadowing*: Metal (e.g. platinum) is evaporated from an overhead electrode and applied to the surface of a biological sample at an angle. This is followed by a dissolution of the biological material in an acid bath leaving only the metallic surface replica intact. This metallic surface replica can then be examined using transmission electron microscopy. Variations in the thickness and angle of the metal surface allows an image to be formed since incident electrons will scatter in different directions rather than pass through it.
- *Sectioning:* Produces thin slices of specimen, semitransparent to electrons. These can be cut on an ultramicrotome with a diamond knife to produce ultra-thin slices about 60–90 nm thick. Disposable glass knives are also used because they can be made in the lab and are much cheaper.
- *Staining:* Uses heavy metals such as lead, uranium or tungsten to scatter imaging electrons and thus give contrast between different structures, since many (especially biological) materials are nearly "transparent" to electrons (weak phase objects). In biology, specimens can be stained "en bloc" before embedding and also later after sectioning. Typically thin sections are stained for several minutes with an aqueous or alcoholic solution of uranyl acetate followed by aqueous lead citrate.
- *Freeze-fracture or freeze-etch:* A preparation method particularly useful for examining lipid membranes and their incorporated proteins in "face on" view. The fresh tissue or cell suspension is frozen rapidly (cryofixation), then fractured by simply breaking or by using a microtome while maintained at liquid nitrogen temperature. The cold fractured surface (sometimes "etched" by increasing the temperature to about −100 °C for several minutes to let some ice sublime) is then shadowed with evaporated platinum or gold at an average angle of 45° in a high vacuum evaporator. A second coat of carbon, evaporated perpendicular to the average surface plane is often performed to improve stability of the replica coating. The specimen is returned to room temperature and pressure, and then the extremely fragile "pre-shadowed" metal replica of the fracture surface is released from the underlying biological material by careful chemical digestion with acids, hypochlorite solution or SDS detergent. The still-floating replica is thoroughly washed free from residual chemicals, carefully fished up on fine grids, dried then viewed in the TEM.
- *Ion beam milling:* Thins samples until they are transparent to electrons by firing ions (typically argon) at the surface from an angle and sputtering material from the surface. A subclass of this is focused ion beam milling, where gallium ions are used to produce an electron transparent membrane in a specific region of the sample, for example through a device within a microprocessor. Ion beam milling may also be used for cross-section polishing prior to SEM analysis of materials that are difficult to prepare using mechanical polishing.

- *Conductive coatings*: An ultrathin coating of electrically conducting material deposited either by high vacuum evaporation or by low vacuum sputters coating of the sample. This is done to prevent the accumulation of static electric fields at the specimen due to the electron irradiation required during imaging. The coating materials include gold, gold/palladium, platinum, tungsten, graphite, etc.
- *Earthing:* To avoid electrical charge accumulation on a conductive coated sample, it is usually electrically connected to the metal sample holder. Often an electrically conductive adhesive is used for this purpose.

Disadvantages

Electron microscopes are expensive to build and maintain, but the capital and running costs of confocal light microscope systems now overlaps with those of basic electron microscopes. Microscopes designed to achieve high resolutions must be housed in stable buildings (sometimes underground) with special services such as magnetic field cancelling systems.

The samples largely have to be viewed in vacuum, as the molecules that make up air would scatter the electrons. One exception is the environmental scanning electron microscope, which allows hydrated samples to be viewed in a low-pressure (up to 20 Torr or 2.7 kPa) and/or wet environment.

Scanning electron microscopes operating in conventional high-vacuum mode usually image conductive specimens; therefore non-conductive materials require conductive coating (gold/palladium alloy, carbon, osmium, etc.). The low-voltage mode of modern microscopes makes possible the observation of non-conductive specimens without coating. Non-conductive materials can be imaged also by a variable pressure (or environmental) scanning electron microscope.

Small, stable specimens such as carbon nanotubes, diatom frustules and small mineral crystals (asbestos fibres, for example) require no special treatment before being examined in the electron microscope. Samples of hydrated materials, including almost all biological specimens have to be prepared in various ways to stabilize them, reduce their thickness (ultrathin sectioning) and increase their electron optical contrast (staining). These processes may result in *artifacts*, but these can usually be identified by comparing the results obtained by using radically different specimen preparation methods. It is generally believed by scientists working in the field that as results from various preparation techniques have been compared and that there is no reason that they should all produce similar artifacts, it is reasonable to believe that electron microscopy features correspond with those of living cells. Since the 1980s, analysis of cry fixed, vitrified specimens has also become increasingly used by scientists, further confirming the validity of this technique.

Applications

• **Semiconductor and data storage**	**Materials research**
• Circuit edit	• Electron beam-induced deposition
• Defect analysis	• Materials qualification
• Failure analysis	• Medical research
• **Biology and life sciences**	• Nanoprototyping
• Diagnostic electron microscopy	• Nanometrology
• Cryobiology	• Device testing and characterization
• Protein localization	**Industry**
• Electron tomography	• High-resolution imaging
• Cryo-electron microscopy	• 2D & 3D micro-characterization
• Toxicology	• Macro sample to nanometer metrology
• Biological production and viral load monitoring	• Particle detection and characterization
	• Direct beam-writing fabrication
• Particle analysis	• Dynamic materials experiments
• Pharmaceutical QC	• Sample preparation
• Structural biology	• Forensics
• 3D tissue imaging	• Mining (mineral liberation analysis)
• Virology	• Chemical/Petrochemical
• Vitrification	• Fractography and failure analysis

6. RADIATION

In physics, radiation is the emission or transmission of energy in the form of waves or particles through space or through a material medium. This includes electromagnetic radiation such as radio waves, visible light, and x-rays, particle radiation such as α, β, and neutron radiation and acoustic radiation such as ultrasound, sound, and seismic waves. Radiation may also refer to the energy, waves, or particles being radiated.

Radiation is often categorized as either ionizing or non-ionizing depending on the energy of the radiated particles. Ionizing radiation carries more than 10 eV, which is enough to ionize atoms and molecules, and break chemical bonds. This is an important distinction due to the large difference in harmfulness to living organisms. A common source of ionizing radiation is radioactive materials that emit α, β, or γ radiation, consisting of helium nuclei, electrons or positrons, and photons, respectively. Other sources include X-rays from medical radiography examinations and muons, mesons, positrons, neutrons and other particles that constitute the secondary cosmic rays that are produced after primary cosmic rays interact with Earth's atmosphere.

Gamma rays, X-rays and the higher energy range of ultraviolet light constitute the ionizing part of the electromagnetic spectrum. The lower-energy, longer-wavelength part of the spectrum including visible light, infrared light, microwaves, and radio waves is all non-ionizing, that mainly cause heating when interacting with tissue. This means that the much higher intensities required to cause excessive heating are needed to damage cells. Ultraviolet radiation has some features of both ionizing and non-ionizing radiation. Although the part of the ultraviolet spectrum that penetrates the Earth's atmosphere is non-ionizing, this radiation does far more damage to many molecules in biological systems than can be accounted for by heating effects, with sunburn being a well-known example. These properties derive from ultraviolet's power to alter chemical bonds, even without having quite enough energy to ionize atoms.

The word radiation arises from the phenomenon of waves radiating (i.e., traveling outward in all directions) from a source. This aspect leads to a system of measurements and physical units that are applicable to all types of radiation. Because such radiation expands as it passes through space, and as its energy is conserved (in vacuum), the intensity of all types of radiation radiating from a point source follows an inverse-square law in relation to the distance from its source. This law does not apply close to an extended source of radiation or for focused beams.

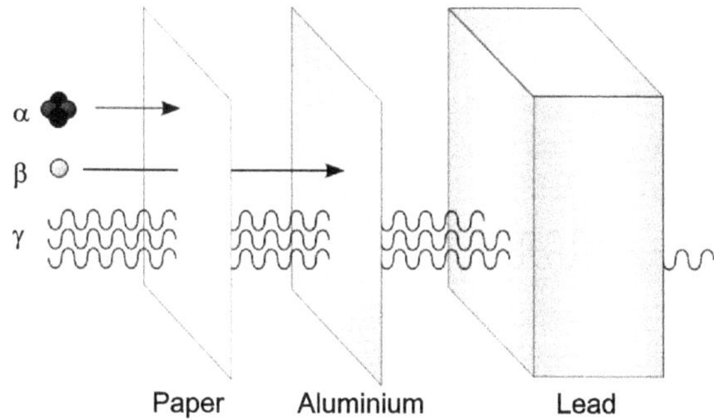

Figure 8.21: Illustration of the relative abilities of three different types of ionizing radiation to penetrate solid matter. Typical alpha particles (α) are stopped by a sheet of paper, while beta particles (β) are stopped by an aluminium plate. Gamma radiation (γ) is damped when it penetrates lead.

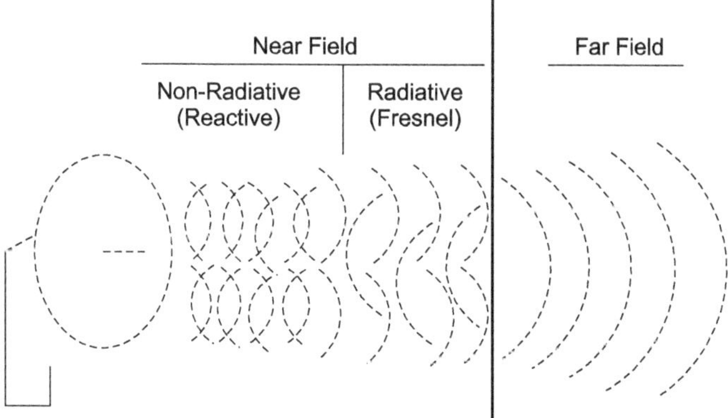

In electromagnetic radiation (such as microwaves from an antenna, shown here) the term "radiation" applies only to the parts of the electromagnetic field that radiate into infinite space and decrease in intensity by an inverse-square law of power so that the total radiation energy that crosses through an imaginary spherical surface is the same, no matter how far away from the antenna the spherical surface is drawn.Electromagnetic radiation includes the far field part of the electromagnetic field around a transmitter. A part of the "near-field" close to the transmitter, is part of the changing electromagnetic field, but does not count as electromagnetic radiation.

Ionizing Radiation

Radiation with sufficiently high energy can ionize atoms; that is to say it can knock electrons off atoms and create ions, as well as lower-energy damage by breaking chemical bonds within molecules. Ionization occurs when an electron is stripped (or "knocked out") from an electron shell of the atom, which leaves the atom with a net positive charge. Because living cells and, more importantly, the DNA in those cells can be damaged by this ionization, exposure to ionizing radiation is considered to increase the risk of cancer. Thus "ionizing radiation" is somewhat artificially separated from particle radiation and electromagnetic radiation, simply due to its great potential for biological damage. While an individual cell is made of trillions of atoms, only a small fraction of those will be ionized at low to moderate radiation powers. The probability of ionizing radiation causing cancer is dependent upon the absorbed dose of the radiation, and is a function of the damaging tendency of the type of radiation (equivalent dose) and the sensitivity of the irradiated organism or the tissue's (effective dose).

If the source of the ionizing radiation is a radioactive material or a nuclear process such as fission or fusion, there is also particle radiation to consider. Particle radiation issubatomic particles accelerated to relativistic speeds by nuclear reactions. Because of their momenta they are also quite capable of knocking out electrons and ionizing materials, but since most have an electrical charge, they don't have the penetrating power of ionizing radiation. The exception is neutron particles; see below. There are several different kinds of these particles, but the majority are alpha particles, beta particles, neutrons, and protons. Roughly speaking, photons and particles with energies above about 10 electron volts (eV) are ionizing (some authorities use 33 eV, the ionization energy for water). Particle radiation from radioactive material or cosmic rays almost invariably carries enough energy to be ionizing.

Much ionizing radiation originates from radioactive materials and space (cosmic rays), and as such is naturally present in the environment, since most rock and soil has small concentrations of radioactive materials. The radiation is invisible and not directly detectable by human senses; as a result, instruments such as Geiger counters are usually required to detect its presence. In some cases, it may lead to secondary emission of visible light upon its interaction with matter, as in the case of Cherenkov radiation and radio-luminescence. Ionizing radiation has many practical uses in medicine, research and construction, but presents a health hazard if used improperly. Exposure to radiation causes damage to living tissue; high doses result in Acute radiation syndrome (ARS), with skin burns, hair loss, internal organ failure and death, while any dose may result in an increased chance of cancer and genetic damage; a particular form of cancer, thyroid cancer, often occurs when nuclear weapons and reactors are the radiation source because of the biological proclivities of the radioactive iodine fission product, iodine-131. However, calculating the exact risk and chance of cancer forming in cells caused by ionizing radiation is still not well understood and currently estimates are loosely determined by population based on data from the atomic bombing in Japan and from reactor accident follow-up, such as with the Chernobyl disaster. The International Commission on Radiological Protection states that "The Commission is aware of uncertainties and lack of precision of the models and parameter values", "Collective effective dose is not intended as a tool for epidemiological risk assessment, and it is inappropriate to use it in risk projections" and "in particular, the calculation of the number of cancer deaths based on collective effective doses from trivial individual doses should be avoided."

Ultraviolet Radiation

Ultraviolet of wavelengths from 10 nm to 125 nm ionizes air molecules, and this interaction causes it to be strongly absorbed by air, ozone (O_3) in particular. Ionizing UV therefore does not penetrate Earth's atmosphere to a significant degree, and is sometimes referred to as vacuum ultraviolet. Although present in space, this part of the UV spectrum is not of biological importance, because it does not reach living organisms on Earth.

There is a zone of the atmosphere in which ozone absorbs some 98% of non-ionizing but dangerous UV-C and UV-B. This so-called ozone layer, starts at about 20 miles (32 km) and extends upward. Some of the ultraviolet spectrum that does reach the ground (the part that begins above energies of 3.1 eV, a wavelength less than 400 nm) is non-ionizing, but is still biologically hazardous due to the ability of single photons of this energy to cause electronic excitation in biological molecules, and thus damage them by means of unwanted reactions. An example is the formation of pyrimidine dimers in DNA, which begins at wavelengths below 365 nm (3.4 eV), which is well below ionization energy. This property gives the ultraviolet spectrum some of the dangers of ionizing radiation in biological systems without actual ionization occurring. In contrast, visible light and longer-wavelength electromagnetic radiation, such as infrared, microwaves, and radio waves, consists of photons with too little energy to cause damaging molecular excitation, and thus this radiation is far less hazardous per unit of energy.

X-Ray

X-rays are electromagnetic waves with a wavelength less than about 10^{-9} m (greater than 3×10^{17} Hz and 1,240 eV). A smaller wavelength corresponds to a higher energy according to the equation $E=hc/\lambda$. ("E" is Energy; "h" is Planck's constant; "c" is the speed of light; "λ" is wavelength.) When an X-ray photon collides with an atom, the atom may absorb the energy of the photon and boost an electron to a higher orbital level or if the photon is very energetic, it may knock an electron from the atom altogether, causing the atom to ionize. Generally, larger atoms are more likely to absorb an X-ray photon since they have greater energy differences between orbital electrons. Soft tissue in the human body is composed of smaller atoms than the calcium atoms that make up bone, hence there is a contrast in the absorption of X-rays. X-ray machines are specifically designed to take advantage of the absorption difference between bone and soft tissue, allowing physicians to examine structure in the human body.

X-rays are also totally absorbed by the thickness of the earth's atmosphere, resulting in the prevention of the X-ray output of the sun, smaller in quantity than that of UV but nonetheless powerful, from reaching the surface.

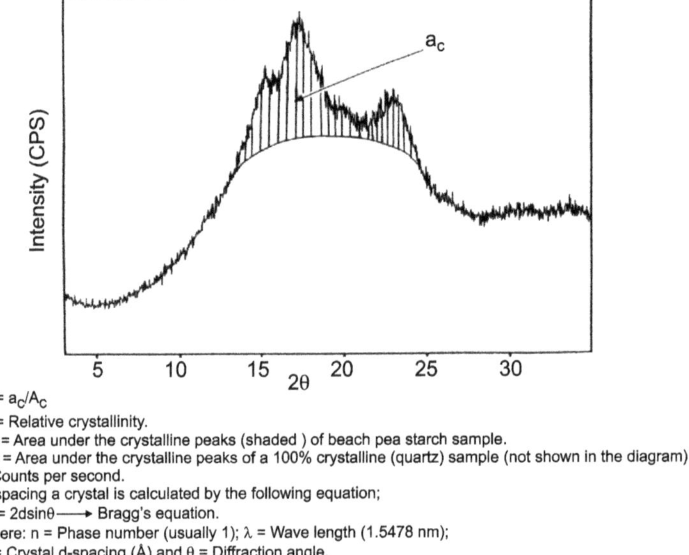

Figure 8.22: X-ray diffractogram for measurement of relative crystallinity of starch recorded by X-ray diffractometer.

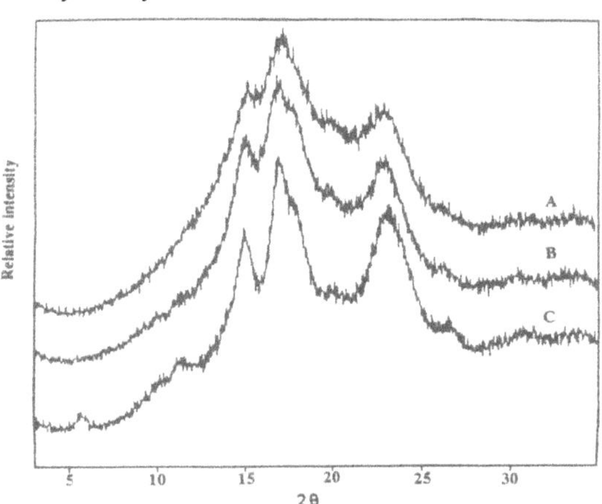

Figure 8.23: X-ray diffraction patterns of (A) beach pea starch; (B) Canadian grass pea starch and (C) green pea starch.

Gamma Radiation

Gamma (γ) radiation consists of photons with a wavelength less than $3x10,^{-11}$ meters (greater than 10^{19} Hz and 41.4 keV). Gamma radiation emission is a nuclear process that occurs to rid an unstable nucleus of excess energy after most nuclear reactions. Both alpha and beta particles have an electric charge and mass, and thus are quite likely to interact with other atoms in their path. Gamma radiation, however, is composed of photons, which have neither mass nor electric charge and, as a result, penetrates much further through matter than either alpha or beta radiation.

Gamma rays can be stopped by a sufficiently thick or dense layer of material, where the stopping power of the material per given area depends mostly (but not entirely) on the total mass along the path of the radiation, regardless of whether the material is of high or low density. However, as is the case with X-rays, materials with high atomic number such as lead or depleted uranium add a modest (typically 20% to 30%) amount of stopping power over an equal mass of less dense and lower atomic weight materials (such as water or concrete). The atmosphere absorbs all gamma rays approaching Earth from space. Even air is capable of absorbing gamma rays, halving the energy of such waves by passing through, on the average, 500 ft (150 m).

Alpha Radiation

Alpha particles are helium-4 nuclei (two protons and two neutrons). They interact with matter strongly due to their charges and combined mass, and at their usual velocities only penetrate a few centimeters of air, or a few millimeters of low density material (such as the thin mica material which is specially placed in some Geiger counter tubes to allow alpha particles in). This means that alpha particles from ordinary alpha decay do not penetrate the outer layers of dead skin cells and cause no damage to the live tissues below. Some very high energy alpha particles compose about 10% of cosmic rays, and these are capable of penetrating the body and even thin metal plates. However, they are of danger only to astronauts, since they are deflected by the Earth's magnetic field and then stopped by its atmosphere.

Alpha radiation is dangerous when alpha-emitting radioisotopes are ingested (breathed or swallowed). This brings the radioisotope close enough to sensitive live tissue for the alpha radiation to damage cells. Per unit of energy, alpha particles are at least 20 times more effective at cell-damage as gamma rays and X-rays. See relative biological effectiveness for a discussion of this. Examples of highly poisonous α-emitters are all isotopes of radium, radon, and polonium, due to the amount of decay that occur in these short half-life materials.

Beta Radiation

Beta-minus (β^-) radiation consists of an energetic electron. It is more penetrating than alpha radiation, but less than gamma. Beta radiation from radioactive decay can be stopped with a few centimeters of plastic or a few millimeters of metal. It occurs when a neutron decays into a proton in a nucleus, releasing the beta particle and an antineutrino. Beta radiation from linac accelerators is far more energetic and penetrating than natural beta radiation. It is sometimes used therapeutically in radiotherapy to treat superficial tumors.

Beta-plus (β^+) radiation is the emission of positrons, which are the antimatter form of electrons. When a positron slows down to speeds similar to those of electrons in the material, the positron will annihilate an electron, releasing two gamma photons of 511 keV in the process. Those two gamma photons will be traveling in (approximately) opposite direction. The gamma radiation from positron annihilation consists of high energy photons, and is also ionizing.

Neutron Radiation

Neutrons are categorized according to their speed/energy. Neutron radiation consists of free neutrons. These neutrons may be emitted during either spontaneous or inducednuclear fission. Neutrons are rare radiation particles; they result in large amounts only where chain reaction fission or fusion reactions are active; this happens for about 10 microseconds in a thermonuclear explosion, or continuously inside an operating nuclear reactor; the neutrons stop almost immediately in the reactor when it goes non-critical.

Neutrons are the only type of ionizing radiation that can make other objects, or material, radioactive. This process, called neutron activation, is the primary method used to produce radioactive sources for use in medical, academic, and industrial applications. Even comparatively low speed thermal neutrons, will cause neutron activation (in fact, they cause it more efficiently). Neutrons do not ionize atoms in the same way that charged particles such as protons and electrons do (by the excitation of an electron), because neutrons have no charge. It is through their absorption by and the creation of unstable nuclei that they cause ionization. Such neutrons are "indirectly ionizing." Even neutrons without significant kinetic energy are indirectly ionizing, and are thus a significant radiation hazard. Not all materials are capable of neutron activation; in water, for example, both of the normal atoms present will capture neutrons and become heavier but still stable forms of those atoms. Only the absorption of more than one neutron, a statistically rare occurrence, can activate a hydrogen atom, while oxygen requires two additional absorptions. Thus water is only very weakly capable of activation. The sodium in salt (as in sea water), on the other hand, need only absorb a single neutron to become Na-24, a very intense source of beta decay, with half-life of 15 hours.

In addition, high-energy (high-speed) neutrons have the ability to directly ionize atoms. One mechanism by which high energy neutrons ionize atoms is to strike the nucleus of an atom and knock the atom out of a molecule, leaving one or more electrons behind as the chemical bond is broken. This leads to production of chemical free radicals. In addition, very high energy neutrons can cause ionizing radiation by "neutron spallation" or knockout, wherein neutrons cause emission of high-energy protons from atomic nuclei (especially hydrogen nuclei) on impact. The last process imparts most of the neutron's energy to the proton, much like one billiard ball striking another. The charged protons, and other products from such reactions are directly ionizing.

High-energy neutrons are very penetrating and can travel great distances in air (hundreds or even thousands of meters) and moderate distances (several meters) in common solids. They typically require hydrogen rich shielding, such as concrete or water, to block them within distances of less than a meter. A common source of neutron radiation occurs inside a nuclear reactor, where a meters-thick water layer is used as effective shielding.

Cosmic Radiation

There are two sources of high energy particles entering the Earth's atmosphere from outer space: the sun and deep space. The sun continuously emits particles, primarily free protons, in the solar wind, and occasionally augments the flow hugely with coronal mass ejections (CME).

The particles from deep space (inter- and extra-galactic) are much less frequent, but of much higher energies. These particles are also mostly protons, with much of the remainder consisting of helions (alpha particles). A few completely ionized nuclei of heavier elements are present. The origin of these galactic cosmic rays is not yet well understood, but they seem to be remnants of supernovae and especially gamma-ray bursts (GRB), which feature magnetic fields capable of the huge accelerations measured from these particles. They may also be generated by quasars, which are galaxy-wide jet phenomena similar to GRBs but for their much larger size, and which seem to be violent part of the universe's early history.

Non-Ionizing Radiation

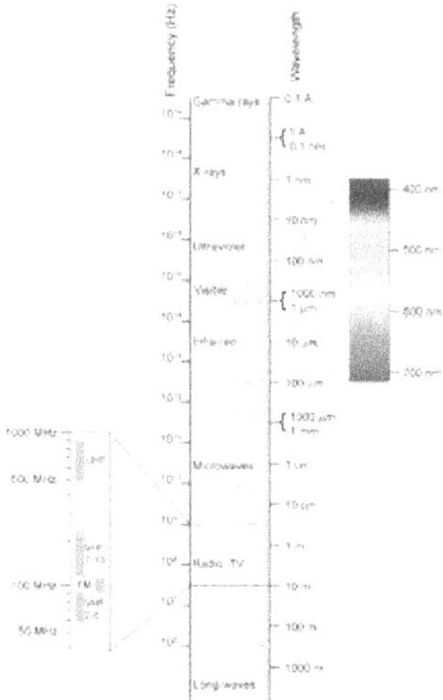

Figure 8.24: The electromagnetic spectrum

The kinetic energy of particles of non-ionizing radiation is too small to produce charged ions when passing through matter. For non-ionizing electromagnetic radiation (see types below), the associated particles (photons) have only sufficient energy to change the rotational, vibrational or electronic valence configurations of molecules and atoms. The effect of non-ionizing forms of radiation on living tissue has only recently been studied. Nevertheless, different biological effects are observed for different types of non-ionizing radiation.

Even "non-ionizing" radiation is capable of causing thermal-ionization if it deposits enough heat to raise temperatures to ionization energies. These reactions occur at far higher energies than with ionization radiation, which requires only single particles to cause ionization. A familiar example of thermal ionization is the flame-ionization of a common fire, and the browning reactions in common food items induced by infrared radiation, during broiling-type cooking.

The electromagnetic spectrum is the range of all possible electromagnetic radiation frequencies. The electromagnetic spectrum (usually just spectrum) of an object is the characteristic distribution of electromagnetic radiation emitted by, or absorbed by, that particular object.

The non-ionizing portion of electromagnetic radiation consists of electromagnetic waves that (as individual quanta or particles) are not energetic enough to detach electrons from atoms or molecules and hence cause their ionization. These include radio waves, microwaves, infrared, and (sometimes) visible light. The lower frequencies of ultraviolet light may cause chemical changes and molecular damage similar to ionization, but is technically not ionizing. The highest frequencies of ultraviolet light, as well as all X-rays and gamma-rays are ionizing.

The occurrence of ionization depends on the energy of the individual particles or waves, and not on their number. An intense flood of particles or waves will not cause ionization if these particles or waves do not carry enough energy to be ionizing, unless they raise the temperature of a body to a point high enough to ionize small fractions of atoms or molecules by the process of thermal-ionization (this, however, requires relatively extreme radiation intensities).

Ultraviolet Light

As noted above, the lower part of the spectrum of ultraviolet, called soft UV, from 3 eV to about 10 eV, is non-ionizing. However, the effects of non-ionizing ultraviolet on chemistry and the damage to biological systems exposed to it (including oxidation, mutation, and cancer) are such that even this part of ultraviolet is often compared with ionizing radiation.

Visible Light

Light, or visible light, is a very narrow range of electromagnetic radiation of a wavelength that is visible to the human eye, or 380–750 nm which equates to a frequency range of 790 to 400 THz respectively. More broadly, physicists use the term "light" to mean electromagnetic radiation of all wavelengths, whether visible or not.

Infrared

Infrared (IR) light is electromagnetic radiation with a wavelength between 0.7 and 300 micrometers, which corresponds to a frequency range between 430 to 1 THz respectively. IR wavelengths are longer than that of visible light, but shorter than that of microwaves. Infrared may be detected at a distance from the radiating objects by "feel." Infrared sensing snakes can detect and focus infrared by use of a pinhole lens in their heads, called "pits". Bright sunlight provides an irradiance of just over 1 kilowatt per square meter at sea level. Of this energy, 53% is infrared radiation, 44% is visible light, and 3% is ultraviolet radiation.

Microwave

Microwaves are electromagnetic waves with wavelengths ranging from as short as one millimeter to as long as one meter, which equates to a frequency range of 300 GHz to 300 MHz. This broad definition includes both UHF and EHF (millimeter waves), but various sources use different other limits. In all cases, microwaves include the entire super high frequency band (3 to 30 GHz, or 10 to 1 cm) at minimum, with RF engineering often putting the lower boundary at 1 GHz (30 cm), and the upper around 100 GHz (3mm).

Radio Waves

Radio waves are a type of electromagnetic radiation with wavelengths in the electromagnetic spectrum longer than infrared light. Like all other electromagnetic waves, they travel at the speed of light. Naturally occurring radio waves are made by lightning, or by certain astronomical objects. Artificially generated radio waves are used for fixed and mobile radio communication, broadcasting, radar and other navigation systems, satellite communication, computer networks and innumerable other applications. In addition, almost any wire carrying alternating current will radiate some of the energy away as radio waves; these are mostly termed interference. Different frequencies of radio waves have different propagation characteristics in the Earth's atmosphere; long waves may bend at the rate of the curvature of the Earth and may cover a part of the Earth very consistently, shorter waves travel around the world by multiple reflections off the ionosphere and the Earth. Much shorter wavelengths bend or reflect very little and travel along the line of sight.

Very Low Frequency

Very low frequency (VLF) refers to a frequency range of 30 Hz to 3 kHz which corresponds to wavelengths of 100,000 to 10,000 meters respectively. Since there is not much bandwidth in this range of the radio spectrum, only the very simplest signals can be transmitted, such as for radio navigation. Also known as the myriameter band or myriameter wave as the wavelengths range from ten to one myriameter (an obsolete metric unit equal to 10 kilometers).

Extremely Low Frequency

Extremely low frequency (ELF) is radiation frequencies from 3 to 30 Hz (10^8 to 10^7 meters respectively). In atmosphere science, an alternative definition is usually given, from 3 Hz to 3 kHz. In the related magnetosphere science, the lower frequency electromagnetic oscillations (pulsations occurring below ~3 Hz) are considered to lie in the ULF range, which is thus also defined differently from the ITU Radio Bands. A massive military ELF antenna in Michigan radiates very slow messages to otherwise unreachable receivers, such as submerged submarines.

Thermal Radiation (Heat)

Thermal radiation is a common synonym for infrared radiation emitted by objects at temperatures often encountered on Earth. Thermal radiation refers not only to the radiation itself, but also the process by which the surface of an object radiates its thermal energy in the form black body radiation. Infrared or red radiation from a common household radiator or electric heater is an example of thermal radiation, as is the heat emitted by an operating incandescent light bulb. Thermal radiation is generated when energy from the movement of charged particles within atoms is converted to electromagnetic radiation.

As noted above, even low-frequency thermal radiation may cause temperature-ionization whenever it deposits sufficient thermal energy to raises temperatures to a high enough level. Common examples of this are the ionization (plasma) seen in common flames, and the molecular changes caused by the "browning" during food-cooking, which is a chemical process that begins with a large component of ionization.

Black-Body Radiation

Black-body radiation is an idealized spectrum of radiation emitted by a body that is at a uniform temperature. The shape of the spectrum and the total amount of energy emitted by the body is a function the absolute temperature of the body. The radiation emitted covers the entire electromagnetic spectrum and the intensity of the radiation (power/unit-area) at a given frequency is described by Planck's law of radiation. For a given temperature of a black-body there is some frequency at which the maximum amount of radiation is emitted. That maximum radiation frequency moves toward higher frequencies as the temperature of the body increases. The frequency at which the black body radiation is at maximum is given by Wien's displacement law and is a function of the body's absolute temperature. A black-body is one that emits at any temperature the maximum possible amount of radiation at any given wavelength. A black-body will also absorb the maximum possible incident radiation at any given wavelength. A black-body with a temperature at or below room temperature would thus appear absolutely black, as it would not reflect any incident light nor would it emit enough radiation at visible wavelengths for our eyes to detect. Theoretically, a black-body emits electromagnetic radiation over the entire spectrum from very low frequency radio waves to x-rays, creating a continuum of radiation.

The colour of a radiating black-body tells the temperature of its radiating surface. It is responsible for the colour of stars, which vary from infrared through red (2,500K), to yellow (5,800K), to white and to blue-white (15,000K) as the peak radiance passes through those points in the visible spectrum. When the peak is below the visible spectrum the body is black, while when it is above the body is blue-white, since all the visible colours are represented from blue decreasing to red.

Discovery

Electromagnetic radiations of wavelengths other than visible light were discovered in the early 19th century. The discovery of infrared radiation is ascribed to William Herschel, the astronomer. Herschel published his results in 1800 before the Royal Society of London. Herschel, like Ritter, used a prism to refract light from the Sun and detected the infrared (beyond the red part of the spectrum), through an increase in the temperature recorded by a thermometer.

In 1801, the German physicist Johann Wilhelm Ritter made the discovery of ultraviolet by noting that the rays from a prism darkened silver chloride preparations more quickly than violet light. Ritter's experiments were an early precursor to what would become photography. Ritter noted that the UV rays were capable of causing chemical reactions.

The first radio waves detected were not from a natural source, but were produced deliberately and artificially by the German scientist Heinrich Hertz in 1887, using electrical circuits calculated to produce oscillations in the radio frequency range, following formulas suggested by the equations of James Clerk Maxwell.

Wilhelm Röntgen discovered and named X-rays. While experimenting with high voltages applied to an evacuated tube on 8 November 1895, he noticed a fluorescence on a nearby plate of coated glass. Within a month, he discovered the main properties of X-rays that we understand to this day.

In 1896, Henri Becquerel found that rays emanating from certain minerals penetrated black paper and caused fogging of an unexposed photographic plate. His doctoral student Marie Curie discovered that only certain chemical elements gave off these rays of energy. She named this behaviour radioactivity.

Alpha rays (alpha particles) and beta rays (beta particles) were differentiated by Ernest Rutherford through simple experimentation in 1899. Rutherford used a generic pitchblende radioactive source and determined that the rays produced by the source had differing penetrations in materials. One type had short penetration (it was stopped by paper) and a positive charge, which Rutherford named *alpha rays.* The other was more penetrating (able to expose film through paper but not metal) and had a negative charge, and this type Rutherford named *beta.* This was the radiation that had been first detected by Becquerel from uranium salts. In 1900, the French scientist Paul Villard discovered a third neutrally charged and especially penetrating type of radiation from radium, and after he described it, Rutherford realized it must be yet a third type of radiation, which in 1903 Rutherford named gamma rays.

Henri Becquerel himself proved that beta rays are fast electrons, while Rutherford and Thomas Royds proved in 1909 that alpha particles are ionized helium. Rutherford and Edward Andrade proved in 1914 that gamma rays are like X-rays, but with shorter wavelengths.

Cosmic ray radiations striking the Earth from outer space were finally definitively recognized and proven to exist in 1912, as the scientist Victor Hess carried an electrometer to various altitudes in a free balloon flight. The nature of these radiations was only gradually understood in later years.

Neutron radiation was discovered with the neutron by Chadwick, in 1932. A number of other high energy particulate radiations such as positrons, muons, and pions were discovered by cloud chamber examination of cosmic ray reactions shortly thereafter, and others types of particle radiation were produced artificially in particle accelerators, through the last half of the twentieth century.

Uses

Medicine

Radiation and radioactive substances are used for diagnosis, treatment, and research. X-rays, for example, pass through muscles and other soft tissue but are stopped by dense materials. This property of X-rays enables doctors to find broken bones and to locate cancers that might be growing in the body. Doctors also find certain diseases by injecting a radioactive substance and monitoring the radiation given off as the substance moves through the body. Radiation used for cancer treatment is called ionizing radiation because it forms ions in the cells of the tissues it passes through as it dislodges electrons from atoms. This can kill cells or change genes so the cells cannot grow. Other forms of radiation such as radio waves, microwaves, and light waves are called non-ionizing. They don't have as much energy and are not able to ionize cells.

Communication

All modern communication systems use forms of electromagnetic radiation. Variations in the intensity of the radiation represent changes in the sound, pictures, or other information being transmitted. For example, a human voice can be sent as a radio wave or microwave by making the wave vary to correspond variations in the voice. Musicians have also experimented with gamma sonification, or using nuclear radiation, to produce sound and music.

Science

Researchers use radioactive atoms to determine the age of materials that were once part of a living organism. The age of such materials can be estimated by measuring the amount of radioactive carbon they contain in a process called radiocarbon dating. Similarly, using other radioactive elements, the age of rocks and other geological features (even some man-made objects) can be determined; this is called Radiometric dating. Environmental scientists use radioactive atoms, known as tracer atoms, to identify the pathways taken by pollutants through the environment.

Radiation is used to determine the composition of materials in a process called neutron activation analysis. In this process, scientists bombard a sample of a substance with particles called neutrons. Some of the atoms in the sample absorb neutrons and become radioactive. The scientists can identify the elements in the sample by studying the emitted radiation.

Food Irradiation

Food irradiation is the process of exposing foodstuffs to ionizing radiation, energy that is transmitted to the food without direct contact capable of stripping electrons from the food.

This treatment is used to preserve food, reduce the risk of food borne illness, prevent the spread of invasive pests, and delay or eliminate sprouting or ripening. The radiation can be emitted by a radioactive substance or generated electrically. Irradiated food does not become radioactive. Food irradiation is permitted by over 60 countries, with about 500,000 metric tons of foodstuffs annually processed worldwide. Irradiation is also used for non-food applications, such as medical devices.

Although there have been concerns about the safety of irradiated food, a large amount of independent research has confirmed it to be safe. One family of chemicals is uniquely formed by irradiation, and this product is nontoxic. When heating food, all other chemicals occur in a lower or comparable frequency. Others criticize irradiation because of confusion with radioactive contamination or because of negative impressions of the nuclear industry. Australia banned irradiated cat food after it was shown to cause paralysis and death in cats. The regulations that dictate how food is to be irradiated, as well as the food allowed to be irradiated, vary greatly from country to country. In Austria, Germany, and many other countries of the European Union only dried herbs, spices, and seasonings can be processed with irradiation and only at a specific dose, while in Brazil all foods are allowed at any dose.

Uses

Irradiation is used to reduce the pathogens in foods. Depending on the dose, some or all of the microorganisms, bacteria, and viruses present are destroyed, slowed down, or rendered incapable of reproduction. This reduces or eliminates the risk of food borne illnesses. Some foods are irradiated at sufficient doses to ensure that the product is sterilized and does not add any spoilage or pathogenic microorganisms into the final product.

Irradiation is used to delay the ripening of fruits and the sprouting of vegetables by slowing down the enzymatic action in foods. By halting or slowing down spoilage and slowing down the ripening of food, irradiation prolongs the shelf life of goods. Irradiation cannot revert spoiled or over ripened food to a fresh state. If this food was processed by irradiation, spoilage would cease and ripening would slow down, yet the irradiation would not destroy the toxins or repair the texture, colour, or taste of the food.

Insect pests are sterilized using irradiation at relatively low doses of irradiation. This stops the spread of foreign invasive species across national boundaries, and allows foods to pass quickly through quarantine and avoid spoilage. Depending on the dose, some or all of the insects present are destroyed, or rendered incapable of reproduction.

PUBLIC PERCEPTION AND IMPACT

Irradiation has been approved by the FDA for over 50 years, but the only major growth area for the commercial sale of irradiated foods for human consumption is fruits and vegetables that are irradiated to kill insects for the purpose of quarantine. In the early 2000s in the US irradiated meat was common at some grocery stores, but because of lack of consumer demand it is no longer common. Because consumer demand for irradiated food is low, reducing the spoilage between manufacture and consumer purchase and reducing the risk of food borne illness is currently not sufficient incentive for most manufactures to supplement their process with irradiation.

It is widely believed that consumer perception of foods treated with irradiation is more negative than those processed by other means, although some industry studies indicate the number of consumers concerned about the safety of irradiated food has decreased in the last 10 years to levels comparable to those of people concerned about food additives and preservatives. "These irradiated foods are not less safe than others," Dr. Tarantino said, "and the doses are effective in reducing the level of disease-causing micro-organisms." "People think the product is radioactive," said Harlan Clemmons, president of Sadex, a food irradiation company based in Sioux City, Iowa.

Some common concerns about food irradiation include the impact of irradiation on food chemistry, as well as the indirect effects of irradiation becoming a prevalent in the food handling process. Irradiation reduces the risk of infection and spoilage, does not make food radioactive, and the food is shown to be safe, but it does cause chemical reactions that alter the food and therefore alters the chemical makeup, nutritional content, and the sensory qualities of the food. Some of the potential secondary impacts of irradiation are hypothetical, while others are demonstrated. These effects include impacts due to the reduction of food quality, the loss of bacteria, and the irradiation process. Because of these concerns and the increased cost of irradiated foods, there is not a widespread public demand for the irradiation of foods for human consumption.

Effect of Irradiation on Food Chemistry

The irradiation source supplies energetic particles or waves. As these waves/ particles pass through a target material they collide with other particles. Around the sites of these collisions chemical bonds are broken, creating short lived radicals (e.g. the hydroxyl radical, the hydrogen atom and solvated electrons). These radicals cause further chemical changes by bonding with and or stripping particles from nearby molecules. When collisions damage DNA or RNA, effective reproduction becomes unlikely; also when collisions occur in cells, cell division is often suppressed.

Irradiated food does not become radioactive as the radioactive source is never in contact with the foodstuffs and energy of radiation is limited below the threshold of induction of radioactivity, but it does reduce the nutritional content and change the flavor (much like cooking), produce radiolytic products, and increase the number of free radicals in the food.

Irradiation causes a multitude of chemical changes including introducing radiolytic products and free radicals. A few of these products are unique, but not considered dangerous. The scale of these chemical changes is not unique. Cooking, smoking, salting, and other less novel techniques, cause the food to be altered so drastically that its original nature is almost unrecognizable, and must be called by a different name. Storage of food also causes dramatic chemical changes, ones that eventually lead to deterioration and spoilage.

Misconceptions

A major concern is that irradiation might cause chemical changes that are harmful to the consumer. Several national expert groups and two international expert groups evaluated the available data and concluded that any food at any dose is wholesome and safe to consume as long as it remains palatable and maintains its technical properties (e.g. feel, texture, or colour).

Irradiated food does not become radioactive, just as an object exposed to light does not start producing light. Radioactivity is the ability of a substance to emit high energy particles. When these particles hit the target materials they may free other highly energetic particles. This ends shortly after the end of the exposure, much like objects stop reflecting light when the source is turned off and warm objects emit heat until they cool down but do not continue to produce their own heat.

It is impossible for food irradiators to induce radiation into a product. Irradiators radiate non-alpha particles and radiation is intrinsically radiated at precisely known strengths (wavelengths). These radiated particles can never be strong enough to split the atoms found in food. Without alpha particles, radioactivity can only be induced if a radiated particle with sufficient strength hits another atom and that atom splits into two or more pieces. If this happens the resulting atom(s) may be radioactive. If the particle is not strong enough, it can never split an atom, no matter how many particles are emitted from the radioactive source. Only in rare materials, such as plutonium and uranium, is the energy released by splitting an atom strong enough to split other atoms, these materials is not found in foods in sufficient quantities, so there can be no chain reaction.

Food Quality

Because of the extent of the chemical reactions, changes to the foods quality after irradiation are inevitable. The nutritional content of food, as well as the sensory qualities (taste, appearance, and texture) is impacted by irradiation. Because of this food advocacy groups consider labelling irradiated food raw as misleading. However, the degradation of vitamins caused by irradiation is similar or even less than the loss caused by other food preservation processes. Other processes like chilling, freezing, drying, and heating also result in some vitamin loss.

The changes in quality and nutrition vary greatly from food to food. The changes in the flavour of fatty foods like meats, nuts and oils are sometimes noticeable, while the changes in lean products like fruits and vegetables are less so. Some studies by the irradiation industry show that for some properly treated fruits and vegetables irradiation is seen by consumers to improve the sensory qualities of the product compared to untreated fruits and vegetables.

Radiolytic Products and Free Radicals

The formation of new, previously unknown chemical compounds (unique radiolytic products) via irradiation is a concern. Most of the substances found in irradiated food are also found in food that has been subjected to other food processing treatments, and are therefore not unique. Furthermore, the quantities in which they occur in irradiated food are lower or similar to the quantities formed in heat treatments.

When fatty acids are irradiated, a family of compounds called 2-alkylcyclobutanones (2-ACBs) are produced. These are thought to be unique radiolytic products. Some studies show that these chemicals may be toxic, while others dispute this.

Potentially damaging compounds known as free radicals form when food is irradiated. Most of these are oxidizers (i.e., accept electrons) and some react very strongly. According to the free-radical theory of aging excessive amounts of these free radicals can lead to cell injury and cell death, which may contribute to many diseases. Though this traditional relates to the free radicals generated in the body, not the free radicals consumed by the individual, as much of these are destroyed in the digestive process.

The radiation doses to cause toxic changes are much higher than the doses needed to accomplish the benefits of irradiation, and taking into account the presence of 2-ABCs along with what is known of free radicals, these results lead to the conclusion that there is no significant risk from radiolytic products.

Side Effects of Irradiation

The side effects of irradiation are the concerns and benefits of irradiation that are not directly related to the chemical changes that occur when food is irradiated, but instead are related to what would occur if food irradiation was a common process.

If the majority of food was irradiated at high enough levels to decrease its nutritional content significantly, there could be an increase in nutritional deficiencies due to a diet composed entirely of irradiated foods. Furthermore, for at least 3 studies on cats, the consumption of irradiated food was associated with a loss of tissue in the myelin sheath, leading to reversible paralysis. Researchers suspect that reduced levels of vitamin A and high levels of free radicals may be the cause. This effect is thought to be specific to cats and has not been reproduced in any other animal. To produce these effects the cats were fed solely on food that was irradiated at a dose at least five times higher than the maximum allowable dose.

If irradiation was to become common in the food handling process there would be a reduction of the prevalence of foodborne illness and potentially the eradication of specific pathogens. However, multiple studies suggest that an increased rate of pathogen growth may occur when irradiated food is cross-contaminated with a pathogen, as the competing spoilage organisms are no longer present. This being said, cross contamination itself becomes less prevalent with an increase in usage of irradiated foods.

The ability to remove bacterial contamination through post-processing by irradiation may reduce the fear of mishandling food which could cultivate a cavalier attitude toward hygiene and result in contaminants other than bacteria. However, concerns that the pasteurization of milk would lead to increased contamination of milk where prevalent when mandatory pasteurization was introduced, but these fears never materialized after adoption of this law. Therefore, it is unlikely for irradiation to cause an increase of illness due to non-bacteria based contamination.

It may seem reasonable to assume that irradiating food might lead to radiation-tolerant strains, similar to the way that strains of bacteria have developed resistance to antibiotics. Bacteria develop a resistance to antibiotics after an individual uses antibiotics repeatedly. Much like pasteurization plants products that pass through irradiation plants are processed once, and are not processed and reprocessed. Cycles of heat treatment have been shown to produce heat tolerant bacteria, yet no problems have appeared so far in pasteurization plants. Furthermore, when the irradiation dose is chosen to target a specific species of microbe, it is calibrated to doses several times the value required to target the species. This ensures that the process randomly destroys all members of a target species. Therefore, the more irradiation tolerant members of the target species are not given any evolutionary advantage. Without evolutionary advantage selection does not occur. As to the irradiation process directly producing mutations that lead to more virulent, radiation resistant, strains the European Commission's Scientific Committee on Food found that there is no evidence, on the contrary, irradiation has been found to cause loss of virulence and infectivity as mutants are usually less competitive and less adapted."

Misconceptions

The argument is made that there is a lack of long-term studies, and therefore the safety of irradiated food is not scientifically proven in spite of the fact that hundreds of animal feeding studies of irradiated food, including multigenerational studies, have been performed since 1950. Endpoints investigated have included sub chronic and chronic changes in metabolism, histopathology, and function of most systems; reproductive effects; growth; teratogenicity; and mutagenicity. A large number of studies have been performed; meta-studies have supported the safety of irradiated food.

- The below experiments are cited by food irradiation opponents, but could be either not verified in later experiments, could not be clearly attributed to the radiation effect, or could be attributed to an inappropriate design of the experiment etc.
- India's National Institute of Nutrition (NIN) found an elevated rate of cells with more than one set of genes (Polyploidy) in humans and animals when fed wheat that was irradiated recently (within 12 weeks). Upon analysis scientist determined that the techniques used by NIN allowed for too much human error and statistical variation, therefore the results where unreliable. After multiple studies by independent agencies and scientists no correlation between polyploidy and irradiation of food could be found.

Change in Chronaxie in Rats

Treatment

Up to the point where the food is processed by irradiation, the food is processed in the same way as all other food. To treat the foodstuffs, they are exposed to a radioactive source, for a set period of time to achieve a desired dose. Radiation may be emitted by a radioactive substance, or by X-ray and electron beam accelerators. Special precautions are taken to ensure the food stuffs never come in contact with the radioactive substances and that the personnel and the environment are protected from exposure radiation. Irradiation treatments are typically classified by dose (high, medium, and low), but are sometimes classified by the effects of the treatment (radappertization, radicidation andradurization). Food irradiation is sometimes referred to as "cold pasteurization" or "electronic pasteurization" because ionizing the food does not heat the food to high temperatures during the process, and the effect is similar to heat pasteurization. The term "cold pasteurization" is controversial because the term may be used to disguise the fact the food has been irradiated and pasteurization and irradiation are fundamentally different processes.

Treatment costs vary as a function of dose and facility usage. A pallet or tote is typically exposed for several minutes to hours depending on dose. Low-dose applications such as disinfestation of fruit range between US$0.01/lbs and US$0.08/lbs while higher-dose applications can cost as much as US$0.20/lbs.

Process

Typically, when the food is being irradiated, pallets of food are exposed a source of radiation for a specific time. Dosimeters are embedded in the pallet (at various locations) of food to determine what dose was achieved. Most irradiated food is processed by gamma irradiation. Special precautions are taken because gamma rays are continuously emitted by the radioactive material. In most designs, to nullify the effects of radiation, the radioisotope is lowered into a water-filled storage pool, which absorbs the radiation but does not become radioactive. This allows pallets of the products to be added and removed from the irradiation chamber and other maintenance to be done. Sometimes movable shields are used to reduce radiation levels in areas of the irradiation chamber instead of submerging the source. For x ray and electron irradiation these precautions are not necessary as the source of the radiation can be turned off.

For x-ray, gamma ray and electron irradiation, shielding is required when the foodstuffs are being irradiated. This is done to protect workers and the environment outside of the chamber from radiation exposure. Typically permanent or movable shields are used. In some gamma irradiators the radioactive source is under water at all times, and the hermetically sealed product is lowered into the water. The water acts as the shield in this application. Because of the lower penetration depth of electron irradiation, treatment to entire industrial pallets or totes is not possible.

Dosimetry

The radiation absorbed dose is the amount energy absorbed per unit weight of the target material. Dose is used because, when the same substance is given the same dose, similar changes are observed in the target material. The SI unit for dose is grays (Gy or J/kg). Dosimeters are used to measure dose, and are small components that, when exposed to ionizing radiation, change measurable physical attributes to a degree that can be correlated to the dose received. Measuring dose (dosimetry) involves exposing one or more dosimeters along with the target material.

For purposes of legislation doses are divided into low (up to 1 kGy), medium (1 kGy to 10 kGy), and high dose applications (above 10 kGy). High dose applications are above those currently permitted in the USA for commercial food items by the FDA and other regulators around the world.[44] Though these doses are approved for non-commercial applications, such as sterilizing frozen meat for NASA astronauts (doses of 44 kGy) and food for hospital patients.

Applications by Overall Average Dose

Low dose (up to 1 kGy)		Medium dose (1 kGy to 10 kGy)		High dose (above 10 kGy)	
Application	**Dose (kGy)**	**Application**	**Dose (kGy)**	**Application**	**Dose (kGy)**
Inhibit sprouting	0.03-0.15 kGy	Delay spoilage of meat	1.50–3.00 kGy	Sterilization of packaged meat	25.00-70.00 kGy
Delay fruit ripening	0.03-0.15 kGy	Reduce risk of pathogens in meat	3.00–7.00 kGy	Increase juice yield	
Stop insect/ parasite infestations	0.07-1.00 kGy	Increase sanitation of spices	10.00 kGy	Improve re-hydration	

Technology

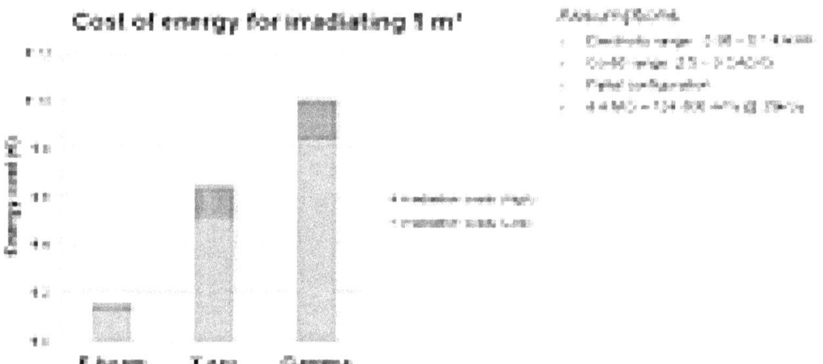

Figure 8.25: Efficiency illustration of the different radiation technologies (electron beam, X-ray, gamma rays).

Electron irradiation uses electrons accelerated in an electric field to a velocity close to the speed of light. Electrons have a charge, and therefore do not penetrate the product beyond a few centimeters, depending on product density.

Gamma irradiation involves exposing the target material to packets of light (photons) that are highly energetic (Gamma rays). A radioactive material (radioisotopes) is used as the source for the gamma rays. Gamma irradiation is the standard because the deeper penetration of the gamma rays enables administering treatment to entire industrial pallets or totes (reducing the need for material handling) and it is significantly less expensive than using an X-ray source. Generally cobalt-60 is used as a radioactive source for gamma irradiation. Cobalt-60 is bred from cobalt-59 using neutron irradiation in specifically designed nuclear reactors. In limited applications caesium-137, a less costly alternative recovered during the processing of spent nuclear fuel, is used as a radioactive source. Insufficient quantities are available for large scale commercial use. An incident where water-soluble caesium-137 leaked into the source storage pool requiring NRC intervention has led to near elimination of this radioisotope outside of military applications.

Irradiation by X-ray is similar to irradiation by gamma rays in that less energetic packets of light (X-rays) are used. X-rays are generated by colliding accelerated electrons with a dense material (this process is known as bremsstrahlung-conversion), and therefore do not necessitate the use of radioactive materials. X-rays ability to penetrate the target is similar to gamma irradiation. X-ray machine produces better dose uniformity then Gamma irradiation but they require much more electricity as only as much as 12% of the input energy is converted into X-rays.

Cost

The cost of food irradiation is influenced by dose requirements, the food's tolerance of radiation, handling conditions, i.e., packaging and stacking requirements, construction costs, financing arrangements, and other variables particular to the situation. Irradiation is a capital-intensive technology requiring a substantial initial investment, ranging from \$1 million to \$5 million. In the case of large research or contract irradiation facilities, major capital costs include a radiation source, hardware (irradiator, totes and conveyors, control systems, and other auxiliary equipment), land (1 to 1.5 acres), radiation shield, and warehouse. Operating costs include salaries (for fixed and variable labour), utilities, maintenance, taxes/insurance, cobalt-60 replenishment, general utilities, and miscellaneous operating costs.

Regulations and International Standards

The Codex Alimentarius represents the global standard for irradiation of food, in particular under the WTO-agreement. Member states are free to convert those standards into national regulations at their discretion; therefore regulations about irradiation differ from country to country.

The United Nations Food and Agricultural Organization (FAO) has passed a motion to commit member states to implement irradiation technology for their national phytosanitaryprograms; the General assembly of the International Atomic Energy Agency (IAEA) has urged wider use of the irradiation technology.

Labeling Regulations and International Standards

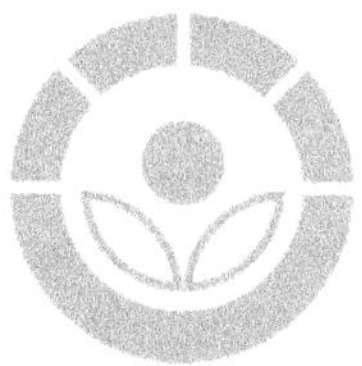

Figure 8.26: The Radura symbol, as required by U.S. Food and Drug Administration regulations to show a food has been treated with ionizing radiation.

The provisions of the Codex Alimentarius are that any "first generation" product must be labelled "irradiated" as any product derived directly from an irradiated raw material; for ingredients the provision is that even the last molecule of an irradiated ingredient must be listed with the ingredients even in cases where the unirradiated ingredient does not appear on the label. The RADURA-logo is optional; several countries use a graphical version that differs from the Codex-version. The suggested rules for labelling is published at CODEX-STAN – 1 (2005), and includes the usage of the Radurasymbol for all products that contain irradiated foods. The Radura symbol is not a designator of quality. The amount of pathogens remaining is based upon dose and the original content and the dose applied can vary on a product by product basis.

The European Union follows the Codex's provision to label irradiated ingredients down to the last molecule of irradiated foodstuffs. The European Community does not provide for the use of the Radura logo and relies exclusively on labelling by the appropriate phrases in the respective languages of the Member States. The European Union enforces its irradiation labelling laws by requiring its member countries to perform tests on a cross section of food items in the market-place and to report to the European Commission. The results are published annually in the OJ of the European Communities.

The US defines irradiated foods as foods in which the irradiation causes a material change in the food, or a material change in the consequences that may result from the use of the food. Therefore, food that is processed as an ingredient by a restaurant or food processor is exempt from the labelling requirement in the US. This definition is not consistent with the Codex Alimentarius. All irradiated foods must bear a slightly modified Radura symbol at the point of sale and use the term "irradiated" or a derivative there of, in conjunction with explicit language describing the change in the food or its conditions of use.

Food Safety Regulations and International Standards

In 2003, the Codex Alimentarius removed any upper dose limit for food irradiation as well as clearances for specific foods, declaring that all are safe to irradiate. Countries such as Pakistan and Brazil have adopted the Codex without any reservation or restriction. Other countries, including New Zealand, Australia, Thailand, India, and Mexico, have permitted the irradiation of fresh fruits for fruit fly quarantine purposes, amongst others.

Standards that describe calibration and operation for radiation dosimetry, as well as procedures to relate the measured dose to the effects achieved and to report and document such results, are maintained by the American Society for Testing and Materials (ASTM international) and are also available as ISO/ASTM standards. All of the rules involved in processing foodstuffs are applied to all foods before they are irradiated.

United States Clearances

In the United States, each new food is approved separately with a guideline specifying a maximum dosage; in case of quarantine applications the minimum dose is regulated. Packaging materials containing the food processed by irradiation must also undergo approval. Food irradiation in the United States is primarily regulated by the FDA since it is considered a food additive. The United States Department of Agriculture (USDA) amends these rules for use with meat, poultry, and fresh fruit.

The United States Department of Agriculture (USDA) has approved the use of low-level irradiation as an alternative treatment to pesticides for fruits and vegetables that are considered hosts to a number of insect pests, including fruit flies and seed weevils. Under bilateral agreements that allows less-developed countries to earn income through food exports agreements are made to allow them to irradiate fruits and vegetables at low doses to kill insects, so that the food can avoid quarantine.

The U.S. Food and Drug Administration (FDA) and the USDA have approved irradiation of the following foods and purposes:

Packaged refrigerated or frozen red meat to control pathogens (*E. Coli* O157:H7 and *Salmonella*), and to extend shelf life.

Packaged poultry control pathogens (*Salmonella* and *Camplylobacter*).

Fresh fruits, vegetables and grains to control insects and inhibit growth, ripening and sprouting.

Pork to control trichinosis.

Herbs, spices and vegetable seasonings to control insects and microorganisms.

Dry or dehydrated enzyme preparations to control insects and microorganisms.

White potatoes to inhibit sprout development.

Wheat and wheat flour to control insects.

Loose or bagged fresh iceberg lettuce and spinach

European Union Clearances

European law dictates that no foods other than dried aromatic herbs, spices and vegetable seasonings are permitted for the application of irradiation. However, any Member State is permitted to maintain previous clearances that are in categories that the EC's Scientific Committee on Food (SCF) had previously approved, or add clearance granted to other Member States. Presently, Belgium, Czech Republic, France, Italy, Netherlands, Poland, and the United Kingdom) have adopted such provisions. Before individual items in an approved class can be added to the approved list, studies into the toxicology of each of such food and for each of the proposed dose ranges are requested. It also states that irradiation shall not be used "as a substitute for hygiene or health practices or good manufacturing or agricultural practice". These regulations only govern food irradiation in consumer products to allow irradiation to be used for patients requiring sterile diets.

Because of the Single Market of the EC any food, even if irradiated, must be allowed to be marketed in any other Member State even if a general ban of food irradiation prevails, under the condition that the food has been irradiated legally in the state of origin. Furthermore, imports into the EC are possible from third countries if the irradiation facility had been inspected and approved by the EC and the treatment is legal within the EC or some Member state.

Nuclear and Employee Safety Regulations

Interlocks and safeguards are mandated to minimize this risk. There have been radiation related accidents, deaths, and injury at such facilities, many of them caused by operators overriding the safety related interlocks. In a radiation processing facility, radiation specific concerns are supervised by special authorities, while "Ordinary" occupational safety regulations are handled much like other businesses.

The safety of irradiation facilities is regulated by the United Nations International Atomic Energy Agency and monitored by the different national Nuclear Regulatory Commissions. The regulators enforce a safety culture that mandates that all incidents that occur are documented and thoroughly analyzed to determine the cause and improvement potential. Such incidents are studied by personnel at multiple facilities, and improvements are mandated to retrofit existing facilities and future design.

In the US the Nuclear Regulatory Commission (NRC) regulates the safety of the processing facility, and the United States Department of Transportation (DOT) regulates the safe transport of the radioactive sources.

Irradiated Food Supply

There are analytical methods available to detect the usage of irradiation on food items in the marketplace. This is used as a tool for government authorities to enforce existing labelling standards and to bolster consumer confidence. Phytosanitary irradiation of fruits and vegetables has been increasing globally. In 2010, 18446 tonnes of fruits and vegetables were irradiated in six countries for export quarantine control; the countries follow: Mexico (56.2%), United States (31.2%), Thailand (5.18%), Vietnam (4.63%), Australia (2.69%), and India (0.05%). The three types of fruits irradiated the most were guava (49.7%), sweet potato (29.3%) and sweet lime (3.27%).

In total, 103 000 tonnes of food products were irradiated on mainland United States in 2010. The three types of foods irradiated the most were spices (77.7%), fruits and vegetables (14.6%) and meat and poultry (7.77%). 17 953 tonnes of irradiated fruits and vegetables were exported to the mainland United States. Mexico, the United States' state of Hawaii, Thailand, Vietnam and India export irradiated produce to the mainland U.S. Mexico, followed by the United States' state of Hawaii, and is the largest exporter of irradiated produce to the mainland U.S.

In total, 7 972 tonnes of food products were irradiated in European Union countries in 2012; mainly in three member state countries: Belgium (64.7%), the Netherlands (18.5%) and France (7.7%). The three types of foods irradiated the most were frog legs (36%), poultry (35%) and dried herbs and spices (15%). The European Union's official site gives information on the regulatory status of food irradiation, the quantities of foods irradiated at authorized facilities in European Union member states and the results of market surveillance where foods have been tested to see if they are irradiated. The Official Journal of the European Union publishes annual reports on food irradiation; the current report covers the period from 1 January 2012 to 31 December 2012 and compiles information from 27 member States.

Timeline of the History of Food Irradiation

1895 Wilhelm Conrad Röntgen discovers X-rays ("bremsstrahlung", from German for radiation produced by deceleration)

1896 Antoine Henri Becquerel discovers natural radioactivity; Minck proposes the therapeutic use

1904 Samuel Prescott describes the bactericide effects Massachusetts Institute of Technology (MIT)

1906 Appleby & Banks: UK patent to use radioactive isotopes to irradiate particulate food in a flowing bed

1918 Gillett: U.S. Patent to use X-rays for the preservation of food

1921 Schwartz describes the elimination of Trichinella from food

1930 Wuest: French patent on food irradiation

1943 MIT becomes active in the field of food preservation for the U.S. Army

1951 U.S. Atomic Energy Commission begins to co-ordinate national research activities

1958 World first commercial food irradiation (spices) at Stuttgart, Germany

1970 Establishment of the International Food Irradiation Project (IFIP), headquarters at the Federal Research Centre for Food Preservation, Karlsruhe, Germany

1980 FAO/IAEA/WHO Joint Expert Committee on Food Irradiation recommends the clearance generally up to 10 kGy "overall average dose"

1981/1983 End of IFIP after reaching its goals

1983 Codex Alimentarius General Standard for Irradiated Foods: any food at a maximum "overall average dose" of 10 kGy

1984 International Consultative Group on Food Irradiation (ICGFI) becomes the successor of IFIP

1998 The European Union's Scientific Committee on Food (SCF) voted "positive" on eight categories of irradiation applications

1997 FAO/IAEA/WHO Joint Study Group on High-Dose Irradiation recommends to lift any upper dose limit

1999 The European Union issues Directives 1999/2/EC (framework Directive) and 1999/3/EC (implementing Directive) limiting irradiation a positive list whose sole content is one of the eight categories approved by the SFC, but allowing the individual states to give clearances for any food previously approved by the SFC.

2000 Germany leads a veto on a measure to provide a final draft for the positive list.

2003 Codex Alimentarius General Standard for Irradiated Foods: no longer any upper dose limit

2003 The SCF adopts a "revised opinion" that recommends against the cancellation of the upper dose limit.

2004 ICGFI ends

2011 The successor to the SFC, European Food Safety Authority (EFSA), reexamines the SFC's list and makes further recommendations for inclusion.

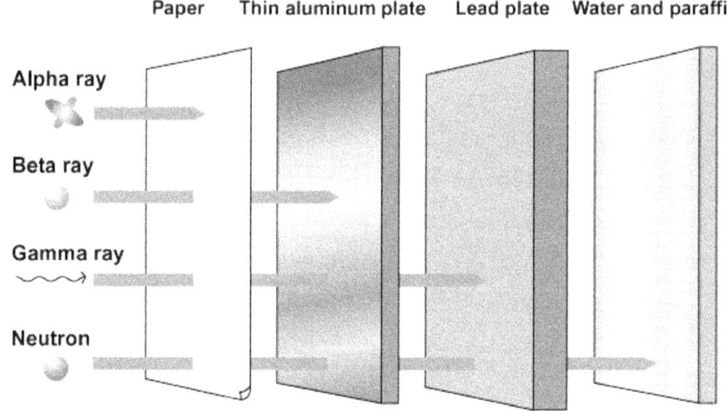

CHAPTER 9

Enzyme Assay and Activity

INTRODUCTION

Enzyme assays are laboratory methods for measuring enzymatic activity. They are vital for the study of enzyme kinetics and enzyme inhibition.

Every enzyme assay involves the use of an enzyme as a catalyst to convert a substrate (and co-substrate in some cases) to product. To detect the reaction, a property (e.g., light absorption) of either the substrate, product, or co-substrate is measured at appropriate times. If none of them has a suitable property, the reaction can be coupled to a second reaction system that has a readily measurable property. Coupling is achieved by making a product of the first reaction serve as a substrate or co-substrate for the second. The stoichiometries of the reactions facilitate calculating the amount of substrate or product catalyzed in the first reaction.

Enzyme assays may be qualitative or quantitative. The qualitative assay seeks to establish the presence or absence of either the enzyme or the substrate in a sample. In contrast, the quantitative assay measures the amount of enzyme or substrate in a sample and requires optimal conditions if accuracy is desired. Quantitative assays can be classified into two broad categories: One category includes those that are aimed at determining the enzyme's activity or kinetic constants, and the other category includes those that are aimed at determining the concentration of substrate, using the enzyme as a reagent.

Applications for enzyme assays include the determination of the activity and kinetic constants for enzymes; determination of substrate or co-substrate concentration; determination of antigen concentration by means of enzyme immunoassays; qualitative detection of biomolecules, cellular components, cells, tissues, or other matrices in which a suitable enzyme or substrate serves as a marker.

CONDITIONS REQUIRED FOR QUANTITATIVE ENZYME ASSAYS

The Michaelis-Menton Equation as a Basis for Assay Conditions

The Michaelis-Menton equation expresses the quantitative aspects of enzyme kinetics. For an enzyme reaction,

$$\frac{[S]v_{max}}{K_m+[S]}$$

where v_i and v_{max} are the initial and maximal velocities, respectively of the reaction [S] is the substrate concentration at the time v_i is measured; and K_m is the Michaelis constant, defined as the substrate concentration at half maximal velocity. The equation relates the initial velocity of the reaction to the maximal velocity and substrate concentration. If the true initial velocities are measured, then [S] = [So] where [So] is the initial substrate concentration. A plot of v_i versus [So] illustrates this relationship. In the figure, the kinetics in region A form the basis for conditions required by assays that determine an enzyme's activity. Likewise, the kinetics in region B forms the basis for conditions required by assays that determine the concentration of a substrate or co-substrate, using an enzyme as a reagent.

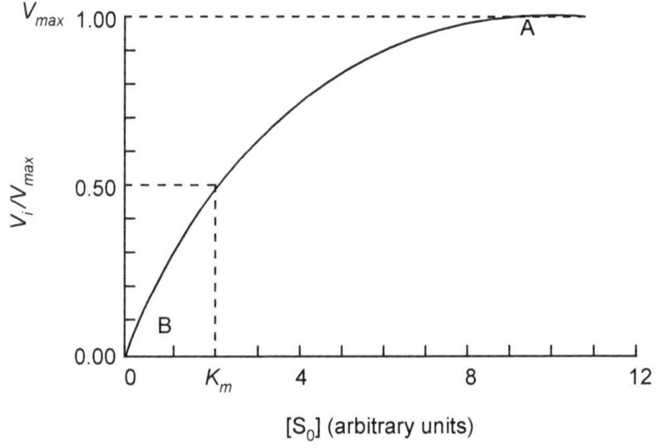

Figure 9.1: Relationship between initial velocity and initial substrate concentration of an enzyme-catalyzed reaction.

Why Study Enzyme Kinetics (Reaction Rates)?

- measurement of velocity = reaction rate
- compare enzymes under different conditions, or from different tissues or organisms – understand how differences relate to physiology/function of organism – e.g., physiological reason for different Km values for hexokinase vs. glucokinase (discussed later in course)
- compare activity of same enzyme with different substrates (understand specificity)
- measure amount or concentration of one enzyme in a mixture by its activity
- measure enzyme purity (specific activity = amount of activity/amount of protein)
- study/distinguish different types of inhibitors info about enzyme active sites and reaction mechanism development of specific drugs (enzyme inhibition).

MICHAELIS-MENTEN KINETICS

The general reaction scheme of an enzyme-catalyzed reaction is as follows:

$$E+S-\rightarrow k_1[ES]-\rightarrow K_2E+P$$

The enzyme interacts with the substrate by binding to its active site to form the enzyme-substrate complex, ES. That reaction is followed by the decomposition of ES to regenerate the free enzyme, E, and the new product, P. For more general information about enzyme-catalyzed reactions.

To begin our discussion of enzyme kinetics, let's define the number of moles of product (P) formed per time as *V*. The variable, *V*, is also referred to as the rate of catalysis of an enzyme. For different enzymes, *V* varies with the concentration of the substrate, S. At low S, *V* is linearly proportional to S, but when S is high relative to the amount of total enzyme, *V* is independent of S. Concentrations is important in determining the initial rate of an enzyme-catalyzed reaction. A more thorough explanation of enzyme rates can be found here: Definition of Reaction Rate.

To understand Michaelis-Menten Kinetics, we will use the general enzyme reaction scheme shown below, which includes the back reactions in addition the forward reactions:

$$E+S-\rightarrow k_1[ES]-\rightarrow K_2E+P$$

$$E+S\rightarrow -k_3[ES]\rightarrow -K_4E+P$$

The table below defines each of the rate constants in the above scheme.

Table 9.1: Model parameters

Rate Constant	Reaction
k_1	The binding of the enzyme to the substrate forming the enzyme substrate complex.
k_2	Catalytic rate; the catalysis reaction producing the final reaction product and regenerating the free enzyme. This is the rate limiting step.
k_3	The dissociation of the enzyme-substrate complex to free enzyme and substrate.
k_4	The reverse reaction of catalysis.

Substrate Complex

$$E+S-\rightarrow k_1ES \qquad vo=k_1[E][S]$$

$$ES-\rightarrow k_2E+S \qquad vo=k_2[ES]$$

$$ES-\rightarrow k_3E+P \qquad vo=k_3[ES]$$

$$E+P-\rightarrow k_4ES \qquad vo=k_4[E][P]=0$$

The ES complex is formed by combining enzyme E with substrate S at rate constant k_1. The ES complex can either dissociate to form E_F(free enzyme) and S, or form product P at rate constant k_2 and k_3, respectively. The velocity equation can be derived in either of the 2 methods that follow:

The Rapid Equilibrium Approximation

E, S, and the ES complex can equilibrate very rapidly. The instantaneous velocity is the catalytic rate that is equal to the product of ES concentration and k_2 the catalytic rate constant.

$$vo = k_2[E\text{–}S]$$

The total enzyme concentration (E_T) is equal to the concentration of free enzyme E (E_F) plus the concentration of the bound enzyme in ES complex:

$$[E]T = [EF]+[ES]$$

$$Ks = k_2k_1=[E][S][ES]$$

$$Ks([Eo]-[ES])[S][ES]$$

$$[ES]=[Eo][S]Ks+[S]$$

$$vo=(dPdt)o = k_3[ES]$$

\[v_o = \left(\dfrac{dP}{dt} \right)_o = \dfrac{k_3[Eo][S]}{Ks + [S]}\]

At high substrate concentrations, [S]>>Ks we get:

vo=(dPdt)o=k3[Eo]=Vmax ...(1)

The Steady-State Approximation

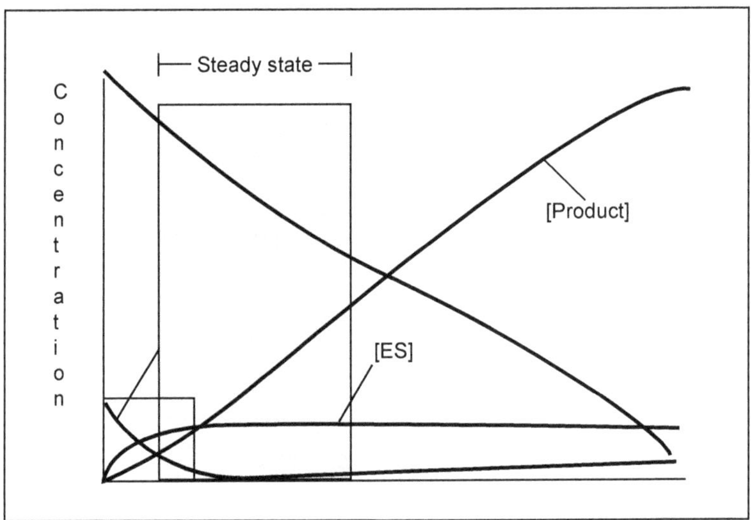

Figure 9.2: The steady-state approximation.

The figure above shows the relatively low and constant concentration of the enzyme-substrate complex due to the complex's slow formation and rapid consumption. Note the falling substrate concentration and the rising product concentration.

The rates of formation and breakdown of the E - S complex are given in terms of known quantities:

- The rate of formation of E-S = $k_1[E][S]$
  (with the assumption that [P] =0)
- The rate of breakdown of E-S = $k_2[ES]+k_3[ES]=(K_2+K_3)[ES]$

At steady state,

$$d[ES]dt=k_1[E][S]+k_2[ES]+k_3[ES]=0$$

Therefore, rate of formation of E-S is equal to the rate of breakdown of E-S

So,

$$k_1[E][S]=(k_2+k_3)[ES]$$

Dividing through by k1:

$$[E][S]=(k_2+k_3)k_1[E{-}S]$$

Substituting $(k_2+k_3)k_1$ with k_M:

$$[E][S]=KM[ES]$$

$$kM = breakdown[ES]formation[ES] \quad ...(2)$$

Km implies that half of the active sites on the enzymes are filled. Different enzymes have different Km values. They typically range from 10^{-1} to 10^{-7} M. The factors that affect Km are:

- pH
- temperature
- ionic strengths
- the nature of the substrate

Substituting $[E_F]$ with $[E_T]$-[ES]:

$$E_T = [ES] + [E_F]$$

$$([E_T] - [ES])\ [S] = k_M\ [ES]$$

$$[E_T]\ [S] - [ES][S] = k_M\ [ES]$$

$$[E_T]\ [S] = [ES]\ [S] + k_M\ [ES]$$

$$[E_T]\ [S] = [ES]\ ([S] + k_M)$$

Solving for [ES]:

$$[ES] = ([ET][S])([S]+kM) \quad ...(3)$$

The rate equation from the rate limiting step is:

$$_{Vo} = dPdt = k_2[ES]$$

Multiplying both sides of the equation by k_2:

$$k_2[ES]=k_2(([ET][S])(KM+[S])$$

$$Vo=k_2(([ET][S])(KM+[S])$$

When $S>>K_{M,}$ v_o is approximately equal to $k_2[E_T]$. When the [S] great, most of the enzyme is found in the bound state ([ES]) and $V_o = V_{max}$

We can then substitue $k_2[E_T]$ with $V_{max}$to get the Michaelis Menten Kinetic Equation:

$$v_o =(vmax[S])(kM+[S]) \quad ...(4)$$

Reaction Order Note

When [S]<<Km,

$$v=Vmax[S]Km$$

This means that the rate and the substrate concentration are directly proportional to each other. The reaction is first-order kinetics.

When [S]>>Km,

$$v=Vmax$$

This means that the rate is equal to the maximum velocity and is independent of the substrate concentration. The reaction is zero-order kinetics.

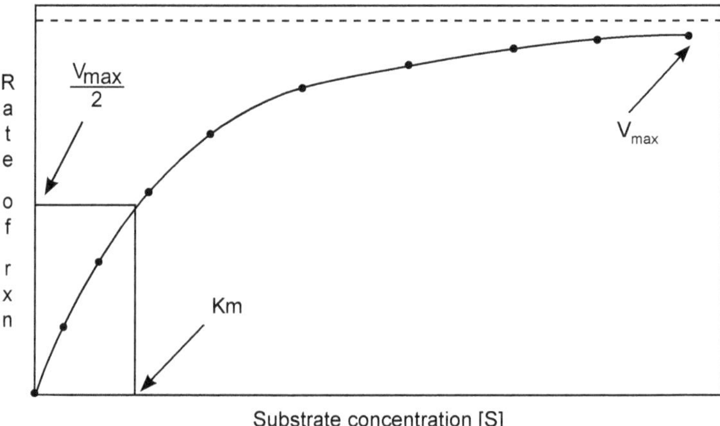

Figure 9.3: The reaction is zero-order kinetics.

Then, at

$$v=Vmax2, Km=[S]$$

$$v=Vmax2=Vmax[S]Km+[S] \quad ...(5)$$

Therefore, Km is equal to the concentration of the substrate when the rate is half of the maximum velocity. From the Michaelis Menten Kinetic equation, we have many different ways to find Km and Vmax such as the Lineweaver-Burk plot, Hanes-Woolf plot, and Eadie-Hofstee plot, etc.

Lineweaver-Burk Plot

For example, by taking the reciprocal of the Michaelis Menten Kinetics Equation, we can obtain the Lineweaver-Burk double reciprocal plot:

$$vo=(Vmax[S])(KM+[S])$$

$$1v=(kM+[S])vmax[S]$$

$$1v=(KmVmax)(1[S])+1VmaxC$$

Apply this to equation for a straight line y=mx+b and we have:

$$y=1v$$

$$x=1[S]$$
$$m=slope=KmVmax$$
$$b=y-intercept=1Vmax$$

When we plot $y=1v$ versus $x=1[S]$, we obtain a straight line.

$$x-intercept=-1Km$$
$$y-intercept=1Vmax$$
$$slope=KmVmax \quad ...(6)$$

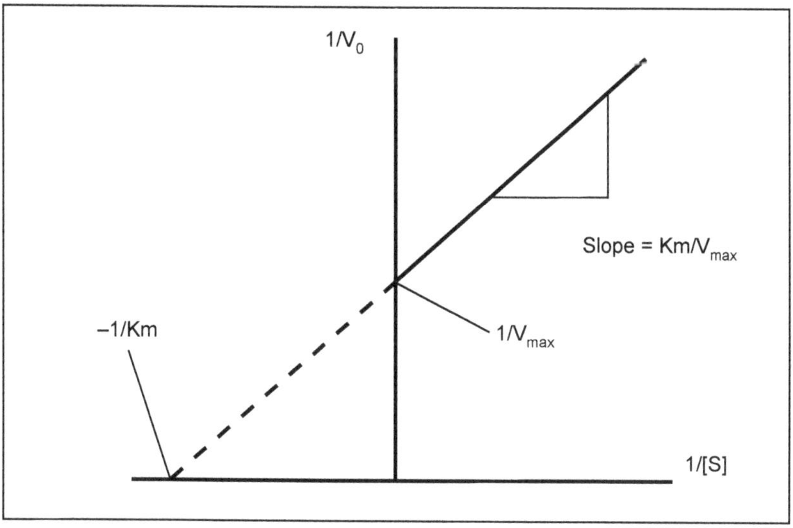

Figure 9.4: Lineweaver-Burk plot.

Eadie-Hofstee

Another way to calculate these values (k_M, V_{max}) and represent enzyme kinetics:

$$Vo=(Vmax[S])(KM+[S])$$
$$v_o (k_M + [S]) = v_{max}[S]$$
$$v_o k_M + v_o[S] = v_{max} [S]$$
$$v_o [S] = -vo\ k_M = vmax\ [S]$$

Dividing through by [S]

$$vo=-kmvo[S]+vmax \quad ...(7)$$

Enzyme Units

Amounts of enzymes can either be expressed as molar amounts, as with any other chemical, or measured in terms of activity, in enzyme units.

Enzyme Activity

Enzyme activity = moles of substrate converted per unit time = rate × reaction volume. Enzyme activity is a measure of the quantity of active enzyme present and is thus dependent on conditions, which should be specified. The SI unit is the katal, 1 katal = 1 mol s^{-1}, but this is an excessively large unit. A more practical and commonly used value is enzyme unit(U) = 1 μmol min^{-1}. 1 U corresponds to 16.67 nanokatals.

Enzyme activity as given in katal generally refers to that of the assumed natural target substrate of the enzyme. Enzyme activity can also be given as that of certain standardized substrates, such as gelatin, then measured in gelatin digesting units (GDU), or milk proteins, and then measured in milk clotting units (MCU). The units GDU and MCU are based on how fast one gram of the enzyme will digest gelatin or milk proteins, respectively. 1 GDU equals approximately 1.5 MCU.

An increased amount of substrate will increase the rate of reaction with enzymes, however once past a certain point; the rate of reaction will level out because the amount of active sites available has stayed constant.

Specific Activity

The specific activity of an enzyme is another common unit. This is the activity of an enzyme per milligram of total protein (expressed in μmol $min^{-1}mg^{-1}$). Specific activity gives a measurement of enzyme purity in the mixture. It is the amount of product formed by an enzyme in a given amount of time under given conditions per milligram of total proteins. Specific activity is equal to the rate of reaction multiplied by the volume of reaction divided by the mass of total protein. The SI unit is katal kg^{-1}, but a more practical unit is μmol mg^{-1} min^{-1}. Specific activity is a measure of enzyme processivity, at a specific (usually saturating) substrate concentration, and is usually constant for a pure enzyme. For elimination of errors arising from differences in cultivation batches and/or misfolded enzyme etc. an active site titration needs to be done. This is a measure of the amount of active enzyme, calculated by e.g. titrating the amount of active sites present by employing an irreversible inhibitor. The specific activity should then be expressed as μmol min^{-1} mg^{-1}active enzyme. If the molecular weight of the enzyme is known, the turnover number, or μmol product sec^{-1} $μmol^{-1}$ of active enzyme, can be calculated from the specific activity. The turnover number can be visualized as the number of times each enzyme molecule carries out its catalytic cycle per second.

Related Terminology

The rate of a reaction is the concentration of substrate disappearing (or product produced) per unit time (mol L^{-1} s^{-1}).

The % purity is 100% × (specific activity of enzyme sample / specific activity of pure enzyme). The impure sample has lower specific activity because some of the mass is not actually enzyme. If the specific activity of 100% pure enzyme is known, then an impure sample will have a lower specific activity, allowing purity to be calculated.

Types of Assay

All enzyme assays measure either the consumption of substrate or production of product over time. A large number of different methods of measuring the concentrations of substrates and products exist and many enzymes can be assayed in several different ways. Biochemists usually study enzyme-catalysed reactions using four types of experiments:

- **Initial rate experiments**: When an enzyme is mixed with a large excess of the substrate, the enzyme-substrate intermediate builds up in a fast initial transient. Then the reaction achieves a steady-state kinetics in which enzyme substrate intermediates remains approximately constant over time and the reaction rate changes relatively slowly. Rates are measured for a short period after the attainment of the quasi-steady state, typically by monitoring the accumulation of product with time. Because the measurements are carried out for a very short period and because of the large excess of substrate, the approximation that the amount of free substrate is approximately equal to the amount of the initial substrate can be made. The initial rate experiment is the simplest to perform and analyze, being relatively free from complications such as back-reaction and enzyme degradation. It is therefore by far the most commonly used type of experiment in enzyme kinetics.
- **Progress curve experiments**: In these experiments, the kinetic parameters are determined from expressions for the species concentrations as a function of time. The concentration of the substrate or product is recorded in time after the initial fast transient and for a sufficiently long period to allow the reaction to approach equilibrium. Progress curve experiments were widely used in the early period of enzyme kinetics, but are less common now.
- **Transient kinetics experiments**: In these experiments, reaction behaviour is tracked during the initial fast transient as the intermediate reaches the steady-state kinetics period. These experiments are more difficult to perform than either of the above two classes because they require specialist techniques (such as flash photolysis of caged compounds) or rapid mixing (such as stopped-flow, quenched flow or continuous flow).
- **Relaxation experiments**: In these experiments, an equilibrium mixture of enzyme, substrate and product is perturbed, for instance by a temperature, pressure or pH jump, and the return to equilibrium is monitored. The analysis of these experiments requires consideration of the fully reversible reaction. Moreover, relaxation experiments are relatively insensitive to mechanistic details and are thus not typically used for mechanism identification, although they can be under appropriate conditions.

Enzyme assays can be split into two groups according to their sampling method: continuous assays, where the assay gives a continuous reading of activity, and discontinuous assays, where samples are taken, the reaction stopped and then the concentration of substrates/products determined.

Continuous assays

Continuous assays are most convenient, with one assay giving the rate of reaction with no further work necessary. There are many different types of continuous assays.

Spectrophotometric

In spectrophotometric assays, you follow the course of the reaction by measuring a change in how much light the assay solution absorbs. If this light is in the visible region you can actually see a change in the color of the assay, and these are called colorimetric assays. The MTT assay, a redox assay using a tetrazolium dye as substrate is an example of a colorimetric assay.

UV light is often used, since the common coenzymes NADH and NADPH absorb UV light in their reduced forms, but do not in their oxidized forms. An oxidoreductase using NADH as a substrate could therefore be assayed by following the decrease in UV absorbance at a wavelength of 340 nm as it consumes the coenzyme.

Direct Versus Coupled Assays

Even when the enzyme reaction does not result in a change in the absorbance of light, it can still be possible to use a spectrophotometric assay for the enzyme by using a coupled assay. Here, the product of one reaction is used as the substrate of another, easily detectable reaction. For example, the coupled assay for the enzyme hexokinase, which can be assayed by coupling its production of glucose-6-phosphate to NADPH production, usingglucose-6-phosphate dehydrogenase.

Fluorometric

Fluorescence is when a molecule emits light of one wavelength after absorbing light of a different wavelength. Fluorometric assays use a difference in the fluorescence of substrate from product to measure the enzyme reaction. These assays are in general much more sensitive than spectrophotometric assays, but can suffer from interference caused by impurities and the instability of many fluorescent compounds when exposed to light.

An example of these assays is again the use of the nucleotide coenzymes NADH and NADPH. Here, the reduced forms are fluorescent and the oxidized forms non-fluorescent. Oxidation reactions can therefore be followed by a decrease in fluorescence and reduction reactions by an increase. Synthetic substrates that release a fluorescent dye in an enzyme-catalyzed reaction are also available, such as 4-methylumbelliferyl-β-D-galactoside for assaying β-galactosidase.

Calorimetric

Calorimetry is the measurement of the heat released or absorbed by chemical reactions. These assays are very general, since many reactions involve some change in heat and with use of a microcalorimeter, not much enzyme or substrate is required. These assays can be used to measure reactions that are impossible to assay in any other way.

Chemiluminescent

Chemiluminescence is the emission of light by a chemical reaction. Some enzyme reactions produce light and this can be measured to detect product formation. These types of assay can be extremely sensitive, since the light produced can be captured by photographic film over days or weeks, but can be hard to quantify, because not all the light released by a reaction will be detected.

The detection of horseradish peroxidase by enzymatic chemiluminescence (ECL) is a common method of detecting antibodies in western blotting. Another example is the enzyme luciferase, this is found in fireflies and naturally produces light from its substrate luciferin.

Light Scattering

Static light scattering measures the product of weight-averaged molar mass and concentration of macromolecules in solution. Given a fixed total concentration of one or more species over the measurement time, the scattering signal is a direct measure of the weight-averaged molar mass of the solution, which will vary as complexes form or dissociate. Hence the measurement quantifies the stoichiometry of the complexes as well as kinetics. Light scattering assays of protein kinetics is a very general technique that does not require an enzyme.

Microscale Thermophoresis

Microscale Thermophoresis (MST) measures the size, charge and hydration entropy of molecules/substrates in real time. The thermophoretic movement of a fluorescently labeled substrate changes significantly as it is modified by an enzyme. This enzymatic activity can be measured with high time resolution in real time. The material consumption of the all optical MST method is very low, only 5 μl sample volume and 10nM enzyme concentration are needed to measure the enzymatic rate constants for activity and inhibition. MST allows measuring the modification of two different substrates at once (multiplexing) if both substrates are labeled with different fluorophores. Thus substrate competition experiments can be performed.

Discontinuous Assays

Discontinuous assays are when samples are taken from an enzyme reaction at intervals and the amount of product production or substrate consumption is measured in these samples.

Radiometric

Radiometric assays measure the incorporation of radioactivity into substrates or its release from substrates. The radioactive isotopes most frequently used in these assays are ^{14}C, ^{32}P, ^{35}S and ^{125}I. Since radioactive isotopes can allow the specific labelling of a single atom of a substrate, these assays are both extremely sensitive and specific. They are frequently used in biochemistry and are often the only way of measuring a specific reaction in crude extracts (the complex mixtures of enzymes produced when you lyse cells).

Radioactivity is usually measured in these procedures using a scintillation counter.

Chromatographic

Chromatographic assays measure product formation by separating the reaction mixture into its components by chromatography. This is usually done by high-performance liquid chromatography (HPLC), but can also use the simpler technique of thin layer chromatography. Although this approach can need a lot of material, its sensitivity can be increased by labelling the substrates/products with a radioactive or fluorescent tag. Assay sensitivity has also been increased by switching protocols to improved chromatographic instruments (e.g. ultra-high pressure liquid chromatography) that operate at pump pressure a few-fold higher than HPLC instruments.

Factors to Control in Assays

- **Salt Concentration**: Most enzymes cannot tolerate extremely high salt concentrations. The ions interfere with the weak ionic bonds of proteins. Typical enzymes are active in salt concentrations of 1-500 mM. As usual there are exceptions such as the halophilic algae and bacteria.
- **Effects of Temperature**: All enzymes work within a range of temperature specific to the organism. Increases in temperature generally lead to increases in reaction rates. There is a limit to the increase because higher temperatures lead to a sharp decrease in reaction rates. This is due to the denaturating (alteration) of protein structure resulting from the breakdown of the weak ionic and hydrogen bonding that stabilizes the three-dimensional structure of the enzyme active site. The "optimum" temperature for human enzymes is usually between 35 and 40 °C. The average temperature for humans is 37 °C. Human enzymes start to denature quickly at temperatures above 40 °C. Enzymes from thermophilic archaea found in the hot springs

are stable up to 100 °C. However, the idea of an "optimum" rate of an enzyme reaction is misleading, as the rate observed at any temperature is the product of two rates, the reaction rate and the denaturation rate. If you were to use an assay measuring activity for one second, it would give high activity at high temperatures, however if you were to use an assay measuring product formation over an hour, it would give you low activity at these temperatures.

- **Effects of pH**: Most enzymes are sensitive to pH and have specific ranges of activity. All have an optimum pH. The pH can stop enzyme activity by denaturating (altering) the three-dimensional shape of the enzyme by breaking ionic, and hydrogen bonds. Most enzymes function between a pH of 6 and 8; however pepsin in the stomach works best at a pH of 2 and trypsin at a pH of 8.
- **Substrate Saturation**: Increasing the substrate concentration increases the rate of reaction (enzyme activity). However, enzyme saturation limits reaction rates. An enzyme is saturated when the active sites of all the molecules are occupied most of the time. At the saturation point, the reaction will not speed up, no matter how much additional substrate is added. The graph of the reaction rate will plateau.
- **Level of crowding**, large amounts of macromolecules in a solution will alter the rates and equilibrium constants of enzyme reactions, through an effect called macromolecular crowding.

Summary

For enzyme-catalyzed reactions, the velocity of product formation can be described by the equation: v = k[ES]. The reaction is therefore first-order in relation to the concentration of ES complex. However, the reaction is not first-order relative to the directly measurable substrate concentration. Instead, under steady state conditions where [ES] is effectively constant, the velocity of an enzyme-catalyzed reaction is a hyperbolic function of [S]: v = Vmax [S] / K m + [S]. The Michaelis-Menten equation has two parameters, Vmax and Km. Vmax = K_{cat} [E] total, and therefore is a function of both the total enzyme concentration and of the catalytic rate constant of the enzyme for the reaction; K_{cat} is an intrinsic property of an enzyme, while Vmax is not. Km is an intrinsic property of an enzyme; it is a measure of the affinity of the enzyme for the substrate. Biological systems often vary velocity by altering Vmax (either by increasing or decreasing the amount of enzyme present); Km is a sensitive measure of changes in the enzyme (either modifications of one enzyme, or the presence of more than one isozymes). The Michaelis-Menten equation is somewhat difficult to analyze directly. One simple method for determining Vmax and Km from a set of velocity versus substrate data is to use the double reciprocal (Lineweaver-Burk) plot, a linear transformation of the Michaelis-Menten equation. A second method, which is generally preferable, is to use non-linear regression techniques to directly fit experimental data to the Michaelis-Menten equation. All biochemists need to be able to interpret the information presented in the Lineweaver-Burk plot, and to understand the implications of K_{cat}, V_{max}, and K_m.

The Michaelis-Menten Model Accounts for the Kinetic Properties of Many Enzymes.

The primary function of enzymes is to enhance rates of reactions so that they are compatible with the needs of the organism. To understand how enzymes function, we need a kinetic description of their activity. For many enzymes, the rate of catalysisV_0, which is defined as the number of moles of product formed per second, varies with the substrate concentration [S] in a manner shown in Figure 9.5. The rate of catalysis rises linearly as substrate concentration increases and then begins to level off and approach a maximum at higher substrate concentrations. Before we can accurately interpret this graph, we need to understand how it is generated. Consider an enzyme that catalyzes the S to P by the following pathway:

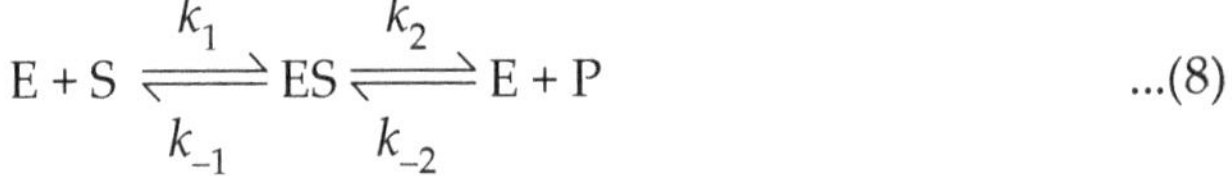

$$E + S \underset{k_{-1}}{\overset{k_1}{\rightleftharpoons}} ES \underset{k_{-2}}{\overset{k_2}{\rightleftharpoons}} E + P \quad ...(8)$$

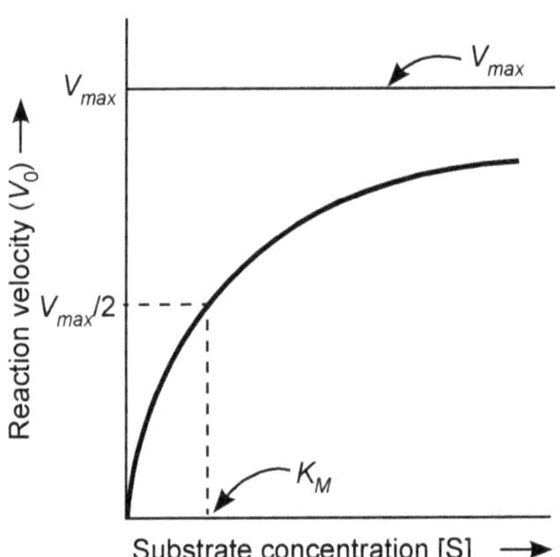

Figure 9.5: Michaelis-Menten Kinetics

Michaelis-Menten Kinetics. A plot of the reaction velocity (V_0) as a function of the substrate concentration [S] for an enzyme that obeys Michaelis-Menten kinetics shows that the maximal velocity (V_{max}) is approached asymptotically. The extent of product formation is determined as a function of time for a series of substrate concentrations (Figure 9.6). As expected, in each case, the amount of product formed increases with time, although eventually a time is reached when there is*no net change* in the concentration of S or P. The enzyme is still actively converting substrate into product and vice versa, but the reaction equilibrium has been attained. Figure 9.7A illustrates the changes in concentration observed in all of the reaction participants with time until equilibrium has been reached.

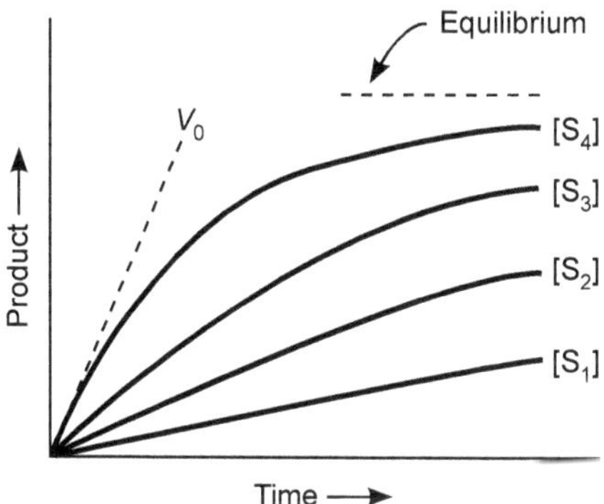

Figure 9.6: Determining Initial Velocity.

Determining Initial Velocity. The amount of product formed at different substrate concentrations is plotted as a function of time. The initial velocity (V_0) for each substrate concentration is determined from the slope of the curve at the beginning.

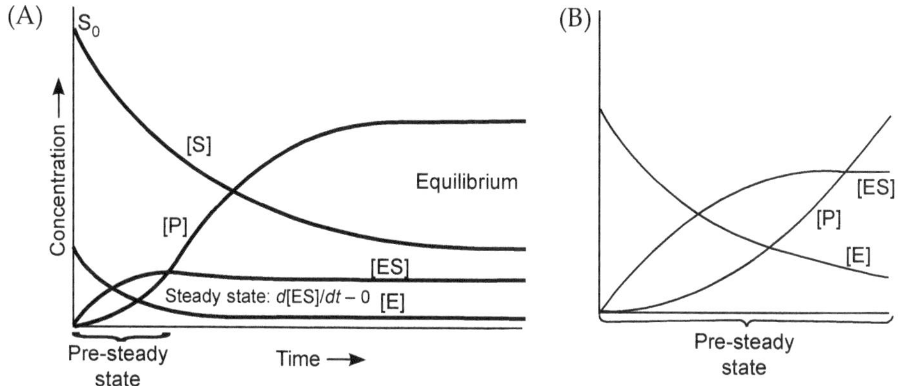

Figure 9.7: Enzyme-catalyzed reaction with time.

Changes in the Concentration of Reaction Participants of an Enzyme-Catalyzed Reaction with Time. Concentration changes under (A) steady-state conditions, and (B) the pre-steady-state conditions.

Enzyme kinetics is more easily approached if we can ignore the back reaction. We define V_0 as the rate of increase in product with time when [P] is low; that is, at times close to zero (hence, V_0) (Figure 9.7B). Thus, for the graph in Figure 9.5, V_0 is determined for each substrate concentration by measuring the rate of product formation at early times before P accumulates (Figure 9.6).

We begin our kinetic examination of enzyme activity with the graph shown in Figure 9.5. At a fixed concentration of enzyme, V_0 is almost linearly proportional to [S] when [S] is small but is nearly independent of [S] when [S] is large. In 1913, Leonor Michaelis and Maud Menten proposed a simple model to account for these kinetic characteristics. The critical feature in their treatment is that a specific ES complex is a necessary intermediate in catalysis. The model proposed, which is the simplest one that accounts for the kinetic properties of many enzymes, is

$$E + S \underset{k_{-1}}{\overset{k_1}{\rightleftharpoons}} ES \overset{k_2}{\rightleftharpoons} E + P \quad ...(9)$$

An enzyme E combines with substrate S to form an ES complex, with a rate constant k_1. The ES complex has two possible fates. It can dissociate to E and S, with a rate constant k_{-1}, or it can proceed to form product P, with a rate constant k_2. Again, we assume that almost none of the product reverts to the initial substrate, a condition that holds in the initial stage of a reaction before the concentration of product is appreciable.

We want an expression that relates the rate of catalysis to the concentrations of substrate and enzyme and the rates of the individual steps. Our starting point is that the catalytic rate is equal to the product of the concentration of the ES complex and

$$k_2.V_{.0}\, k_2[ES] \quad ...(10)$$

Now we need to express [ES] in terms of known quantities. The rates of formation and breakdown of ES are given by:

$$\text{Rate of formation of ES} = k_1[E][S] \quad ...(11)$$

$$\text{Rate of formation of ES} = (k_{-1} + k_2)\ [ES] \quad ...(12)$$

To simplify matters, we will work under the steady-state assumption. In a steady state, the concentrations of intermediates, in this case [ES], stay the same even if the concentrations of starting materials and products are changing. This occurs when the rates of formation and breakdown of the ES complex are equal. Setting the right-hand sides of equations 11 and 12 equal gives

$$k_1[E][S] = (k_{-1} + k_2)[ES] \quad ...(13)$$

By rearranging equation 13, we obtain

$$[E][S]/[ES] = (k_{-1} + k_2)/k_1 \quad ...(14)$$

Equation 14 can be simplified by defining a new constant, K_M, called the *Michaelis constant:*

$$K_M = \frac{k_{-1} + k_2}{k_1} \quad ...(15)$$

Note that K_M has the units of concentration. K_M is an important characteristic of enzyme-substrate interactions and is independent of enzyme and substrate concentrations.

Inserting equation 15 into equation 14 and solving for [ES] yields

$$[ES] = \frac{[E][S]}{K_M} \quad ...(16)$$

Now let us examine the numerator of equation 16. The concentration of uncombined substrate [S] is very nearly equal to the total substrate concentration, provided that the concentration of enzyme is much lower than that of substrate. The concentration of uncombined enzyme [E] is equal to the total enzyme concentration $[E]_T$ minus the concentration of the ES complex.

$$[E] = [E]_T - [ES] \qquad ...(17)$$

Substituting this expression for [E] in equation 16 gives

$$[ES] = \frac{([E]_T - [ES])[S]}{K_M} \qquad ...(18)$$

Solving equation 18 for [ES] gives

$$[ES] = \frac{([E]_T [S])/K_M}{1+[S]K_M} \qquad ...(19)$$

or

$$[ES] = [E]_T \frac{[S]}{[S]+K_M} \qquad ...(20)$$

By substituting this expression for [ES] into equation 10, we obtain

$$V_0 = k_2[E]_T \frac{[S]}{[S]+K_M} \qquad ...(21)$$

The maximal rate, V_{max}, is attained when the catalytic sites on the enzyme are saturated with substrate—that is, when $[ES] = [E]_T$. Thus,

$$V_{max} = k_2[E]_T \qquad ...(22)$$

Substituting equation 22 into equation 21 yields the *Michaelis-Menten equation:*

$$V_0 = V_{max} \frac{[S]}{[S]+K_M} \qquad ...(23)$$

This equation accounts for the kinetic data given in Figure 9.5. At very low substrate concentration, when [S] is much less than K_M, $V_0 = (V_{max}/K_M)[S]$; that is, the rate is directly proportional to the substrate concentration. At high substrate concentration, when [S] is much greater than K_M, $V_0 = V_{max}$; that is, the rate is maximal, independent of substrate concentration.

The meaning of K_M is evident from equation 23. When $[S] = K_M$, then $V_0 = V_{max}/2$. Thus, K_M *is equal to the substrate concentration at which the reaction rate is half its maximal value.* K_M is an important characteristic of an enzyme-catalyzed reaction and is significant for its biological function.

The physiological consequence of K_M is illustrated by the sensitivity of some individuals to ethanol. Such persons exhibit facial flushing and rapid heart rate (tachycardia) after ingesting even small amounts of alcohol. In the liver, alcohol dehydrogenase converts ethanol into acetaldehyde.

$$CH_3CH_2OH + NAD^+ \underset{}{\overset{\text{Alchohol dehydrogenase}}{\rightleftharpoons}} CH_3CHO + H^+ + NADH$$

Normally, the acetaldehyde, which is the cause of the symptoms when present at high concentrations, is processed to acetate by acetaldehyde dehydrogenase.

$$CH_3CHO + NAD^+ \xrightleftharpoons[]{\text{Alchohol dehydrigebase}} CH_3CHO^- + NADH + 2H^+$$

Most people have two forms of the acetaldehyde dehydrogenase, a low K_M mitochondrial form and a high K_M cytosolic form. In susceptible persons, the mitochondrial enzyme is less active due to the substitution of a single amino acid, and acetaldehyde is processed only by the cytosolic enzyme. Because this enzyme has a high K_M, less acetaldehyde is converted into acetate; excess acetaldehyde escapes into the blood and accounts for the physiological effects.

The Significance of K_M and V_{max} Values

The Michaelis constant, K_M, and the maximal rate, V_{max}, can be readily derived from rates of catalysis measured at a variety of substrate concentrations if an enzyme operates according to the simple scheme given in equation 23. The derivation of K_M and V_{max} is most commonly achieved with the use of curve-fitting programs on a computer (see the appendix to this chapter for alternative means of determining K_M and V_{max}). The K_M values of enzymes range widely (Table 9.2). For most enzymes, K_M lies between 10^{-1} and 10^{-7} M. The K_M value for an enzyme depends on the particular substrate and on environmental conditions such as pH, temperature, and ionic strength. The Michaelis constant, K_M, has two meanings. First, K_M is the concentration of substrate at which half the active sites are filled. Thus, K_M provides a measure of the substrate concentration required for significant catalysis to occur. In fact, for many enzymes, experimental evidence suggests that K_M provides an approximation of substrate concentration in vivo. When the K_M is known, the fraction of sites filled, f_{ES}, at any substrate concentration can be calculated from

$$f_{ES} = \frac{V}{V_{max}} = \frac{[S]}{[S] + K_M} \quad \text{...(24)}$$

Table 9.2: K_M values of some enzymes.

Enzyme	Substrate	K_M(μM)
Chymotrypsin	Acetyl-L-tryptophanamide	5000
Lysozyme	Hexa-*N*-acetylglucosamine	6
β-Galactosidase	Lactose	4000
Threonine deaminase	Threonine	5000
Carbonic anhydrase	CO_2	8000
Penicillinase	Benzylpenicillin	50
Pyruvate carboxylase	Pyruvate	400
	HCO_3^-	1000
	ATP	60
Arginine-tRNA synthetase	Arginine	3
	tRNA	0.4
	ATP	300

Second, K_M is related to the rate constants of the individual steps in the catalytic scheme given in equation 9. In equation 15,K_M is defined as $(k_{-1} + k_2)/k_1$. Consider a limiting case in which k_{-1} is much greater than k_2. Under such circumstances, the ES complex dissociates to E and S much more rapidly than product is formed. Under these conditions ($k_{-1} >> k_2$),

$$K_M = \frac{k_{-1}}{k_1} \quad ...(25)$$

The dissociation constant of the ES complex is given by

$$K_{ES} = \frac{[E][S]}{[ES]} = \frac{k_{-1}}{k_1} \quad ...(26)$$

In other words, K_M is equal to the dissociation constant of the ES complex if k_2 is much smaller than k_{-1}. When this condition is met, K_M is a measure of the strength of the ES complex: a high K_M indicates weak binding; a low K_M indicates strong binding. It must be stressed that K_M indicates the affinity of the ES complex only when k_{-1} is much greater than k_2.

The maximal rate, V_{max}, reveals the turnover number of an enzyme, which is the number of substrate molecules converted into product by an enzyme molecule in a unit time when the enzyme is fully saturated with substrate. It is equal to the kinetic constant k_2, which is also called k_{cat}. The maximal rate, V_{max}, reveals the turnover number of an enzyme if the concentration of active sites $[E]_T$ is known, because

$$V_{max} = k_2[E]_T$$

and thus

$$k_2 = V_{max}/[E]_T \quad ...(27)$$

For example, a 10^{-6} M solution of carbonic anhydrase catalyzes the formation of 0.6 M H_2CO_3 per second when it is fully saturated with substrate. Hence, k_2 is 6×10^5 s^{-1}. This turnover number is one of the largest known. Each catalyzed reaction takes place in a time equal to $1/k_2$, which is 1.7 μs for carbonic anhydrase. The turnover numbers of most enzymes with their physiological substrates fall in the range from 1 to 10^4 per second (Table 9.3).

Table 9.3: Maximum turnover numbers of some enzymes.

Enzyme	Turnover number (per second)
Carbonic anhydrase	600,000
3-Ketosteroid isomerase	280,000
Acetylcholinesterase	25,000
Penicillinase	2,000
Lactate dehydrogenase	1,000
Chymotrypsin	100
DNA polymerase I	15
Tryptophan synthetase	2
Lysozyme	0.5

Kinetic Perfection in Enzymatic Catalysis: The k_{cat}/K_M Criterion

When the substrate concentration is much greater than K_M, the rate of catalysis is equal to k_{cat}, the turnover number; most enzymes are not normally saturated with substrate. Under physiological conditions, the $[S]/K_M$ ratio is typically between 0.01 and 1.0. When $[S] << K_M$, the enzymatic rate is much less than k_{cat} because most of the active sites are unoccupied. Is there a number that characterizes the kinetics of an enzyme under these more typical cellular conditions? Indeed there is, as can be shown by combining equations 10 and 16 to give

$$V_0 = \frac{k_{cat}}{K_M}[E][S] \qquad ...(28)$$

When $[S] << K_M$, the concentration of free enzyme, [E], is nearly equal to the total concentration of enzyme $[E_T]$, so

$$V_0 = \frac{k_{cat}}{K_M}[S][E]_T \qquad ...(29)$$

Thus, when $[S] << K_M$, the enzymatic velocity depends on the values of k_{cat}/K_M, [S], and $[E]_T$. Under these conditions, k_{cat}/K_M is the rate constant for the interaction of S and E and can be used as a measure of catalytic efficiency. For instance, by using k_{cat}/K_M values, one can compare an enzyme's preference for different substrates. Table 9.4 show the k_{cat}/K_M values for several different substrates of chymotrypsin. Chymotrypsin clearly has a preference for cleaving next to bulky, hydrophobic side chains.

Table 9.4: Substrate preferences of chymotrypsin.

Amino acid in ester	Amino acid side chain	$k_{cat}/K_M (s^{-1}M^{-1})$
Glycine	—H	1.3×10^{-1}
Valine	$-CH(CH_3)_2$	2.0
Norvaline	$-CH_2CH_2CH_3$	3.6×10^{2}
Norleucine	$-CH_2CH_2CH_2CH_3$	3.0×10^{3}
Phenylalanine	$-CH_2-C_6H_5$	1.0×10^{5}

Source: After A. Fershet, Structure and s Mechanism in Protein Science: A Guide to Enzyme Catalysis and Protein Folding (W.H. Freeman and Company, Company, 1999).

How efficient can an enzyme be? We can approach this question by determining whether there are any physical limits on the value of k_{cat}/K_M. Note that this ratio depends on k_1, k_{-1}, and k_{cat}, as can be shown by substituting for K_M.

$$\frac{k_{cat}}{K_M} = \frac{k_{cat}}{(k_{-1} + k_{cat})/k_1} = \frac{k_{cat}}{k_{cat} + k_{-1}} k_1 < k_1 \qquad ...(30)$$

Suppose that the rate of formation of product (k_{cat}) is much faster than the rate of dissociation of the ES complex (k_{-1}). The value of k_{cat}/K_M then approaches k_1. Thus, the ultimate limit on the value of k_{cat}/K_M is set by k_1, the rate of formation of the ES complex. This rate cannot be faster than the diffusion-controlled encounter of an enzyme and its substrate. Diffusion limits the value of k_1 so that it cannot be higher than between 10^8 and 10^9 s^{-1} M^{-1}. Hence, the upper limit on k_{cat}/K_M is between 10^8 and 10^9 s^{-1} M^{-1}.

The k_{cat}/K_M ratios of the enzymes superoxide dismutase, acetylcholinesterase, and triose phosphate isomerase are between 10^8 and 10^9 s^{-1} M^{-1}. Enzymes such as these that have k_{cat}/K_M ratios at the upper limits have attained kinetic perfection. Their catalytic velocity is restricted only by the rate at which they encounter substrate in the solution (Table 9.5). Any further gain in catalytic rate can come only by decreasing the time for diffusion. Remember that the active site is only a small part of the total enzyme structure. Yet, for catalytically perfect enzymes, every encounter between enzyme and substrate is productive. In these cases, there may be attractive electrostatic forces on the enzyme that entice the substrate to the active site. These forces are sometimes referred to poetically as *Circe effects*.

Circe Effect

The utilization of attractive forces to lure a substrate into a site in which it undergoes a transformation of structure, as defined by William P. Jencks, an enzymologist, who coined the term.

Table 9.5: Enzymes for which k_{cat}/K_M is close to the diffusion-controlled rate of encounter.

Enzyme	k_{cat}/K_M **($s^{-1}M^{-1}$)**
Acetylcholinesterase	1.6×10^8
Carbonic anhydrase	8.3×10^7
Catalase	4×10^7
Crotonase	2.8×10^8
Fumarase	1.6×10^8
Triose phosphate isomerase	2.4×10^8
β-Lactamase	1×10^8
Superoxide dismutase	7×10^9

The limit imposed by the rate of diffusion in solution can also be partly overcome by confining substrates and products in the limited volume of a multienzyme complex. Indeed, some series of enzymes are associated into organized assemblies so that the product of one enzyme is very rapidly found by the next enzyme.

In effect, products are channeled from one enzyme to the next, much as in an assembly line.

Most Biochemical Reactions Include Multiple Substrates

Most reactions in biological systems usually include two substrates and two products and can be represented by the bisubstrate reaction:

$$A + B \rightleftharpoons P + Q$$

The majority of such reactions entail the transfer of a functional group, such as a phosphoryl or an ammonium group, from one substrate to the other. In oxidation-reduction reactions, electrons are transferred between substrates. Multiple substrate reactions can be divided into two classes: sequential displacement and double displacement.

Sequential Displacement

In the sequential mechanism, all substrates must bind to the enzyme before any product is released. Consequently, in a bisubstrate reaction, a ternary complex of the enzyme and both substrates forms. Sequential mechanisms are of two types: ordered, in which the substrates bind the enzyme in a defined sequence, and random.

Many enzymes that have NAD^+ or NADH as a substrate exhibit the sequential ordered mechanism. Consider lactate dehydrogenase, an important enzyme in glucose metabolism. This enzyme reduces pyruvate to lactate while oxidizing NADH to NAD^+.

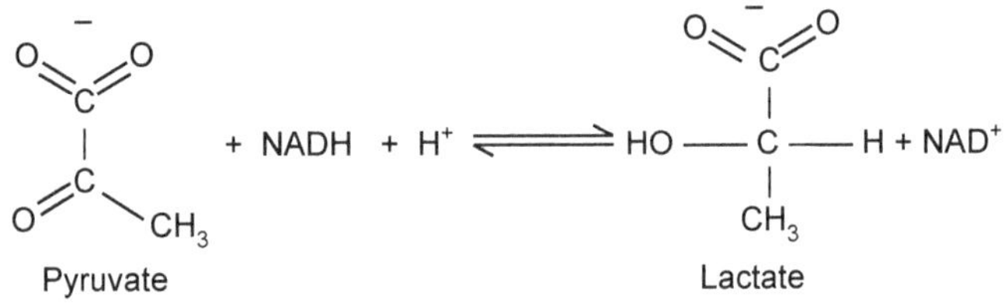

$$\text{Pyruvate} + NADH + H^+ \rightleftharpoons \text{Lactate } (HO{-}CH(CH_3){-}COO^-) + NAD^+$$

Pyruvate Lactate

In the ordered sequential mechanism, the coenzyme always binds first and the lactate is always released first. This sequence can be represented as follows in a notation developed by W. Wallace Cleland:

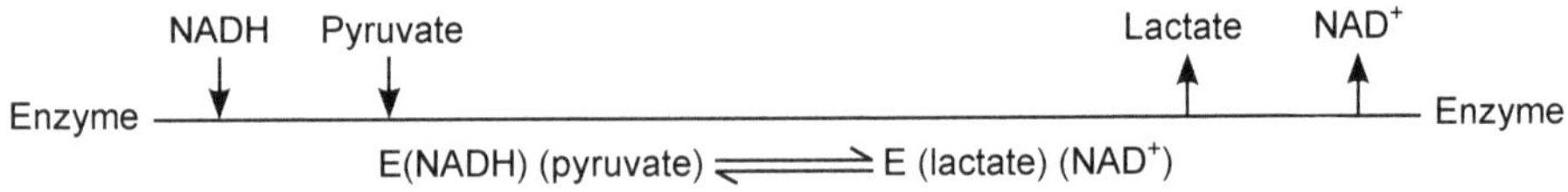

Enzyme — NADH ↓ — Pyruvate ↓ — E(NADH) (pyruvate) ⇌ E (lactate) (NAD^+) — Lactate ↑ — NAD^+ ↑ — Enzyme

The enzyme exists as a ternary complex: first, consisting of the enzyme and substrates and, after catalysis, the enzyme and products.

In the random sequential mechanism, the order of addition of substrates and release of products is random. Sequential random reactions are illustrated by the formation of phosphocreatine and ADP from ATP and creatine, a reaction catalyzed by creatine kinase.

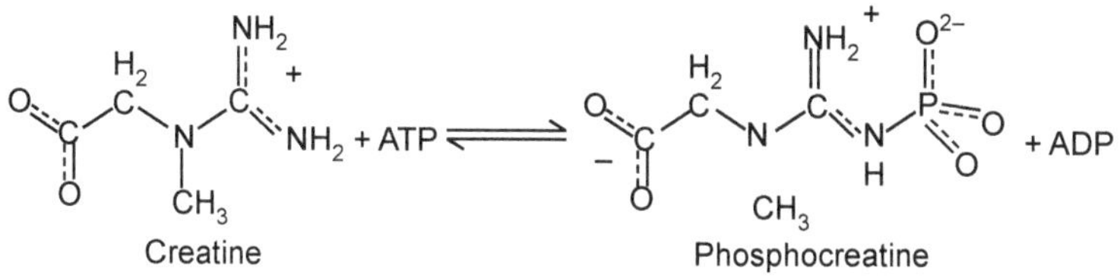

Creatine + ATP ⇌ Phosphocreatine + ADP

Phosphocreatine is an important energy source in muscle. Sequential random reactions can also be depicted in the Cleland notation.

ATP Creatine | Phosphocreatine ATP

Enzyme — E(creatine)(ATP) ⇌ E(phosphocreatine)(ADP) — Enzyme

Creatine ATP | ATP Phosphocreatine

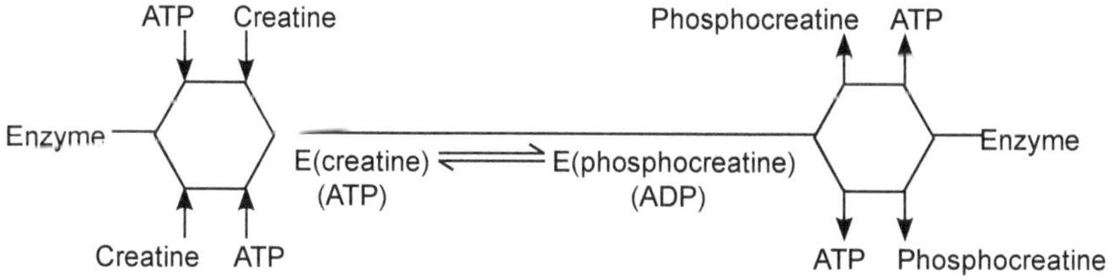

Although the order of certain events is random, the reaction still passes through the ternary complexes including, first, substrates and, then, products.

Double-Displacement (Ping-Pong) Reactions

In double-displacement, or Ping-Pong, reactions, one or more products are released before all substrates bind the enzyme. The defining feature of double-displacement reactions is the existence of a substituted enzyme intermediate, in which the enzyme is temporarily modified. Reactions that shuttle amino groups between amino acids and α-keto acids are classic examples of double-displacement mechanisms. The enzyme aspartate aminotransferase catalyzes the transfer of an amino group from aspartate to α-ketoglutarate.

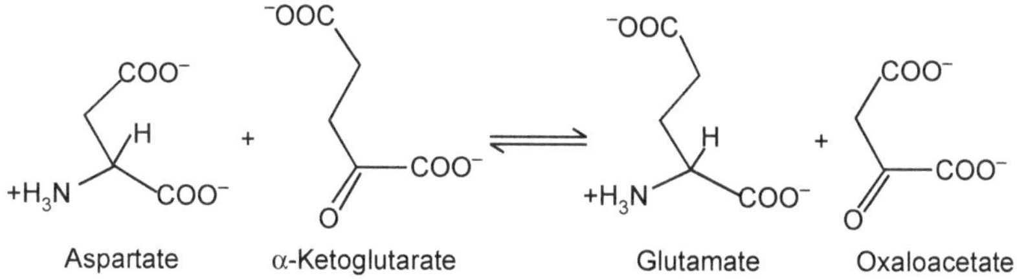

Aspartate + α-Ketoglutarate ⇌ Glutamate + Oxaloacetate

The sequence of events can be portrayed as the following diagram.

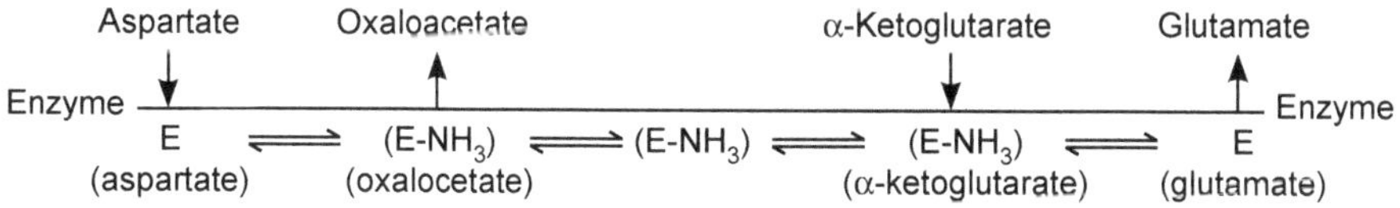

Aspartate ↓ Oxaloacetate ↑ α-Ketoglutarate ↓ Glutamate ↑

Enzyme — E (aspartate) ⇌ ($E\text{-}NH_3$) (oxalocetate) ⇌ ($E\text{-}NH_3$) ⇌ ($E\text{-}NH_3$) (α-ketoglutarate) ⇌ E (glutamate) — Enzyme

After aspartate binds to the enzyme, the enzyme removes aspartate's amino group to form the substituted enzyme intermediate. The first product, oxaloacetate, subsequently departs. The second substrate, α-ketoglutarate, binds to the enzyme, accepts the amino group from the modified enzyme, and is then released as the final product, glutamate. In the Cleland notation, the substrates appear to bounce on and off the enzyme analogously to a Ping-Pong ball bouncing on a table.

Allosteric Enzymes Do Not Obey Michaelis-Menten Kinetics

The Michaelis-Menten model has greatly assisted the development of enzyme chemistry. Its virtues are simplicity and broad applicability. However, the Michaelis-Menten model cannot account for the kinetic properties of many enzymes. An important group of enzymes that do not obey Michaelis-Menten kinetics comprises the allosteric enzymes. These enzymes consist of multiple subunits and multiple active sites.

Allosteric enzymes often display sigmoidal plots (Figure 9.8) of the reaction velocity V_0 versus substrate concentration [S], rather than the hyperbolic plots predicted by the Michaelis-Menten equation (equation 23). In allosteric enzymes, the binding of substrate to one active site can affect the properties of other active sites in the same enzyme molecule. A possible outcome of this interaction between subunits is that the binding of substrate becomes cooperative; that is, the binding of substrate to one active site of the enzyme facilitates substrate binding to the other active sites. As will be considered such cooperativity results in a sigmoidal plot of V_0 versus [S]. In addition, the activity of an allosteric enzyme may be altered by regulatory molecules that are reversibly bound to specific sites other than the catalytic sites. The catalytic properties of allosteric enzymes can thus be adjusted to meet the immediate needs of a cell. For this reason, allosteric enzymes are key regulators of metabolic pathways in the cell.

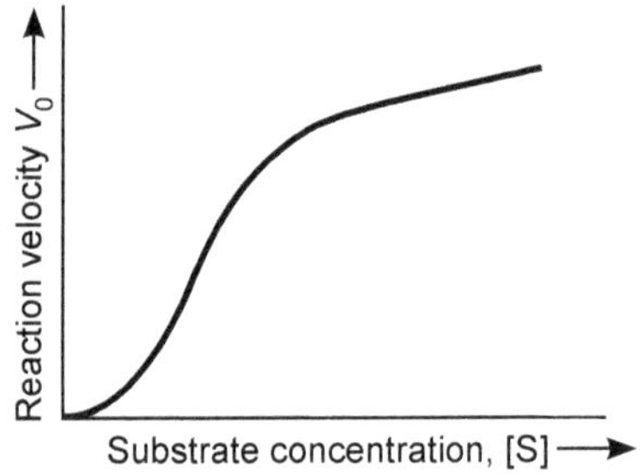

Figure 9.8: Kinetics for an Allosteric Enzyme. Allosteric enzymes display a sigmoidal dependence of reaction velocity on substrate concentration.

Spectrophotometric Kinase Activity Assays

Biaffin provides a comprehensive kinase activity analysis by the use of a spectrophotometric assay. The method couples the phosphorylation of substrates by PKA or PKG and the resulting conversion of ATP to ADP with a reaction catalyzed by pyruvate kinase and lactate dehydrogenase in the presence of phosphoenol pyruvate and NADH which restores the pool of ATP in the assay. For each mole of ADP generated one mole of NADH is oxidized to NAD. Due to a shift in absorbance from the reduced to the oxidized form of NAD the kinase specific activity is determined from the slope obtained by plotting the initial decrement in absorbance with time. The assay will be performed in 96 well formats in kinetic mode.

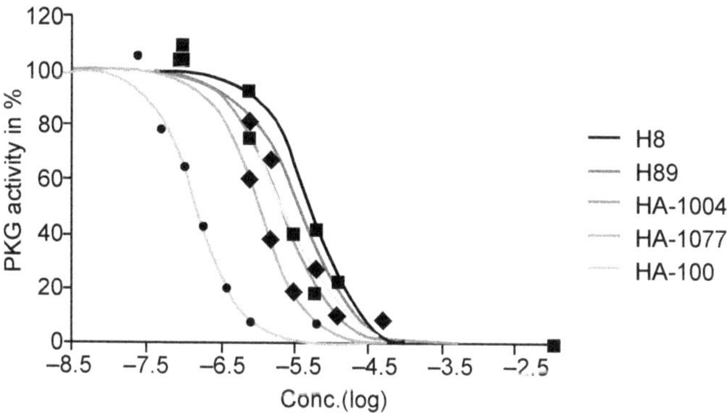

Radiometric Assay

A method for analyzing the chemical composition of substances based on the use of radioisotopes and nuclear radiation. Radiometric instruments are used in these assays for a qualitative and quantitative determination of the composition of substances. There are several different types of assays. A direct radiometric assay is based on the precipitation of the ion to be determined through an excess of a reagent containing a radioisotope. Both the concentration of the reagent and the radioactivity of the isotope are known, and after precipitation the radioactivity of the precipitate or of the excess reagent can be measured.

Radiometric titration is based on the combination of the ion to be determined with the reagent to form a compound that is either poorly soluble or easily extractable. During titration, the change in the radioactivity of the solution with the addition of a reagent serves as an indicator in those cases where a poorly soluble compound is formed; where an easily extractable compound is formed, the indicators are the changes in radioactivity with added reagent of both the solution and the extract. The equivalence point is determined by a break in the titration curve,which expresses the relationship between the volume of reagent introduced and the radioactivity of the titrated solution (or precipitate). The radioisotope either can be introduced into the reagent or the substance being determined or can be introduced into both.

Isotope dilution is based on the identical nature of the chemical reactions of the isotopes of a given element. In this method, some amount of the substance to be determined m_0 is added to the mixture under analysis. The added substance contains a radioisotope whose radioactivity I_0 is known. A portion of the substance to be determined is then separated in a pure state by any convenient method, for example,precipitation, extraction, or electrolysis, and the mass m_1 and radioactivity I_1 of the separated portion are measured. The total amount of the unknown substance in the mixture can be found from the equality of two ratios. The ratio between the radioactivities of the separated portion and that of the added substance is equal to the ratio between the mass of the separated portion and the sum of the masses of the addedsubstance and the substance originally in the mixture. Thus, $I_1/m_1 = I_0/(m + m_0)$, from which $m = (I_0/I_1)m_1 - m_0$.

In activation analysis, the substance being analyzed is irradiated (activated) with nuclear particles or hard gamma rays, and the radioactivity of the resulting radioisotopes is then determined. This radioactivity is proportional to the number of atoms of the element to be determined,the amount of activated isotope, the intensity of the flux of nuclear particles or photons, and the cross section for the nuclear reaction producing the radioisotope.

The photoneutron method is based on the emission of neutrons upon the action of high- energy photons (gamma quanta) on the nuclei of atoms. The number of neutrons, which is determined by neutron detectors, is proportional to the content of the element being analyzed. The energy imparted by the photons must exceed the binding energy of the nucleons in the nucleus, which for most elements is about 8 mega electron volts (MeV). (For beryllium and deuterium, however, the binding energy is only 1.666 and 2.226 MeV, respectively. Thus if the isotope ^{124}Sb having $£_\gamma$ equal to 1.7 and 2.1 MeV is used as a source of gamma quanta, beryllium can be determined against a background of all other elements).

Radiometric assays also employ methods based on the absorption of neutrons, gamma rays, beta particles, and quanta of characteristic X- ray emissions of radioisotopes. In the method of analysis based on the reflection of electrons or positrons, the intensity of the reflected beamis measured. Since the energy of particles reflected from light elements is several times less than that of particles reflected from heavy elements, the content of heavy elements in alloys with light elements and in ores can be determined.

ELECTROCHEMICAL APPROACH

Electrode Fabrication

The screen-printed electrode devices (rhodinised-carbon working electrode, carbon counter electrode and silver/ silver chloride reference electrode) used in this study have been described in detail elsewhere (Kr¨oger and Turner, 1997). Reagents for Electrochemical Tests The basic electrochemical measurement solution consisted of 0.1 M phosphate buffer incorporating 0.1M KCl and 0.5M glucose.

Glucose Oxidase Immobilisation

Four ml aliquots of appropriately diluted enzyme in buffer were dried onto the aqueous-polymer based rhodinised-carbon circular working electrode and left to dry at room temperature. Electrodes were stored at room temperature until used.

Test Format

Equilibration protocol: Devices were equilibrated into stirred glucose/buffer/KCl measurement solution for 2 min. and the current output noted. Addition protocol: Devices were first equilibrated in stirred buffer/KCl for 2 min. prior to glucose addition to a final concentration of 0.1 M. Response values were calculated by subtracting the current from the initial steady state current 1 min. after the addition step.

Apparatus And Measurement Procedure

All electrochemical measurements were performed amperometrically using an Autolab Electrochemical Analyser with the GPES 3 operating system (Ecochemie, Utrecht, NL). Hydrogen peroxide activity was determined amperometrically at a working electrode potential of 1300 mV versus the silver/silver chloride reference electrode.

Electrophoretic Enzyme Assay

An electrophoretic mobility shift assay (EMSA) or mobility shift electrophoresis, also referred as a gel shift assay, gel mobility shift assay, band shift assay, or gel retardation assay, is a common affinity electrophoresis technique used to study protein–DNA or protein–RNA interactions. This procedure can determine if a protein or mixture of proteins is capable of binding to a given DNA or RNA sequence, and can sometimes indicate if more than one protein molecule is involved in the binding complex. Gel shift assays are often performed in vitro concurrently with DNase footprinting, primer extension, and promoter-probe experiments when studying transcription initiation, DNA replication, DNA repair or RNA processing and maturation.

Principle

A mobility shift assay is electrophoretic separation of a protein–DNA or protein–RNA mixture on a polyacrylamide or agarose gel for a short period (about 1.5-2 hr for a 15- to 20-cm gel). The speed at which different molecules (and combinations thereof) move through the gel is determined by their size and charge, and to a lesser extent, their shape (see gel electrophoresis). The control lane (DNA probe without protein present) will contain a single band corresponding to the unbound DNA or RNA fragment. However, assuming that the protein is capable of binding to the fragment, the lane with protein present will contain another band that represents the larger, less mobile complex of nucleic acid probe bound to protein which is 'shifted' up on the gel (since it has moved more slowly).

Under the correct experimental conditions, the interaction between the DNA (or RNA) and protein is stabilized and the ratio of bound to unbound nucleic acid on the gel reflects the fraction of free and bound probe molecules as the binding reaction enters the gel. This stability is in part due to a caging effect, in that the protein, surrounded by the gel matrix, is unable to diffuse away from the probe before they recombine. If the starting concentrations of protein and probe are known, and if the stoichiometry of the complex is known, the apparent affinity of the protein for the nucleic acid sequence may be determined. Unless the complex is very long lived under gel conditions, or dissociation during electrophoresis is taken into account, the number derived is an apparent Kd. If the protein concentration is not known but the complex stoichiometry is, the protein concentration can be determined by increasing the concentration of DNA probe until further increments do not increase the fraction of protein bound. By comparison with a set of standard dilutions of free probe run on the same gel, the number of moles of protein can be calculated.

An antibody that recognizes the protein can be added to this mixture to create an even larger complex with a greater shift. This method is referred to as a supershift assay, and is used to unambiguously identify a protein present in the protein nucleic acid complex.

Often, an extra lane is run with a competitor oligonucleotide to determine the most favorable binding sequence for the binding protein. The use of different oligonucleotides of defined sequence allows the identification of the precise binding site by competition (not shown in diagram). Variants of the competition assay are useful for measuring the specificity of binding and for measurement of association and dissociation kinetics.

Once DNA-protein binding is determined *in vitro*, a number of in silico algorithms can narrow the search for identification of the transcription factor. Consensus sequence oligonucleotides for the transcription factor of interest will be able to compete for the binding, eliminating the shifted band, and must be confirmed by supershift. If the predicted consensus sequence fails to compete for binding, identification of the transcription factor may be aided by Multiplexed Competitor EMSA (MC-EMSA), whereby large sets of consensus sequences are multiplexed in each reaction, and where one set competes for binding, the individual consensus sequences from this set are run in a further reaction.

For visualization purposes, the nucleic acid fragment is usually labelled with a radioactive, fluorescent or biotin label. Standard ethidium bromide staining is less sensitive than these methods and can lack the sensitivity to detect the nucleic acid if small amounts of nucleic acid or single-stranded nucleic acid(s) are used in these experiments. When using a biotin label, streptavidin conjugated to an enzyme such as horseradish peroxidase is used to detect the DNA fragment (Non-radioactive EMSA review). While isotopic DNA labeling has little or no effect on protein binding affinity, use of non-isotopic labels including flurophores or biotin can alter the affinity and/or stoichiometry of the protein interaction of interest. Competition between fluorophore or biotin-labeled probe and unlabeled DNA of the same sequence can be used to determine whether the label alters binding affinity or stoichiometry.

Electrophoresis

- Many biological molecules carry an electrical charge, the magnitude of which depends on the particular molecule and also the pH and composition of the suspending medium. These charged molecules migrate in solution to the electrodes of opposite polarity when an electric field is applied and this principle is used in electrophoresis to separate molecules of differing charges.
- The electrophoretic mobility depends mainly on the ionizable groups present on the surface of the particle and the sign and magnitude of the charge carried by the ionizing groups varies according to the ionic strength and pH of the medium in a characteristic mannar. Separation of molecules can therefore be effected by selecting the appropriate medium.
- Proteins are separated under the influence of electric field based on differences mainly in their total charge and also to some extent in their size. Proteins in mixture carrying either negative or positive charge are allowed to migrate through transparent polyacrylamide gels. The proteins with higher magnitude of charge migrate faster and thus get separated from proteins with lesser charge.

Rf = Distance migrated by each protein

Distance migrated by tracking dye from top of separating gel

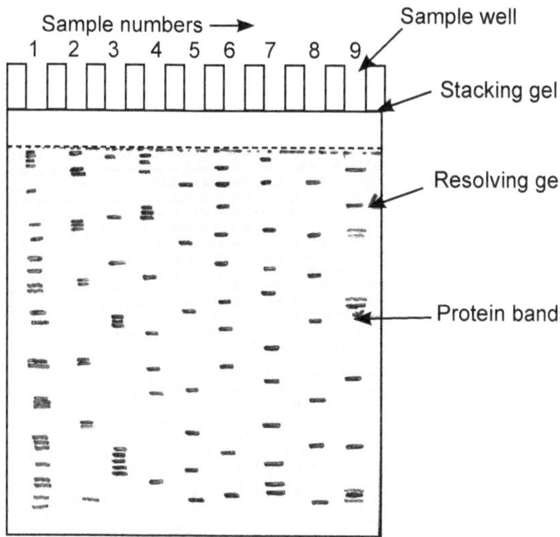

Figure 9.9: Diagrammatic representation of gel electrophoresis apparatus and samples.

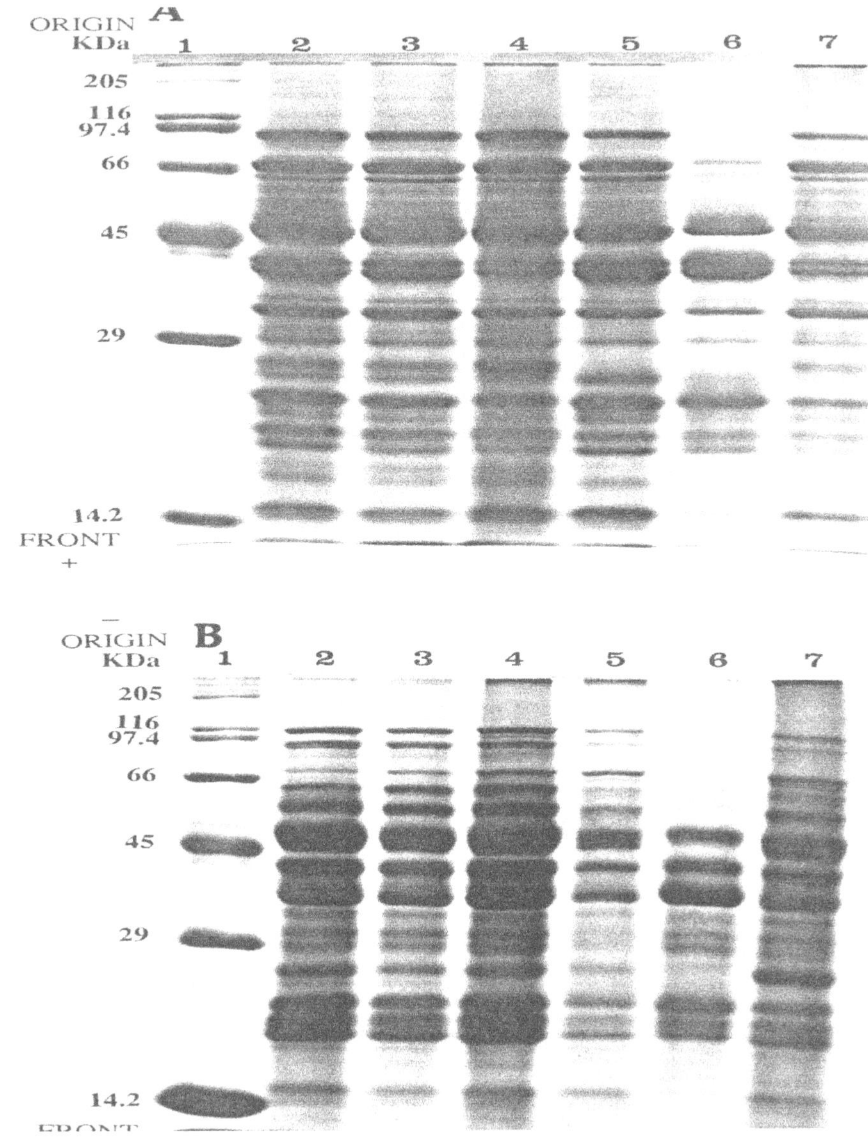

Figure 9.10: **A:** The NPAGE of pea proteins (1, molecular weight markers; 2, beach pea NaOH protein isolate; 3, beach pea SHMP protein isolate; 4, green pea NaOH protein isolate; 5, green pea SHMP protein isolate; 6, Canadian grass pea NaOH protein isolate; 7, Canadian grass pea SHMP protein isolate).

B: The SDS-PAGE of beach pea proteins (1, molecular weight markers; 2, NaOH protein isolate; 3, SHMP protein isolate; 4, albumin; 5, globulin; 6, prolamine; 7, glutelin).

DNA Technology

Recombinant DNA Technology: A recombinant DNA molecule is a vector (e.g. a plasmid, phage or virus) into which the desired DNA fragment has been inserted to enable its cloning in an appropriate host.

Chimaeric gene means a gene from one organism joined to regulatory sequences from another organism.

Gene and gene function: Transcription Translation Termination stapes occur in this technology.

Gene transmission: Smiconservative replication of DNA ensures transmission of genes from parents to progeny without change (Spontaneous mutation 14^{-4} to 10^{-7} per gene/generation). Transformation of DNA from cell to cell directly. Transduction means transformation of necessary genetic information from virus's cell to another cell. Conjugation means sexual transmission process.

Genetic Engineering of Crop Plants

Biotechnology involves the use of molecular genetic tools to give the economically important systems (crop plants and animals) new characteristics that cannot be achieved through the conventional breeding techniques. To put it simple words in genetic engineering we take pieces of DNA (deoxyribonucleic acid) from here and there and put them together to produce something better (recombinant DNA technology) than what is found in nature.

The 19th century monk, Gregor Mendel, through breeding experiments with pea plants, laid the early foundations of genetics. He found that plants contain factors, which contribute to the inheritance of specific characteristics. Later scientists found these factors to be genes, which are contained in the chromosomes of every cell. In the 1940s a Canadian scientist Dr. Oswald Avery discovered that genes were made of deoxyribonucleic acid, a long thin string of chemicals. In 1953 at Cambridge University, dr. James Watson and Dr. Francis Crick found that DNA consisted of two inter twisted strands, each composed of chains of four different chemical basis called adenine (A), guanine (G), cytosine (C) and thymine (T). This discovery has paved the way for recombing or engineering DNA to suite human purposes.

Researchers during the early 1970s developed the recombinant DNA technology required to manipulate and transfer genes from one cell to another. They learned how to use a variety of enzymes to cut genes apart and splice them back together. Today we can take a gene from just about any organism, study it, understand it, modify it, and make more of it, return it to its original host or transfer it to cells in completely different organisms.

By the end of the 1970s biotechnology was becoming a major business as the scientists, aware of the commercial potential of this technology, began setting up companies. Existing drug and chemical companies such as Monsanto, Biotechnical International and Eli Lilly, began spending enormous sums on biotechnological research, forging their links with university laboratories. To date their greatest successes have occurred with bacteria. These simple single-celled organisms contain plasmids, small loops of self-replicating DNA, which float about in the cell and are ideal for the insertion of new genes. In the late 1970s Genentech isolated the gene for human insulin inserted it into an *Escherichia coli* bacterium and left the altered organism in a fermentation tank to maturity. As the bacterium multiplied it mass-produced human insulin, which was purified and sold under the brand, name Humulin.

Bacteria have also been turned into industrial and agricultural products, capable of among other things, digesting crude oil or fertilizing plants. Dr. Aladar Szalay at the University of Alberta, Canada is currently attempting to develop multi-purpose microbes by transferring desirous genes onto already useful bacteria. It may be thus possible to give fertilizing bacteria the ability to kill plant-threating microbes like fungi and nematodes.

Plants and higher animals are more difficult to engineer genetically, because their cells lack plasmids. Hence, more sophisticated methods are needed to insert new genetic material into them. The new genes must also be properly controlled to switch on and off at the right time and place. For example, an insect-repelling gene should produce its toxin only when the insect is in season and only in those plant parts that are likely to be attacked. Although we can put only gene into only plant, gene expression varies from organ to organ. Not all genes are active in every cell. We must therefore learn how to control the signals that turn genes on and off in order to engineer them intelligently. Identifying and isolating "switches" and hooking them to appropriate genes are a major task ahead for the biotechnological researchers.

Virtually any known gene can be chemically assembled in the laboratory with a computerized DNA synthesizer. The switch-gene combination is chemically connected to marker genes (luciferase) plus another gene resistant to particular drug. This is all accomplished in a test tube (*in vitro*) by a variety of enzymes that cut paste DNA into the desired sequence. Once the genetic material has been "designed" it is inserted into bacteria, which quickly produce, copies of the stuff thus giving the scientist plenty of material with which to experiment. Next the genetic material is transferred into selected plant cells, which can be done in one of several ways. The cell membranes must be opened to allow the foreign DNA inside where it is incorporated into the chromosomes and passed on to subsequent generations of cells.

The success of gene transfer can be ascertained by putting the Petridis of cells into the chamber of a computerized "lowlight video image analyzing system" where the cells are scanned by an extremely sensitive camera capable of detecting the light emitted by the marker luciferase genes. Plant cells, which have taken up the foreign luciferase-containing DNA will give off light and show up clearly on the computer screen connected to the photo chamber. The cells are placed into a nutrient medium where they develop into a callus a cluster of undifferentiated cells resembling colored sugar crystals. The callus is placed in another medium containing hormones that encourage leaves and roots to grow. Finally the plant let is potted and grow to maturity. Every cell in the "regenerated" plant contains a copy of the transferred gene. These plants are then observed for the new gene's effect. Apart from genetic engineering, several other molecular marker techniques such as Restriction Fragment Length Polymorphism (RFLP), Random Amplified Polymorphic DNA (RAPD) are being used successfully in agriculture, in addition to gene transfer, tissue culture and hormonal bio-regulation of crops composition. Using these techniques scientists at ICRISAT are trying to improve crop plants like groundnut by transferring genes from wild *Arachis* spp. into the cultivated ones.

Steps in Gene Cloning

1. Identification and isolation of the desired gene or DNA fragment to be cloned.
2. Insertion of the isolated gene in a suitable vector.
3. Introduction of this vector into a suitable organism/cell called host (transformation).
4. Selection of the transformed host cells and
5. Multiplication/expression/integration followed by expression of the introduced gene in the host.

Isolation of the desired gene: The identification and isolation of the desired gene or DNA fragment called DNA insert to be cloned is a critical step in gene cloning.

This can be obtained from:

1. cDNA libraries, 2. Genomic library 3. Chemical (or enzymatic) synthesis and 4. Amplification through polymerase chain reaction (PCR).

Preparation of cDNA

cDNA is the copy or complementary DNA produced by using mRNA (usually) as a template. DNA copy of an RNA molecule is produced by the enzyme reverse transcriptase (RNA-dependent DNA polymerase; discovered by Temin and Baltimore in 1970) from avian mycloblastosis virus (AMV). This enzyme performs similar reactions as DNA polymerase and has an absolute requirement for a primer with a free 3′ –OH.

Gene Amplification Through Polymerase Chain Reaction

The polymerase chain reaction (PCR) technique, developed by Kary Mullis in 1985 is extremely powerful. It generates microgram (μg) quantities of DNA copies (upto billion copies) of the desired DNA (or RNA) segment, present even as single copy in the initial preparation, in a matter of few hours.

The PCR is carried out *in vitro*. It utilizes 1. A DNA preparation containing the desired segment to be amplified. 2. Two nucleotide primers (about 20 bases long), specific, *i.e.* complementary to the two 3′ borders (the sequences present at the

3′ ends of the two strands) of the desired segment. 3. The four-deoxynucleoside triphosphates viz., TTP (thymidine triphosphate), dCTP (deoxycyctidine triphosphate), dATP (deoxyadenosine triphosphate) and dGTP (deoxyguanosine triphosphate) and a heat stable DNA polymerase e.g. Tag (isolated from bacterium the *Thermus acquaticus*), Pfu (from *Pyrococcus furiosus*) and Vent (from *Thermococcus litoralis*) polymerases. Pfu and Vent polymerases are more efficient than the Tag polymerase.

Multiplication, Expression and Integration of The DNA Insert in Host Genome:

Once the clone containing the desired DNA insert is identified, it is multiplied in *E. coli* to obtain sufficient number of copies to be used in one or more of the following ways.

1. It can be used for a structural analysis of the insert, e.g. DNA sequencing, chromosome walking etc.
2. It may be introduced into a bacterium like *B. subtilis* for production of the protein encoded by the insert sine this host secretes proteins into the medium, which allows easy purification.
3. It can be introduced into a eukaryotic host e.g. yeast, animal cells, plants etc. either to investigate the function of the insert or
4. To integrate it into the host genome to achieve one of many diverse objectives.

Southern hybridization: The name of this technique is derived from the name of its inventor E. M. Southern and the DNA-DNA hybridization that forms its basis. It is also called Southern blotting since the procedure for transfer of DNA from the get to the nitrocellulose filter resembles blotting. This technique has since been extended to the analysis of RNA (northern blotting) and proteins (western blotting); these names are only jargon terms.

Dot blot technique: This technique is used to detect the presence of a given sequence of DNA/RNA in the non-fractionated (not subjected to gel electrophoresis) DNA.

Northern hybridization: RNAs are separated by gel electrophoresis; the RNA bands are transferred onto a suitable membrane e.g. diazobenzyloxymethyl (DBM) paper or nylon membranes and immobilized; the bands are hybridized with radioactive single-stranded DNA by autoradiography. It is an extension of the Southern blotting technique.

Southern blotting technique	Northern blotting technique
DNA is separated by gel electrophoresis	RNAs are separated by gel electrophoresis
DNA has to be denatured before blotting	Not needed in this protocol
Nitrocellulose membrane is used in this system	Diazobenzyloxymethyl (DBM) paper is used in this system
Hybridization with the probe produces DNA-DNA hybrid molecules	RNA : DNA molecules produces in this system

- ➔ Recently developed nylon membranes have superceded the use of DBM paper as they are robust, reusable and bind (by cross linking) to RNA on a brief exposure to UV light.
- ➔ Northern hybridization is useful in the identification and separation of the RNA that is complementary to a specific DNA probe; this is a sensitive test for the detection of transcription of a DNA sequence that is used as probe.

Western blotting: Proteins are electrophoresed in polyacrylamide gel transferred onto a nitrocellulose or nylon membrane (to which they bind strongly), and the protein bands are detected by their specific interaction with antibodies, lectins or some other compounds.

The specific protein bands are identified in a variety of ways: Antibodies are the most commonly used as probes for detecting specific antigens. Lectins are used as probes for the identification of glycoproteins. These probes may themselves be radioactive or a radioactive molecule may be tagged to them. Often the identification process is based on a "Sandwich" reaction.

Probes: Probes are small (15-30 bases long) nucleotide sequences used to detect the presence of complementary sequences in nucleic acid samples. This is achieved by permitting the probes to base pair with the sample nucleic acids and then identifying the samples that show base pairing with the probes i.e. hybridization.

Both DNA and RNA are used as probes. Single-stranded DNA probes are more convenient and preferable, but denatured double stranded DNA molecules can also be used.

Nick translation: This is the oldest method of nucleic acid labeling and is still the most commonly used. This technique is quite flexible with respect to probe size, specific activity and concentration; it is particularly suited for the production of large quantities of probes for use in multiple hybridization reactions and/or where a high probe concentration is required.

Enzyme-linked immunosorbent assay [ELISA]: An antibody (Ab) reacts with the concerned antigen (Ag) in a highly specific manner (i.e. an antibody reacts with that determinant or region of an antigen for which it is specific) to produce an Ag-Ab complex. When soluble proteins react with an antibody, the Ag-Ab complex forms a precipitate, while in case of particulate antigens the Ag-Ab complex agglutinates. In either case, either the amount of Ag-Ab complex formed or the rate of its formation is used to determine either quantity of the antigen or that of the antibody involved in the interaction. The various assays used for the following purposes:

Precipitation reaction, the ouchterlony assay, the mancini assay, immuno electrophores is, western blotting, rocket electrophoresis, agglutination reactions, labeled antibody techniques, radioimmune assay (RIA), enzyme-linked immunosorbent assay, fluorescent labels, electron dense labels, nonspecific binding to immunoglobulin and flow cytometry.

In Situ Hybridization: In situ hybridization has been used to establish the location of sat-DNA in chromosomes. For this purpose, radioactive copies of sat-DNA or its complementary RNA (using sat-DNA as template) are prepared. Chromosomes in squash preparations are specially pretreated to expose and denature their DNA without affecting their structural integrity. These chromosomes are then loaded with the radioactive single-stranded sat-DNA or its complementary RNA-after an appropriate interval, the squash preparations are washed to remove the non hybridized radioactive DNA (or RNA) probe and the location of radioactivity in the chromosomes is determined through radio autographic technique.

In Situ or cytological hybridization is also used to locate specific genes in chromosomes, especially in giant chromosomes. For this purpose, a radioactive clone representing a gene, most often labeled cDNA copies of the mRNA produced by the gene, is used as probe. Colony hybridization is also a form of Situ hybridization. This technique is also useful in disease diagnosis, particularly for the detection of viruses in tissues and cells.

Cloning: Cells derived from a single cell through mitosis constitute a clone and the process of obtaining clones is called cloning. (A sexual progeny of a single individual make up a clone). In simple term, cloning consists of trypsinisation of a monolayer culture to prepare a cell suspension, 3-4 dilution steps to achieve a suitable cell density (10-200 cells/ml), and seeding in petri dishes or flasks or multi-well dishes. The culture vessels are incubated for 1-3 weeks with a medium change after 1 wee; by this time colonies will develop.

Cloning is used to:

1. Obtain homogeneous cell lines from heterogeneous cell cultures.
2. To isolate biochemical mutants
3. Cell strains with marker chromosomes and
4. To develop hybridoma clones.

Cloning is generally applied to continuous cell lines, but often their clones become considerably heterogeneous by the time they are sufficiently multiplied for use. The problem with finite cell lines is that of life span; by the time the clone is sufficiently multiplied, the cells may be approaching senescence.

DNA Fingerprinting: DNA fingerprinting or DNA profiling is generally used for the identification of criminals from blood strains, semen etc. and for establishing parentage in cases of dispute. The data from this approach are extremely reliable as compared to the conventional analysis of serum proteins and erythrocyte antigens and proteins. DNA fingerprint of an individual is essentially a Southern blot of this DNA digested with an endonuclease and probed with a radioactive DNA probe.

Molecular Markers: Isozymes (electrophoretic variants of enzymes) and DNA sequences are used as molecular markers in chromosome mapping. Therefore, for all practical purposes, a molecular marker may be defined as a DNA sequence used for chromosome mapping, as it can be located at a specific site in a chromosome.

A molecular marker may be either anonymous or defined. An anonymous marker is a cloned random DNA fragment whose function or specific features are not known. Defined marker may contain a gene or some other specific feature e.g. Restriction sites for rare cutting restriction enzymes etc.

Molecular Markers

1. Restriction fragment length polymorphism (RFLP)
2. Random amplified polymorphic DNAs (RAPD)
3. Variable number of tandem repeats (VNTRs) DNA
   a. Minisatellite DNAs
   b. Microsatellite DNAs
4. CPG islands: About 1% of the human chromosomal DNA is stably unmethylated; these regions are called CPG islands since they contain more than 50% of C + G.
5. Isozymes
6. Short tandem repeat (STR) DNA.

A Comparison Between RFLP and RAPD Markers For Genome Mapping in Plants

Feature	RFLP	RAPD
Inheritance pattern	Codominant	Dominant
Detection of multiple alleles of a marker	Yes	No
Quality of DNA needed for study	Pure	Crude
Amount of DNA needed	2-10 mg	>10 ng
Radio isotopes	Must be used (in probes)	Not used
Restriction enzymes	Must be used	Not used
Type of probe used	Species specific probes, generally low copy genomic or DNA	Random base sequence 9-12 base nucleotides
Time required	About 5 times more than RAPDs	0.20 % of that for RFLPs

Calculations of Enzyme Activity

Unit of Enzyme Activity: Used to measure total units of activity in a given volume of solution.

Specific Activity: Used to follow the increasing purity of an enzyme through several procedural steps.

Molecular Activity: Used to compare activities of different enzymes. Also called the turn-over number (TON = k_{cat})

Classical Units

Unit of enzyme activity:

mmol substrate transformed/min = unit

Specific activity:

mmol substrate/min-mg E = unit/mg E

Molecular activity:

mmol substrate/min- mmol E = units/mmol E

New International Units

Unit of enzyme activity:

mol substrate/sec = katal

Specific activity:

mol substrate/sec-kg E = katal/kg E

Molecular activity:

mol substrate/sec-mol E = katal/mol E

Example 1: The rate of an enzyme catalyzed reaction is 35 μmol/min at [S] = 10^{-4} M, ($K_M = 2 \times 10^{-5}$). Calculate the velocity at [S] = 2×10^{-6} M.

First calculate V_M using the Michaelis-Menton eqn:

$$V = \frac{V_M [S]}{K_M [S]}, \text{ so: } 35 = \frac{V_M (10^{-4})}{2\times10^{-5} + 10^{-4}} = \frac{V_M (10^{-4})}{1.2\times0^{-4}}$$

$V_M = 1.2(35) = 42$ mmol/min; then calculate V:

$$V = \frac{42(2\times10^{-6})}{2\times10^{-5} + 2\times10^{-6}} = \frac{84\times10^{-6}}{22\times10^{-6}} = 3.8 \text{ mmol/min}$$

Example 2: An enzyme (1.84 μgm, MW = 36800) catalyzes a reaction in presence of excess substrate at a rate of 4.2 μmol substrate/min. What is the TON ?

$$\mu \text{ mol E} = \frac{1.84 \propto \text{gm}}{36800 \propto \text{gm}/\propto \text{mol}} = 5\times10^{-5} \ \mu \text{ mol E}$$

$$\text{TON} = \frac{4.2 \propto \text{mol}/\text{min}}{5\times10^{5} \propto \text{mol}} = 84000 \text{ min}^{-1}$$

What is the value of this TON (84000 min^{-1}) in units of sec^{-1} ?

$$\text{TON E} = 84000 \text{ min}^{-1} \times \frac{1 \text{ sec}^{-1}}{60 \text{ min}^{-1}} = 1400 \text{ sec}^{-1}$$

Example 3: Ten micrograms of carbonic anhydrase (MW = 30000) in the presence of excess substrate exhibits a reaction rate of 6.82×10^{3} μmol/min.

At [S] = 0.012 M the rate is 3.41×10^{3} μmol/min.

a. What is Vm ?

b. What is K_M ?

c. What is k_2 (kcat) ?

Work these.

a. The rate in presence of excess substrate is Vmax

so: Vmax = 6.86×10^3 μmol/min.

b. At [S] = 0.012 M the rate is 3.41×10^3 μmol/min which is ½ Vmax so:

$$K_M = 0.012 \text{ M.}$$

This may also be determined using the

Michaelis-Menton equation.

c. Divide Vmax by μmol of E_T to find kcat.

$$\text{kcat} = 2.05 \times 10^7 \text{ min}^{-1}.$$

CHAPTER 10

Radioactivity and Related Calculations

There are three measurement units for radioactivity: the Becquerel measures radioactivity, the Gray measures the absorbed dose and the Sievert measures the biological effects.

Measuring Radioactivity: The Becquerel

The Becquerel (Bq) measures the activity of a radioactive source, giving the number of atoms which, within a particular time frame, transform and emit radiation.

1 Bq = 1 emission of radiation per second.

This is a very small unit, and multiples are often used:

- 1 MBq = 1 mega Becquerel = 1,000,000 Bq
- 1 GBq = 1 giga Becquerel = 1,000,000,000 Bq
- 1 TBq = 1 tera Becquerel = 1,000,000,000,000 Bq

The radioactivity of an environment, a material or a foodstuff is given in Becquerels per kilogram or per liter.

Measuring The Absorbed Dose: The Gray

The Gray (Gy) measures the absorbed dose, giving the energy transferred by ionizing radiations to the material upon encountering it.

1 Gy = 1 joule per kilogram

Sub-multiples are often used:

- 1 mGy = 1 milligray = 0.001 Gy
- 1 μGy = 1 microgray = 0.000001 Gy
- 1 nGy = 1 nanogray = 0.000000001 Gy

Measuring The Biological Effect: The Sievert

The Sievert (Sv) evaluates the effects of ionizing radiation on living material. At equal doses, the effects of radioactivity on living tissue depends on the type of radiation (alpha, beta, gamma, etc.), on the organ concerned and also on the length of exposure.

Contrary to the Becquerel, the sievert is a very large unit, and we often use sub-multiples:

- 1 mSv = 1 millisievert = 0.001 Sv
- 1 μSv = 1 microsievert = 0.000001 Sv

Activity: How much is present?

The size or weight of a container or shipment does not indicate how much radioactivity is in it. The amount of radioactivity in a quantity of material can be determined by noting how many curies of the material are present. This information should be found on labels and/or shipping papers.

More curies = a greater amount of radioactivity

A large amount of material can have a very small amount of radioactivity; a very small amount of material can have a lot of radioactivity.

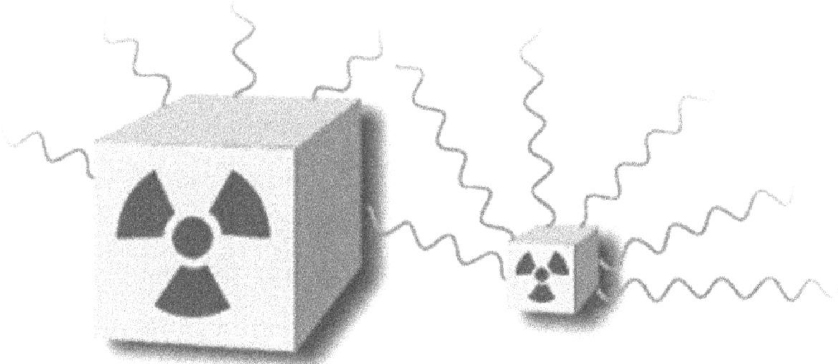

For example, uranium-238 has 0.00015 curies of radioactivity per pound (0.15 millicuries), while cobalt-60 has nearly 518,000 curies per pound.

In the International System of units (SI), the becquerel (Bq) is the unit of radioactivity. One Bq is 1 disintegration per second (dps). One curie is 37 billion Bq. Since the Bq represents such a small amount, you are likely to see a prefix used with Bq, as shown below:

- 1 MBq (27 microcuries)
- 1 GBq (27 millicuries)
- 37 GBq (1 curie)
- 1 TBq (27 curies)

SI Units and Prefixes

The International System of Units has been given official status and recommended for universal use by the General Conference on Weights and Measures.

Radiation Measurements

	Radioactivity	Absorbed Dose	Dose Equivalent	Exposure
Common Units	curie (Ci)	rad	rem	roentgen (R)
SI Units	becquerel (Bq)	gray (Gy)	sievert (Sv)	coulomb/ kilogram (C/kg)

Following is a list of prefixes and their meanings that are often used in conjunction with SI units:

Multiple	Prefix	Symbol
10^{12}	tera	T
10^{9}	giga	G
10^{6}	mega	M
10^{3}	kilo	k
10^{-2}	centi	c
10^{-3}	milli	m
10^{-6}	micro	μ
10^{-9}	nano	n

CONVERSIONS

Conversion Equivalence

1 curie = 3.7 x 10^{10} disintegrations per second

1 becquerel = 1 disintegration per second

1 millicurie (mCi) = 37 megabecquerels (MBq)

1 rad = 0.01 gray (Gy)

1 rem = 0.01 sievert (Sv)

1 roentgen (R) = 0.000258 coulomb/kilogram (C/kg)

1 megabecquerel (MBq) = 0.027 millicuries (mCi)

1 gray (Gy) = 100 rad

1 sievert (Sv) = 100 rem

1 coulomb/kilogram (C/kg) = 3,880 roentgens

Conversion Factors

To convert from	To	Multiply by
Curies (Ci)	becquerels (Bq)	3.7×10^{10}
millicuries (mCi)	megabecquerels (MBq)	37
microcuries (μCi)	megabecquerels (MBq)	0.037
millirads (mrad)	milligrays (mGy)	0.01
millirems (mrem)	microsieverts (μSv)	10
milliroentgens (mR)	microcoulombs/kilogram (μC/kg)	0.258
becquerels (Bq)	curies (Ci)	2.7×10^{-11}
megabecquerels (MBq)	millicuries (mCi)	0.027
megabecquerels (MBq)	microcuries (μCi)	27
milligrays (mGy)	millirads (mrad)	100
microsieverts (μSv)	millrems (mrem)	0.1
microcoulombs/kilogram (μC/kg)	milliroentgens (mR)	3.88

Measuring Radiation

There are four different but interrelated units for measuring radioactivity, exposure, absorbed dose, and dose equivalent. These can be remembered by the mnemonic **R-E-A-D**, as follows, with both common (British, e.g., Ci) and international (metric, e.g., Bq) units in use:

- Radioactivity refers to the amount of ionizing radiation released by a material. Whether it emits alpha or beta particles, gamma rays, x-rays, or neutrons, a quantity of radioactive material is expressed in terms of its radioactivity (or simply its activity), which represents how many atoms in the material decay in a given time period. The units of measure for radioactivity are the curie (Ci) and becquerel (Bq).
- Exposure describes the amount of radiation traveling through the air. Many radiation monitors measure exposure. The units for exposure are the roentgen (R) and coulomb/kilogram (C/kg).
- Absorbed dose describes the amount of radiation absorbed by an object or person (that is, the amount of energy that radioactive sources deposit in materials through which they pass). The units for absorbed dose are the radiation absorbed dose (rad) and gray (Gy).
- Dose equivalent (or effective dose) combines the amount of radiation absorbed and the medical effects of that type of radiation. For beta and gamma radiation, the dose equivalent is the same as the absorbed dose. By contrast, the dose equivalent is larger than the absorbed dose for alpha

and neutron radiation, because these types of radiation are more damaging to the human body. Units for dose equivalent are the roentgen equivalent man (rem) and sievert (Sv), and biological dose equivalents are commonly measured in 1/1000th of a rem (known as a millirem ormrem).

For practical purposes, 1 R (exposure) = 1 rad (absorbed dose) = 1 rem or 1000 mrem (dose equivalent).

Measurement of Radioactivity

Radioactive decay is a random process and therefore fluctuations are expected in the radioactivity measurement. That is why measurement of radioactivity must be treated by statistical methods.

In every measurement a deviation from the true value or error is likely to occur. There are two types of errors - systematic and random. The accuracy of a measurement indicates how closely it agrees with the true value. The precision of a series of measurements describes the reproducibility and indicates the deviation from the average or mean value. The closer the measurement is to the average value, the higher the precision, whereas the closer the measurement is to the true value, the more accurate is the measurement. It is important to keep in mind, which a series of measurements may be quite precise but their value may be far from the true value. Precision can be improved by eliminating the random errors; better accuracy is obtained by removing both the random and systematic errors.

The average or mean value is obtained by adding the values of all measurements divided by the number of measurements. The standard deviation indicates the deviation from the mean value and is a measure of precision. The standard deviation in radioactive measurements indicates the statistical fluctuations in radioactive disintegration. If the number of measurements is large, the distribution can be approximated by a Gaussian distribution even if the radioactive decay follows the Poisson distribution law. For practical reasons, only single measurement is obtained on radioactive sample instead of multiple repeat counts to determine the mean value. The precision of a count of a radioactive sample can be increased by accumulating a large number of counts in a single measurement because of decreasing the standard deviation.

Interaction of Radiation with Matter

All radiations may interact with the atoms of the matter during their passage through it producing ionization and excitation of the atoms. These radiations are called ionizing radiation. The mechanism of interaction differs for particulate and electromagnetic type of radiation.

The interaction of beta particles as a charged particles and gamma radiation as an electromagnetic radiation is the most important from the point of view of using them in nuclear medicine.

Beta particles interact primarily with the electrons of the absorber atoms and rarely with the nucleus.

Ionization occurs when beta particle transfers sufficient amount of its energy to the orbital electron and ejects it from the atom. As a result ion pair is formed. This process may rupture chemical bonds in the molecules. Ionization is used namely in the radiation therapy and also serves as a mean of the detection of charged particles in ion chambers.

When energetic beta particles, namely electrons, pass close to the nucleus of the atom, they lose energy as a result of deceleration. This loss of energy appears as an x ray and is called bremsstrahlung. Bremsstrahlung production increases with the kinetic energy of the beta particles and the atomic number of the absorber. That is why high energy beta particles are stored in plastic rather than shielding by lead.

Beta plus particles, positrons, combine with the orbital electrons and produce two 511 keV photons of gamma radiation, so called annihilation radiation, that are emitted in exactly opposite directions. This is the basis of positron emission tomography.

Gamma rays interact with orbital electrons and if their energy is very high they may also interact with the nucleus of the absorber atoms. They travel a long path in the absorber before losing all energy and so they are called *penetrating radiations*.

There are three mechanisms by which gamma rays interact with absorber atoms from which two are important for nuclear medicine.

Photoelectric effect means transfer of all energy of gamma photon to an orbital electron, called photoelectron, and ejecting it from the atom. The photoelectron then loses its energy by ionization and excitation.

Compton scattering means transfer of only a part of energy of gamma photon to an electron and ejecting it. The gamma photon with less energy is deflected from its original direction. The scattered photon may then undergo further photoelectric or Compton interaction and the Compton electron may cause ionization or excitation.

Depending on the photon energy and the density and thickness of the absorber, some photons may pass through the absorber without any interaction.

Attenuation of gamma radiations by means of their interaction with absorber is an important factor in radiation protection. The term half-value layer is defined as the thickness of the absorber that reduces the intensity of a photon beam by one half. It depends on the energy of the radiation and the atomic number of the absorber.

Radiation Detection

Interaction of ionizing radiations with the matter is also used for their detection and measurement. There are several principles of radiation detection in nuclear medicine. Some of them are used in radiation protection, others in measurement and imaging.

The oldest principle is darkening of photographic emulsion. This principle is used in the personnel dosimetry. The film badge is most popular and cost-effective for personnel monitoring and gives reasonably accurate readings of exposures from beta, gamma and *x* radiations. The film badge consists of a radiation sensitive film held in a plastic holder. Filters of copper and lead are attached to the holder to differentiate exposure from different types and energies of radiation.

Another principle is thermoluminiscence. Several inorganic crystals (e.g. LiF) can accumulate radiation energy and hold it. If the crystal is heated from 300 to 400 degrees of Celsius, it emits light in amount proportional to the absorbed energy. Thermoluminiscent dosimeters, so called TLD, are mostly used as a finger dosimeters, so inorganic crystals are held in a plastic holders and plastic rings. It gives an accurate exposure reading and can be reused.

Another principle is converting the energy of radiation to electric current. There are two basic principles based on ionization and excitation.

First is ionization of gas molecules, the second is excitation and ionization of solid, liquid or plastic material, called scintilator, which emits photons of light after absorbing radiation. Light is then converted to the electric current by means of photomultiplier tube.

Gas-filled detectors collect the ion pairs as a current with the application of a voltage between two electrodes. The measured current is proportional to the applied voltage and the amount of radiation.

At lower voltages from 50 to 300 V, only the primary ion pairs formed by the initial radiation are collected. Ionization chambers operate in this region. The detector is a cylindrical chamber with a central wire filled with air or different gases. These detectors are primarily used for measuring high intensity radiation. Dose calibrators and pocket dosimeters are the common ionization chambers used in nuclear medicine.

The dose calibrator is one of the most essential instruments in nuclear medicine for measuring the activity of radio nuclides and radiopharmaceuticals. It must be regularly checked for constancy, accuracy, linearity and geometry.

At higher voltages from 1000 to 1200 V, the current becomes identical regardless of how many ion pairs are produced by the incident radiation. Geiger-Müller counters operate in this region. Geiger-Müller counters are used to monitor the radiation level in different work areas and they are called area monitors or survey meters. They are more sensitive than ionization chambers but they cannot discriminate between energies. They are almost 100% efficient for counting alpha and beta particles but have only 1 to 2% efficiency for counting gamma and *x* rays.

Scintillation detectors consist of scintilator emitting flashes of light after absorbing gamma or *x* radiation. The light photons produced are then converted to an electrical pulse by means of a photomultiplier tube. The pulse is amplified by a linear amplifier, sorted by a pulse-height analyzer and then registred as a count. Different solid or liquid scintillators are used for different types of radiation. In nuclear medicine, sodium iodide solid crystals with a trace of thallium NaI(Tl) are used for gamma and *X*-ray detection.

The basic solid scintillation counter consists of na NaI(Tl) crystal or detector, a photomultiplier (PM) tube , a preamplifier, a linear amplifier, a pulse-height analyzer (PHA) and a recording device.

NaI (Tl) crystals are hermetically sealed in aluminium containers. They are fragile and must be handled with care. Room temperature should not be changed suddenly because of possibility of cracks in the crystal. In well counters and thyriod probes smaller and thicker crystals are used, whereas larger and thinner crystals are employed in imaging devices like gamma cameras.

PM tube consists of a light-sensitive photocathode facing the crystal, series of *dynodes* in the middle and an *anode* at the other end - all enclosed in a vacuum glass tube. A high voltage about 1000 V is applied between the photocathode and the anode of the PM tube. The electron pulse reaching the anode is delivered to the preamplifier. The amplitude of the pulse is proportional to the number of light photons received by the photocathode and in turn to the energy of gamma ray photon absorbed in the crystal. The applied voltage must be very stable.

A linear amplifier amplifies further the signal from the preamplifier and delivers it to the pulse height analyzer for analysis of its amplitude.

A pulse height analyzer is a device that selects for counting only those pulses falling within preselect voltage intervals and rejects all others. Desired pulses are ultimately delivered to the recording devices such as scalers, computers, films and so on.

In the output of scintillation counter a distribution of pulse heights will be obtained depicting a spectrum of gamma ray energies. In an ideal situation each gamma ray would be seen as a line on the gamma ray spectrum. In reality, the photopeak is broder, which is due to various statistical fluctuations in the process of forming the pulses.

When gamma rays interact with the scintillation crystal by means of Compton scattering, the Compton electrons of variable energies result in a pulse height smaller than that of photopeak. Thus the gamma ray spectrum will show a continuum of pulses corresponding to Compton electron energies between zero and photopeak, so called Compton continuous spectrum. The relative hights of the photopeak and the Compton scattering depend on the photon energy as well as the size of the crystal.

There are several basic characteristics of counters important from the point of view of using them in nuclear medicine procedures.

Background of the detector means registered count rate without presence of any measured specimen. It is caused namely by cosmic radiation, natural radioactivity, radioactivity of building material and of the material the detecting system consists of. It can be minimized by shielding detector in lead cover, by using special material for its construction or by means of pulse-height analyzer to exclude inappropriate radiation energy from detection.

The energy resolution simply means the width or the sharpness of the photo peak or the ability to discriminate the gamma ray photons of similar energies.

The detection efficiency is given by the observed count rate divided by the disintegration rate of a radioactive sample. It depends on the type and energy of the detected radiation, size and thickness of the detector crystal and geometric efficiency of the measuring.

The dead time is the time period during which the counter is insensitive for the radiation detection. This time enclosed time needed to process a radiation event starting from interaction in the crystal all the way up to forming and recording pulse. Dead time for Geiger-Müller detectors is from 100 to 500 microseconds, for NaI(Tl) crystal from 0,5 to 5 microseconds. Dead time loss of counts is a serious problem at high count rates. Either count rates must be lowered or corrections must be made to the observed count rates.

Scintillation detectors can be used as a part of both non imaging and imaging devices. From the non imaging devices, scintillation well counters and thyroid probes are used.

The gamma well counter consists of a scintillation detector with a hole in the center, for a sample to be placed inside for increasing the geometric efficiency and hence the counting efficiency of the counter, and other associated electronics. Well counters are used namely for in vitro measurements of different samples. They are usually available with automatic sample changers and are mostly programmable with computers. Their major advantage is high detection efficiency which is from 50% to 70% for 140 keV gamma photons.

The thyroid probe is a scintillation counter used for measuring radioacitivity above the thyroid gland to assess the uptake of 131I after its oral administration. In contrast to well counter the thyroid probe must be equipped with collimator, which limits the field of view. This is a cylindrical barrel made of lead and it covers all the detector including PM tube. It prevents the gamma radiations from other organs to reach the detector.

Radionuclide Imaging Devices

Radionuclide imaging is based on the ability to detect electromagnetic radiation emitted from an injected radioactive tracer that has been taken up by the organ to be studied. The electromagnetic radiation used is in the form of gamma rays or *x* rays. The radiation absorbed by the detector is used to generate a digital image by the computer, which is then interpreted by the physician. This imaging device is called scintillation camera or gamma camera. It also employs sodium iodide scintillation detector and the associated electronics like nonimaging systems do.

The most frequently used scintillation camera is of Anger type (Hal O. Anger invented it in the 1960), it means it has a large scintillation crystal which makes possible to detect radiation from the entire field of view simultaneously and therefore it is capable of recording dynamic as well as static images of the area of interest in the patient. Many sophisticated improvements have been made of the cameras over the years, but the basic principles of the operation are essentially the same.

Like nonimaging probe also scintillation camera consists of a collimator, a scintillation crystal, PM tubes, a preamplifier, an amplifier, a pulse-height analyser and recording or display devices. In addition it must have an *X,Y* positioning circuit to localize the point of interaction of gamma ray with the crystal. The operation of a camera is performed by a computer built in it and is very convenient for the staff. The detector head (collimator, scintillation crystal, PM tubes and amplifiers) is mounted on a stand called gantry, which moves the head to the appropriate position for patient imaging.

Detectors have usually large (about 50 cm in diameter) circular or rectangular NaI(Tl) crystal with about 1 cm thickness. In front of the crystal, a collimator is attached to limit the field of view so that gamma radiations from outside the field of view cannot reach the crystal.

Collimator is usually a plate of lead with many holes. Most frequently used are *parallel-hole* colimators with holes parallel to each other's and perpendicular to the detector face. They are of different types according to energy of radionuclides used for imaging and according to their spatial resolution. Thus we can distinguish high resolution, high sensitivity and all purpose (with compromise parameters) types or low, medium and high energy types. The spatial resolution of the parallel-hole collimators decreases with the increasing distance of the object from the front of the collimator but the sensitivity is the same. That is why every data collection must be performed with the minimal space between collimator forhead and the patient body surface.

The collimator of conical shape with one up to three holes on the top is called pinhole and is used for imaging of small and near to the surface lying organs, such as a thyroid gland, tight join or infant kidneys. It has very good resolution but very poor sensitivity. Nowadays also collimators with special converging holes called fan-beam are made for small organs imaging, such as a brain. Also collimators with diverging holes can be used, namely in cameras with small crystal to make possible imaging of large organs. Collimators designed for higher energy are thicker with thicker septa between holes to prevent penetration of photons through them.

Gamma cameras have many photomultiplier tubes (up to 90) mounted to the back of the crystal with optical grease. They are used to be of hexagonal shape and the output from each is used to define the X and Y coordinate of the point of interaction of the gamma ray in the crystal by the use of an X,Y positioning circuit. The X and Y pulses are than projected on a cathode ray tube or oscilloscope to create image or can be stored in the computer in a square matrix for further processing. The larger the number of PM tubes, the better the spatial resolution on the image.

The use of digital computers in nuclear medicine has considerably increased and today all nuclear medicine studies are being analyzed by the computers. Data from a gamma camera must be digitized by the analog-to-digital converter. The computer memory approximates the area of the detector as a square matrix from 32x32 up to 1024x1024 size. Each element of this matrix is called pixel and corresponds to a specific X and Y location in the detector. The number in each pixel corresponds to the number of pulses detected in this specific location of the crystal. In this manner of storing data in computer memory, called frame mode (the most common mode in nuclear medicine), we must preset the matrix size, the number of images (frames) in the study, and the time of collection of data per frame or total counts to be collected per frame.

Computers are very important part of imaging devices, current cameras cannot operate without it, and namely ECT is impossible without computers. The basic function of computers during image construction is to correct and maintain cameras performance parameters, such as high voltage in the PM tubes and photopeak setting in pulse-height analyzer.

Another improvement of image quality is achieved by images smoothing and filtering, mathematical operation with images, background subtraction, creation of parametric and tomographic images, regions of interest (ROI) creation, dynamic curves creation and their mathematical processing with computing quantitative data of physiological processes, by using of interpolation to reduce digital raster effect on matrix image, smoothing images by means of temporal and spatial filters or by color coding according to number of counts in each pixel.

Very important camera parameter, field of view uniformity, can be effectively improved by means of computers. Detector uniformity means a uniform response throughout the field of view. Even properly tuned and adjusted gamma cameras produce nonuniform images with count density variation of up to 10%. There are several possibilities of using computer for nonuniformity correction. These are: correction of number of counts in each pixel of image matrix to an average value, setting of the own photo peak for each pixel in image matrix, different gain of high voltage for each photomultiplier tube and spatial distortion correction.

To ensure a high quality of images, quality control tests must be performed routinely on these devices. The most common tests are the positioning of the photo peak, field of view uniformity and background check, which must be performed daily. The spatial resolution of the camera should be checked weekly.

This type of Anger gamma camera provides two dimensional images and that is why it is also called planar camera. According to the type of metabolic processes and the type of data recording we can distinguish two basal type of collecting data.

During static acquisition of images we can evaluate distribution of radio pharmaceuticals in the organs, which does not change in time. To achieve good information density of images, we must preset proper acquisition time according to registered count rate or we must preset needed number of collected counts. Except acquiring images with the same size and shape as detector has we can also acquire a so called *whole body* images. In this type of data collection patient on the examining table passes under or over the detector and the image of radioactivity distribution in the whole body can be obtained. The velocity of the patient movement is again done by the registered count rate to ensure good image information density. Since radioactivity distribution does not change significantly, we can collect data for a longer time period and thus high resolution collimator should be used.

The second type of collecting data, during which we can evaluate differently fast metabolic or functioning processes in the body (blood flow), is called dynamic study. According to velocity of assessing processes we must preset number of images (frames) and duration of one image. Because distribution of radio pharmaceuticals changes rapidly and duration of one frame acquisition is limited (up to split second), high sensitivity collimators should be used to achieve sufficient image information density.

A special kind of collecting data is gated or synchronized method. It is used for acquiring a periodical organ activity, such as heart mechanical function. In this example ECG signal is used for synchronization and by this way to collect data with very high temporal resolution is possible. In principle, computer divides each R to R interval into several intervals, for example twenty. Each interval has its own number, in this example from one to twenty, is presented as a frame in the computer memory and its duration is of tens milliseconds. After R interval detection by computer, data are stored into the frame number one, after the time of one frame duration is over data are stored into frame number two and so forth till the further R wave is detected. From this point all the process is repeated and by this way several hundred heart cycles are summed into one, so image information density is sufficient for further processing.

On planar images, the third dimension of displayed objects is obscured by superimposition of data. Therefore tomographic devices have been developed. Primarily, so called longitudinal tomography was used, which display sharply only one slice parallel to the face of detector. The images as not of good quality and thus nowadays only transversal tomography are used. In this technique multiple views are obtained at many agles around the long axis of the patient and images in the slices perpendicular to the detector face, transversal slices (each element of this slice is in the form of cube in the computer memory and is called voxel), are constructed by the computer. Since in nuclear medicine the source of radioactivity is in the patient body, and the gamma photons or x rays are emitted from it, we talk about emission computed tomography (ECT). This technique improves images quality and by this way physician interpretation by means of a better contrast between target organ and background, better topography of pathological sites and higher detection efficiency of pathological lesions, which is done by better spatial resolution predominantly.

According to the type of radionuclide used we can distinguish two types of ECT. Single photon emission computed tomography (SPECT), which uses gamma emitting radio nuclides (most of today used) and positron emission tomography (PET), which uses positron emitting radio nuclides.

The SPECT cameras have in principle the same detector as planar cameras have, but the gantry makes possible to rotate the detector around the patient. The minimal angle of rotation is 180 degrees at small angle increments. The path around the patient can be circular or elliptical and current cameras have the possibility of so-called *body contouring* pathway to minimize the distance between detector for head and patient body surface. The data are stored in the computer for further processing and image reconstruction in the form of slices in three perpendicular planes of transverse, coronal (frontal) and sagittal direction. There are different designs of SPECT cameras with one, two or three detectors. SPECT image is a type of static image, so sufficient image information density must be achieved. That is why about 20 to 30 minutes of time is needed to collect sufficient data. We must preset angle of rotation, angular step and time for one frame acquisition according to count rate detected.

There are several mathematical algorithms to reconstruct images from acquired data. The most frequently used is so called filtered back projection. Filters are mathematical functions, which increase image quality and suppress artifacts. Various types of filters are commercially available in the form of software packages. Another methods for image reconstruction are Fourier transform or iterative methods.

PET is based on the detection of coincidence of the two annihilation gamma photons that are emitted after interaction of positron with electron in the patient body. These two photons, which arise at the same time, have the same energy of 511 keV and are emitted in the angle of 180 degrees, are detected by the two detectors connected in coincidence. Data collected around the body axis are then used for image reconstruction.

In current PET systems, many detectors (hundreds to thousands) are arranged in circular rings. The number of rings can be up to sixteen and are arranged in arrays. Each detector is connected to the opposite detector in the same ring by a coincidence circuit. The field of view is defined by the width of the array of detectors. For this device no collimator is needed. Data are collected in the computer in the frame mode. Image reconstruction is accomplished by the same method as in the SPECT does.

The isotopes of an element contain the same number of protons but different numbers of neutrons in the atomic nucleus. However, they have identical chemical properties because the number of protons is what determines the chemical properties of the element. Whether or not an isotope is stable depends on the relative numbers of protons and neutrons in its nucleus. When an isotope is unstable, it disintegrates to another isotope of the same or different element by emitting α, β, γ or other particles. Such an isotope is termed radioactive, and those that emit β or γ particles are widely used in biological work.

A β particle has a continuous range of energy values characteristic of the emitting isotope, and this is exploited in liquid scintillation to discriminate between different isotopes in a sample. A γ ray is a photon and has discrete energy values, in contrast to the continuous energy spectrum of the β particle. A given isotope emits γ photons of one or more discrete energy values characteristic of the isotope. This is also exploited to discriminate between different γ-emitting isotopes in a sample. To measure the amount of radioactivity, either liquid scintillation or the Geiger-Muller counting technique is used to measure the rate of particle emission. The underlying principles for these techniques are briefly discussed as follows:

Liquid Scintillation and Geiger-Muller Techniques for Radioactivity Measurements

The general principle underlying these techniques for radioactivity measurement is as follows: When a β particle collides with an atom, the atom absorbs the particle's energy and becomes either ionized or excited to a higher energy state. Liquid scintillation counting is based on detecting the fluorescence that accompanies the return of the excited atom to ground state, whereas the Geiger-Müller technique is based on detecting the ionized atom.

1. Geiger-Müller Technique

This technique counts mostly β particles. In general, a β particle enters a gas-filled tube (Geiger tube) in which an electric field has been applied. Upon collision with an atom of the gas, the particle's energy is absorbed by the atom which then loses an electron and produces an ion pair-an electron that is attracted to the anode, and a positively charged ion of the gas that is attracted to the cathode. The electrodes detect and record these ions as electrical pulses, representing counts.

2. Liquid Scintillation Technique

This is used to count both Band y particles, but the detector used for each type of particle differs.

1. **β Counting:** The overall strategy is to set up an assay medium in which its components will efficiently transfer the energy of a β particle to fluorescence compounds that emit light of a wavelength suitable for detection by a photodetector.

In practice, the radioactive sample is mixed with a liquid scintillation "cocktail" that contains an excitable solvent (usually toluene) and one or more fluorescent compounds short-named "fluors." A β particle emitted by a radioactive sample collides with and transfers some or all of its energy to a solvent molecule which becomes excited. The excited solvent molecule either transfers its energy to another solvent molecule, or phosphoresces and emits the excitation energy as light having a wavelength that is usually too short for detection by the instrument's phototube. This photon is absorbed by a primary fluor (F_1), which becomes excited, fluoresces, and emits a photon of longer wavelength. If its wavelength is sufficiently long, the photon is detected and counted by the phototube; otherwise, it is reabsorbed by a secondary fluor, which subsequently fluoresces and emits a photon with a longer wavelength for a subsequent detection. If the wavelength is still too short, additional fluors with suitable characteristics are added to the cocktail. A summary of the net reaction is as follows:

$$\text{Solvent} + \beta \longrightarrow \beta\ (\text{lower energy}) + \text{solvent}$$

$$\text{Solvent}^* + F_1 \longrightarrow \text{solvent} + F^*_1$$

$$F^*_1 \longrightarrow F + (hv)_1$$

or $F^*_1 + F_2 \longrightarrow F_1 + F^*_2$

$F^*_2 \longrightarrow F_2 + (h\upsilon)_2$

where *(hv)* is the photon emitted by the fluorescent compounds, which is detected by the phototube and reported as counts per minute.

2. **γ Counting:** The liquid scintillation fluid described above for β particles is unsuitable for counting γ photons. This is because a γ photon does not have mass; hence, it penetrates matter deeply and, therefore, requires a medium denser than a liquid to be absorbed efficiently. A fluorescent NaI crystal cell is the medium commonly used. The sample (usually a solid in a vial) is placed in the NaI cell. The γ photon leaving the sample penetrates and interacts with the NaI crystal producing β particles which excite adjacent portions of the crystal and cause fluorescence. Light photons from the fluorescence are detected and counted by the phototube.

Applications of radioactivity to studies in the life sciences of labeling biomolecules with atoms of a radioactive element such as ^3H, ^{14}C, ^{32}P or ^{35}S and using the labeled material to assay various cellular and biochemical functions. The quantity of radioactivity used is critical to the success of the assay and the quantity recovered enables the experimenter to transform raw data to desired results. Basic calculations for experiments involving radioactivity are presented in this chapter.

Calculations Involving Radioactivity

Basic calculations involving radioactivity are performed on the basis of the quantitative descriptions of radioactive decay and the definitions of radioactivity units and specific radioactivity.

1. Quantitative Description of Radioactive Decay

For a given radioactive substance the number of decaying atoms (*dN*) per unit time interval (*dt*) is proportional to the initial number of radioactive atoms (N_0). When expressed mathematically,

$$\frac{dN}{dt} = \lambda N_0$$

2. Units of Radioactivity

Common units of radioactivity are listed below (Table 10.1) along with their equivalents in other units. Many calculations relating to radioactivity can be done based on these definitions.

Table 10.1: Units of radioactivity and their equivalents

Unit	Definition	Equivalent
Curie (Ci)	The amount of a radioactive substance decaying at a rate of 3.7 x 10^{10} disintegrations per second (dps).	1 Ci = 3.7 x 10^{10} dps 1Ci = 2.22 x 10^{12} dpm
Microcurie (μCi)	One millionth of a curie	1 μCi = 2.22 x 10^{6} dpm
Disintegrations per minute (dpm)	The number of radioactive atoms disintegrating per minute.	
Counts per minute (cpm)	The number of disintegrations detected per minute. If the counting device is 100% efficient then cpm is equal to dpm.	Cpm = dpm x counting efficiency
Becquerel (Bq)	The SI unit of radioactivity defined as the quantity of a radioactive substance decaying at a rate of 1 dps.	1 Bq = 1 dps = 60 dpm = 2.7 x 10^{-11} Ci 1 Ci = 3.7 x 10^{10} Bq 1 mCi = 3.7 x 10^{7} Bq 1 μCi = 3.7 x 10^{4} Bq

3. Specific Radioactivity and the Calculation of Concentrations

In a labeling process, atoms of a specific element in a molecule are randomly replaced by radioactive atoms of the same element. Replacing too many atoms can adversely affect the function of the molecule because of high radiation effects; replacing too few can affect the sensitivity of the assay because the radiation signal would be too low for accurate detection. In practice, the proper amount is determined experimentally for particular molecules. To enable the experimenter to determine what quantity of the labeled material contains a given count rate and vice versa, the radioactivity is expressed per unit amount of the labeled material. The quantity of radioactivity per unit amount of labeled material is termed specific radioactivity or, simply, specific activity. Examples of specific radioactivity units include *μCi/mg, mCi/μmol,* cpm/mol, *μCi/mL* and *Bq/mg.* To calculate specific activity, the following equation is used:

$$\text{Specific radioactivity} = \frac{\text{radioactivity of a sample}}{\text{amount of the sample}}$$

Specific radioactivity can be used to calculate the amount of a radioactive substance needed to produce a given count rate, the concentration of a biological receptor that has been labeled with a radioactive ligand, or the intracellular concentration of solutes.

Summary of the Various Analytical Techniques Used in the Various Students' Practical and Research Laboratories

Analytical Techniques and their Uses

Analytical techniques	Purpose/Determination
Colorimetry	Quantitative determination of diff components from fruits, vegetables and their processed products
Spectrophotometry	Identification and quantification of specific component from fruits & vegetables
Spectroscophy	It will give spectra of the compound at one or several wavelength range. *e.g.* Proteins, amino acids, phenolics, tannins, nucleic acids
Column chromatography	Separation of ions/molecules on the basis of size, charge, MWt.
Thin layer chromatography	Separation of compounds on the basis of their movement *e.g.* Amino acids, proteins, phenolics, tannins, pigments *etc.*
Ion-exc. Chromatography	Ionizable ions/molecules can be separated. *e.g.* Salts, amino acids, proteins *etc.*
Gel filtration	Separation of compound on the basis of their size, MWt. *e.g.* proteins, pigments, sugars *etc.*
Electrophoresis	Separate molecules of differing in charges *e.g.* Proteins. carbohydrates *etc.*
Dialysis	Separate small and large molecules. *e.g.* Proteins
Fourier transform Infrared Spectroscophy	Protein conformation
Flame photometry	Mineral elements, *e.g.* Ca, K, P
Atomic absorption	Mineral elements, *e.g.* Mg, Mn, Fe, Zn, Cu, Cl, *etc.*
Inductively coupled plasma	All mineral elements, macro-, micro- and trace elements
Fluorimeter	Fluorescence compounds, *e.g.* Vitamins, pigments etc.
NIR	Identification of functional groups present on the molecule
IEF	Separation of amino acids, proteins on the basis of their isoelectric point/pH
HSA (GC)	Volatile compounds from solid, liquid & gases material
HPLC	Compounds those are soluble in organic solvents. *e.g.* Proteins, amino acids, tocopherols, tannins, alkaloids, sugars, phenolics, tannins *etc.*
GC	Compounds those are volatile under thermal condition, e.g. Fatty acids, essential oils, sugars *etc.*

Contd...

Analytical techniques	Purpose/Determination
MS	Separation and identification of unknown compound from all sources of materials
NMR	Identification of molecular structure, MWt. any compound
SEM	Microscopic structure of any compound/molecule/ biological matter *etc.*
BVA	Rheological properties of proteins, starch, gels and several food products
DSC	Measure energy components, Gross energy, enthalpy, entropy of different food/food products
X-ray diffraction	Conformation of compound (α- helix; and β- helix)

References

Addess, Kenneth J. and Feigon, Juli (1996). "Introduction to ^{1}H NMR Spectroscopy of DNA". In Hecht, Sidney M. *Bioorganic Chemistry: Nucleic Acids*. New York: Oxford University Press. ISBN 0-19-508467-5.

Adrian, Marc; Dubochet, Jacques; Lepault, Jean; McDowall, Alasdair W. (1984). "Cryo-electron microscopy of viruses". *Nature* 308 (5954): 32–36.

Alan J. Rocke, *Chemical Atomism in the Nineteenth Century: From Dalton to Cannizzaro* (Ohio State University Press, 1984).

Alderighi, L.; Gans, P.; Ienco, A.; Peters, D.; Sabatini, A.; Vacca, A. (1999). Hyperquad simulation and speciation (HySS): a utility program for the investigation of equilibria involving soluble and partially soluble species. *Coordination Chemistry Reviews* 184 (1): 311–318.

Alon, T.; Amirav, A. (2006). "Isotope Abundance Analysis Method and Software for Improved Sample Identification with the Supersonic GC-MS". *Rapid Communications in Mass Spectrometry* 20 (17): 2579–2588.

Amirav, A.; Gordin, A. Poliak, M. Alon, T. and Fialkov, A. B.; Poliak, Marina; Fialkov, Alexander B. (2008). "Gas Chromatography Mass Spectrometry with Supersonic Molecular Beams". *Journal of Mass Spectrometry* 43 (2): 141–163.

Analytical Methods for Graphite Tube Atomizers (PDF). *http://www.agilent.com*. Agilent Technologies.

Andreas, B. (2011). An accurate determination of the Avogadro constant by counting the atoms in a ^{28}Si crystal. *Phys. Rev. Lett.* 106 (3): 030801-030804.

Anfinsen, Christian B.; Edsall, John Tileston and Richards, Frederic Middlebrook, ed. (1976). *Advances in Protein Chemistry*. pp. 6–7. ISBN 978-0-12-034230-3.

Antonovsky, A. (1984). "The application of colour to sem imaging for increased definition". *Micron and Microscopica Acta* 15 (2): 77–84.

Appleby, J. and Banks, A. J. Improvements in or relating to the treatment of foodstuffs, more especially cereals and their products. British patent GB 1609 (1906).

Apte A, Meitei NS (2009). "Bioinformatics in Glycomics: Glycan Characterization with Mass Spectrometric Data Using SimGlycan". *Methods in molecular biology*. Methods in Molecular Biology 600: 269–281.

Ashcroft, Neil; Mermin, N. David (1976). *Solid State Physics*. Ithaca: Thomson Learning.ISBN 0-03-049346-3.

Atkins, Peter and de Paula, Julio. *Physical Chemistry for the Life Sciences*. New York, NY: W. H. Freeman and Company, 2006. pp. 309-313.

Atome Grand dictionnaire universel du XIXe siècle (editeur Pierre Larousse, Paris 1866, vol.1, pp. 868-73).

Aue, W. P. and Bartholdi, E. and Ernst, R. R., Two-dimensional spectroscopy. Application to nuclear magnetic resonance; *The Journal of Chemical Physics*, 64, 2229-2246 (1976)

Avogadro, Amedeo (1811). Essai d'une maniere de determiner les masses relatives des molecules elementaires des corps, et les proportions selon lesquelles elles entrent dans ces combinaisons. *Journal de Physique* 73: 58–76. English translation.

Baaske P, Wienken C, Duhr S (2009). "Optisch erzeugte Thermophorese für die Bioanalytik" [Optically generated thermophoresis for bioanalysis]. *Biophotonik* (in German): 22–24.

Background and Theory Page of Nuclear Magnetic Resonance Facility. Mark Wainwright Analytical Centre - University of Southern Wales Sydney. 9 December 2011. Retrieved 9 February 2014.

Bailon, Pascal; Ehrlich, George K.; Fung, Wen-Jian and Berthold, Wolfgang (2000) An Overview of Affinity Chromatography, Humana Press. ISBN 978-0-89603-694-9.

Ball, David W. (2001). *Basics of Spectroscopy*. Bellingham, Washington: Society of Photo-Optical Instrumentation Engineers. pp. 24, 28.

Barden, S.C.; Arns, J.A.; Colburn, W.S. (1998). d'Odorico, Sandro, ed. "Volume-phase holographic gratings and their potential for astronomical applications". *Proc. SPIE*. Optical Astronomical Instrumentation 3355: 866–876.

Becker, P. (2006). Large-scale production of highly enriched 28Si for the precise determination of the Avogadro constant. *Meas. Sci. Technol.* 17 (7): 1854–60.

Becker, Peter (2003). Tracing the definition of the kilogram to the Avogadro constant using a silicon single crystal. *Metrologia* 40 (6): 366–75.

Beer (1852) "Bestimmung der Absorption des rothen Lichts in farbigen Flüssigkeiten" (Determination of the absorption of red light in colored liquids), *Annalen der Physik und Chemie,* vol. 86, pp. 78–88.

Bergmeyer, H.U. (1974). *Methods of Enzymatic Analysis* 4. New York: Academic Press. pp. 2066–72. ISBN 0-89573-236-X.

Blow, Nathan (2009). "Glycobiology: A spoonful of sugar". *Nature* 457 (7229): 617–620. Bibcode: 2009 Natur. 457. 617B.

Boyd, Robert K. (1994). "Linked-scan techniques for MS/MS using tandem-in-space instruments". *Mass Spectrometry Reviews* 13 (5–6): 359–410.

Bray, John J. (1999). Estimating plasma pH in *Lecture notes on human physiology.* Malden, Mass.: Blackwell Science. ISBN 978-0-86542-775-4.

Briggs, David; Martin P. Seah (1983). *Practical Surface Analysis by Auger and X-ray Photoelectron Spectroscopy*. Chichester: John Wiley & Sons. ISBN 0-471-26279-X.

Brock, David C. (2008). "Detecting Success". *Chemical Heritage Magazine* 26 (2): 31.

Brock, David C. (2011). "A Measure of Success". *Chemical Heritage Magazine* 29(1).

Bruins, A. P. (1991). "Mass spectrometry with ion sources operating at atmospheric pressure". *Mass Spectrometry Reviews* 10 (1): 53–77.

Buffer Reference Center. Sigma-Aldrich. Retrieved. 2009-04-17.

Burgess, Jeremy (1987). Under the Microscope: A Hidden World Revealed. CUP Archive. p. 11. ISBN 0521399408.

Carmody, Walter R. (1961). "Easily prepared wide range buffer series". *J. Chem. Educ.* 38 (11): 559–560.

Cassini Plasma Spectrometer. Southwest Research Institute. Retrieved 2008-01-04.

Cazaux, Jacques (1992). "Mechanisms of charging in electron spectroscopy". *Journal of Electronic Spectroscopy and Related Phenomena* 105 (2–3): 155–185.

Chang, Raymond. *Physical Chemistry for the Biosciences*. Sansalito, CA: University Science, 2005. pp. 363-371.

Chao, Liang-Chiun; Shih-Hsuan Yang (2007). "Growth and Auger electron spectroscopy characterization of donut-shaped ZnO nanostructures". *Applied Surface Sciences* 253 (17): 7162–7165. Bibcode:2007ApSS..253.7162C. doi:10.1016/j.apsusc.2007.02.184.

Churchwell, M; Twaddle, N; Meeker, L; Doerge, D. (2005). "Improving Sensitivity in Liquid Chromatography-Mass Spectrometry". *Journal of Chromatography B* 825 (2): 134–143.

Comisarow, M. B. and Marshall, A. G. (1974). "Fourier transforms ion cyclotron resonance spectroscopy". *Chemical Physics Letters* 25 (2): 282–283.

Cool Cosmos - Infrared Astronomy. California Institute of Technology. *Retrieved 23 October 2013.*

Cottrell, John S and Greathead, Roger J (1986). "Extending the Mass Range of a Sector Mass Spectrometer". *Mass Spectrometry Reviews* 5 (3): 215–247.

Covey, T.R.; Lee, E.D.; Henion, J.D. (1986). "Mass Spectrometry for the Determination of Drugs in Biological Samples". *Anal. Chem.* 58 (12): 2453–2460.

Covey, Tom R.; Crowther, Jonathan B.; Dewey, Elizabeth A.; Henion, Jack D. (1985). "Mass Spectrometry Determination of Drugs and Their Metabolites in Biological Fluids". *Anal. Chem.* 57 (2): 474–81.

Cowan DA (1997). "Thermophilic proteins: stability and function in aqueous and organic solvents". *Comp. Biochem. Physiol. A Physiol.* 118 (3): 429–38.

Critical Mass: A History of Mass Spectrometry". *Chemical Heritage Foundation.* Retrieved 23 January 2015.

Daniel RM, Peterson ME, Danson MJ. (2010). "The molecular basis of the effect of temperature on enzyme activity". *Biochem. J.* 425 (2): 353–60.

Danilatos, G.D. (1986). "Colour micrographs for back scattered electron signals in the SEM". *Scanning* 9 (3): 8–18.

Danilatos, G.D. (1986). "Environmental scanning electron microscopy in colour". *J. Microscopy* 142: 317–325.

Dannen, Gene (1998) Leo Szilard the Inventor: A Slideshow (1998, Budapest, conference talk). dannen.com

Dass, Chhabil (2007). *Fundamentals of Contemporary Mass Spectrometry.* John Wiley & Sons. p. 5. ISBN 978-0-470-11848-1.

Davis, L. E. (ed.) (1980). Modern Surface Analysis: Metallurgical Applications of Auger Electron Spectroscopy (AES) and X-ray Photoelectron Spectroscopy (XPS). Warrendale: The Metallurgical Society of AIME. ISBN 0-89520-358-8.

de Bièvre, P.; Peiser, H.S. (1992). Atomic Weight. The Name, Its History, Definition, and Units. *Pure and Applied Chemistry* 64 (10): 1535–43.

de Levie, Robert (2002). "The Henderson Approximation and the Mass Action Law of Guldberg and Waage". *The Chemical Educator* 7 (3): 132–135.

de Levie, Robert. (2003). "The Henderson–Hasselbalch Equation: Its History and Limitations". *J. Chem. Educ.* 80 (2): 146.

Definition of spectrograph. Merriam Webster. Accessed 13 June 2008.

Density of Blood *The Physics Factbook*. Edited by Glenn Elert. Retrieved on 26 Mars, 2009

Devyatykh, G. G. (2008). *Dokl. Akad. Nauk* 421 (1): 61–64. Missing or empty `title`; Devyatykh, G. (2008). High-Purity Single-Crystal Monoisotopic Silicon-28 for Precise Determination of Avogadro's Number. *Dokl. Chem.* 421 (1): 157–60.

Dietz, R. J. B., B. Globisch; M. Gerhard (2013). "64 μW pulsed terahertz emission from growth optimized InGaAs/InAlAs heterostructures with separated photoconductive and trapping regions". *Applied Physics Letters* 103 (6).

Displacement Chromatography 101. Sachem, Inc. Austin, TX 78737

Downard, K.M. (2007). "Francis William Aston – the man behind the mass spectrograph".*European Journal of Mass Spectrometry* 13 (3): 177–190.

Downard, Kevin (2007). "Historical Account: Francis William Aston: the man behind the mass spectrograph". *European Journal of Mass Spectrometry* 13 (1): 177–90.

Dubois, F.; Knochenmuss, R.; Zenobi, R.; Brunelle, A.; Deprun, C.; Le Beyec, Y. (1999). "A comparison between ion-to-photon and microchannel plate detectors". *Rapid Communications in Mass Spectrometry* 13 (9): 786–791.

Duhr S, Braun D (2006). "Why molecules move along a temperature gradient". *Proc. Natl. Acad. Sci. U.S.A.* 103 (52): 19678–82.

Dunn, Peter (2014). "Making Nuclear Music". Slice of MIT. Retrieved 25 Aug 2014.

Duvillaret, L. F. Garet; J.-F. Roux; J.-L. Coutaz (2001). "Analytical modeling and optimization of terahertz time-domain spectroscopy experiments, using photoswitches as antennas". *Selected Topics in Quantum Electronics, IEEE Journal of* 7 (4): 615–623.

Earley, LE; Sanders, CA (1959). The Effect of Changing Serum Osmolality on the Release of Antidiuretic Hormone in Certain PAtients with Decompensated Cirrhosis of the Liver and Low Serum Osmolality. *Journal of Clinical Investigation* 38 (3): 545–550.

Eiceman, G.A. (2000). Gas Chromatography. In R.A. Meyers (Ed.), *Encyclopedia of Analytical Chemistry: Applications, Theory, and Instrumentation*, pp. 10627. Chichester: Wiley. ISBN 0-471-97670-9.

Erni, Rolf; Rossell, MD; Kisielowski, C; Dahmen, U (2009). "Atomic-Resolution Imaging with a Sub-50-pm Electron Probe". *Physical Review Letters* 102 (9): 096101.

Ettre, L. S. (1993). "Nomenclature for chromatography (IUPAC Recommendations 1993)". *Pure and Applied Chemistry* 65 (4) 132-136.

Feldman, Leonard C.; James W. Mayer (1986). *Fundamentals of Surface and Thin Film Analysis*. Upper Saddle River: Prentice Hall. ISBN 0-13-500570-1.

Fenn, J. B.; Mann, M.; Meng, C. K.; Wong, S. F.; Whitehouse, C. M. (1989). "Electrospray ionization for mass spectrometry of large biomolecules". *Science* 246 (4926): 64–71.

Foukal, Peter V. (2004). *Solar Astrophysics*. Weinheim: Wiley VCH. p. 69.

Franchetti V, Solka BH, Baitinger WE, Amy JW, Cooks RG (1977). "Soft landing of ions as a means of surface modification". *Mass Spectrom. Ion Phys.* 23 (1): 29–35.

Fraunhofer, Joseph (1817). "Bestimmung des Brechungs- und des Farben-Zerstreuungs - Vermögens verschiedener Glasarten, in Bezug auf die Vervollkommnung achromatischer Fernröhre". *Annalen der Physik* 56 (7): 282–287.

Fujii, K. (2005). Present State of the Avogadro Constant Determination from Silicon Crystals with Natural Isotopic Compositions. *IEEE Trans. Instrum. Meas.* 54(2): 854–59.

Fürtig, Boris; Richter, Christian; Wöhnert, Jens; Schwalbe, and Harald (2003). "NMR Spectroscopy of RNA". *ChemBioChem* 4 (10): 936–62.

Ghigo, F. "Karl Jansky". National Radio Astronomy Observatory. Associated Universities, Inc. Retrieved 24 October 2013.

Gillet, D. C. (1918). Apparatus for preserving organic materials by the use of x-rays, US Patent No. 1,275,417.

Goesmann, F.; Rosenbauer, H.; Roll, R.; Böhnhardt, H. (2005). "COSAC Onboard Rosetta: A Bioastronomy Experiment for the Short-Period Comet 67P/Churyumov-Gerasimenko". *Astrobiology* 5 (5): 622.

Gondran, Carolyn F. H.; Charlene Johnson; Kisik Choi (September 2006). "Front and back side Auger electron spectroscopy depth profile analysis to verify an interfacial reaction at the HfN/SiO_2 interface". *Journal of Vacuum Science and Technology B* 24 (5): 2457.

Gothard, J.W.W.; Busst, C.M.; Branthwaite, M.A.; Davies, N.J.H.; Denison, D.M. (1980). "Applications of respiratory mass spectrometry to intensive care". *Anaesthesia* 35 (9): 890–895.

Grant, John T.; David Briggs (2003). *Surface Analysis by Auger and X-ray Photoelectron Spectroscopy*. Chichester: IM Publications. ISBN 1-901019-04-7.

Harper, Douglas. "Spectrum." Online Etymology Dictionary. Nov. 2001. Accessed 07-12-2007.)

Harvey, D.; Dwek, R.A.; Rudd, P.M. (2000). "Determining the Structure of Glycan Moieties by Mass Spectrometry". *Current Protocols in Protein Science*. Chapter 12: 12.7–12.7.15.

Harwood, Laurence M. and Moody, Christopher J. (1989). *Experimental organic chemistry: Principles and Practice* (Illustrated ed.). WileyBlackwell. pp. 180–185. ISBN 978-0-632-02017-1.

Hasselbalch, K. A. (1917). "Die Berechnung der Wasserstoffzahl des Blutes aus der freien und gebundenen Kohlensäure desselben, und die Sauerstoffbindung des Blutes als Funktion der Wasserstoffzahl". *Biochemische Zeitschrift* 78: 112–144.

Hearnshaw, J.B. (1986). The analysis of starlight. Cambridge: Cambridge University Press. ISBN 0-521-39916-5.

Hoffman, J; Chaney, R; Hammack, H (2008). "Phoenix Mars Mission The Thermal Evolved Gas Analyzer". *Journal of the American Society for Mass Spectrometry* 19 (10): 1377–83.

Hsieh, Yunsheng; Korfmacher, WA (2006). "Systems for Drug Metabolism and Pharmacokinetic Screening, Y. Hsieh and W.A. Korfmacher, Current Drug Metabolism".*Current Drug Metabolism* 7 (5): 479–489.

Hu, Qizhi; Noll, Robert J.; Li, Hongyan; Makarov, Alexander; Hardman, Mark; Graham Cooks, R. (2005). "The Orbitrap: a new mass spectrometer". *Journal of Mass Spectrometry*40 (4): 430–443.

Hulanicki, A. (1987). *Reactions of acids and bases in analytical chemistry*. Horwood. ISBN 0-85312-330-6.

ICRP Publication 103 The 2007 Recommendations of the International Commission on Protection. ICRP. Retrieved 12 December 2013.

Ilyin, A (2003). "New class of electrostatic energy analyzers with a cylindrical face-field".*Nuclear Instruments and Methods in Physics Research Section A: Accelerators, Spectrometers, Detectors and Associated Equipment* 500: 62.

In the event that the ions do not start at identical kinetic energies, some ions may lag behind higher kinetic energy ions decreasing resolution. Reflectron geometries are commonly employed to correct this problem. Wollnik, H. (1993). "Time-of-flight mass analyzers". *Mass Spectrometry Reviews* 12 (2): 89–114. doi:10.1002/mas.1280120202.

Ingle, J. D. J.; Crouch, S. R. (1988). *Spectrochemical Analysis*. New Jersey: Prentice Hall.

International Bureau of Weights and Measures (2006). *The International System of Units (SI)* (PDF) (8th ed.), pp. 114–15, ISBN 92-822-2213-6.

International Union of Pure and Applied Chemistry (1998). *Compendium of Analytical Nomenclature* (definitive rules 1997, 3rd. ed.). Oxford: Blackwell Science. ISBN 0-86542-6155.section 6.3.

International Union of Pure and Applied Chemistry Commission on Atomic Weights and Isotopic Abundances, P.; Peiser, H. S. (1992). Atomic Weight: The Name, Its History, Definition and Units. *Pure and Applied Chemistry* 64 (10): 1535–43.

International Union of Pure and Applied Chemistry Commission on Quantities and Units in Clinical Chemistry, H. P.; International Federation of Clinical Chemistry Committee on Quantities and Units (1996). Glossary of Terms in Quantities and Units in Clinical Chemistry (IUPAC-IFCC Recommendations 1996) 68 (4). pp. 957–1000.

Introduction to Electron Microscopy (PDF). FEI Company. p. 15. Retrieved 12 December 2012.

Isaac Asimov, Isaac Asimov's Book of Facts. Hastingshouse/Daytrips Publ., 1992. p. 389.

IUPAC, *Compendium of Chemical Terminology*, 2nd ed. (the "Gold Book") (1997). Online corrected version: (2006) "amount concentration, *c*".

IUPAC, *Compendium of Chemical Terminology*, 2nd ed. (the "Gold Book") (1997). Online corrected version: (2006–) "Beer–Lambert law".

Jabbour, Zeina J. (2009). Getting Closer to Redefining the Kilogram. *Weighing & Measurement Magazine* (October): 24–26.

James Hillier. *Inventor of the Week: Archive*. 2003-05-01. Retrieved 2010-01-31.

James Keeler. "Chapter 2: NMR and energy levels" (REPRINTED AT UNIVERSITY OF CAMBRIDGE). *Understanding NMR Spectroscopy*. University of California, Irvine. Retrieved 2007-05-11.

James, A. T.; Martin, A. J. (1952). "Gas-liquid partition chromatography; the separation and micro-estimation of volatile fatty acids from formic acid to dodecanoic acid". *The Biochemical journal* 50 (5): 679–90.

Jeener, J., (2007). Jeener, Jean: Reminiscences about the Early Days of 2D NMR; John Wiley & Sons, Ltd: *Encyclopedia of Magnetic Resonance.*

JeromeJeyakumar, J. (2013). "A Study of Phytochemical Constituents in Caralluma Umbellata By Gc – Ms Anaylsis" (PDF). *International Journal of Pharmaceutical Science Invention*: 37–41. Retrieved 23 January 2015.

Karas, M.; Bachman, D.; Bahr, U.; Hillenkamp, F. (1987). "Matrix-Assisted Ultraviolet Laser Desorption of Non-Volatile Compounds". *Int J Mass Spectrom Ion Proc* 78: 53–68.

Kasas, S.; Dumas, G.; Dietler, G.; Catsicas, S.; Adrian, M. (2003). "Vitrification of cryoelectron microscopy specimens revealed by high-speed photographic imaging". *Journal of Microscopy* 211 (1): 48–53.

Kaufman, Myron (2002). Principles of thermodynamics. CRC Press. p. 213. ISBN 0-8247-0692-7.

Kitchin, C.R. (1995). Optical Astronomical Spectroscopy. Bristol: Institute of Physics Publishing. pp. 127, 143.

Kittel, Charles (1996). Introduction to Solid State Physics (7th ed.). New York: John Wiley & Sons. ISBN 81-265-1045-5.

Koirtyohann, S. R. (1991). "A History of atomic absorption spectrometry". *Analytical Chemistry* 63 (21): 1024A–1031A.

Kotz, John C.; Treichel, Paul M.; Townsend, John R. (2008). *Chemistry and Chemical Reactivity* (7th Ed.). Brooks/Cole. ISBN 0-495-38703-7.

Krasnopolsky, V. A.; Parshev, V. A. (1981). "Chemical composition of the atmosphere of Venus". *Nature* 292 (5824): 610.

Kruger DH; Schneck P; Gelderblom HR (2000). "Helmut Ruska and the visualisation of viruses". *Lancet* 355 (9216): 1713–7.

Kryzhevoi, Nikolai V., and Lorenz S. Cederbaum. "Exploring Protonation and Deprotonation Effects with Auger Electron Spectroscopy." *The Journal of Physical Chemistry Letters*. 3.18 (2012): 2733-737.

Kwan-Hoong Ng (20–22 October 2003). "Non-Ionizing Radiations – Sources, Biological Effects, Emissions and Exposures" (PDF). *Proceedings of the International Conference on Non-Ionizing Radiation at UNITEN ICNIR2003 Electromagnetic Fields and Our Health.*

Lambert, J. H. (1760). Photometria sive de mensura et gradibus luminis, colorum et umbrae [Photometry, or, On the measure and gradations of light, colors, and shade] (Augsburg ("Augusta Vindelicorum"), Germany: Eberhardt Klett, 1760). See especially p. 391.

Lammert SA, Rockwood AA, Wang M, and ML Lee (2006). "Miniature Toroidal Radio Frequency Ion Trap Mass Analyzer". *Journal of the American Society for Mass Spectrometry* 17 (7): 916–922.

Lawrence J. Henderson (1908). "Concerning the relationship between the strength of acids and their capacity to preserve neutrality" (ABSTRACT). *Am. J. Physiol.* 21(4): 173–179.

Leonard, B. P. (2007). On the role of the Avogadro constant in redefining SI units for mass and amount of substance. *Metrologia* 44 (1): 82–86.

Loo JA, Udseth HR, Smith RD (June 1989). "Peptide and protein analysis by electrospray ionization-mass spectrometry and capillary electrophoresis-mass spectrometry". *Anal. Biochem.* 179 (2): 404–12.

Loschmidt, J. (1865). Zur Grösse der Luftmoleküle. *Sitzungsberichte der kaiserlichen Akademie der Wissenschaften Wien* 52 (2): 395–413. English translation.

Luft, J.H. (1961). "Improvements in epoxy resin embedding methods". *The Journal of biophysical and biochemical cytology* 9 (2). p. 409.

L'vov, Boris (1990). Recent advances in absolute analysis by graphite furnace atomic absorption spectrometry. Spectrochimica Acta Part B: Atomic Spectroscopy 45 (7). pp. 633–655.

Maher S, Jjunju FPM, Taylor S (2015). "100 years of mass spectrometry: Perspectives and future trends". *Rev. Mod. Phys.* 87 (1): 113–135. Bibcode: 2015RvMP...87..113M.doi:10.1103/RevModPhys.87.113.

March, R. E. (2000). "Quadrupole ion trap mass spectrometry: a view at the turn of the century". *International Journal of Mass Spectrometry* 200 (1–3): 285–312.

Marshall, A. G.; Hendrickson, C. L.; Jackson, G. S. (1998). "Fourier transform ion cyclotron resonance mass spectrometry: a primer". *Mass Spectrometry Reviews* 17 (1): 1–34.

Martin, Alfred N.; Patrick J Sinko (2006). Martin's physical pharmacy and pharmaceutical sciences: physical chemical and biopharmaceutical principles in the pharmaceutical sciences. Phila: Lippincott Williams and Wilkins. ISBN 0-7817-5027-X.

Martin, G.E; and Zekter, A.S., (1988). *Two-Dimensional NMR Methods for Establishing Molecular Connectivity*; VCH Publishers, Inc: New York, (p.59).

Mathys, Daniel, Zentrum für Mikroskopie, University of Basel: *Die Entwicklung der Elektronenmikroskopie vom Bild über die Analyse zum Nanolabor*, p. 8.

Matz, Laura M.; Asbury, G. Reid; Hill, Herbert H. (2002). "Two-dimensional separations with electrospray ionization ambient pressure high-resolution ion mobility spectrometry/quadrupole mass spectrometry". *Rapid Communications in Mass Spectrometry*16 (7): 670–675.

Maurer, K. F. (1958). Zur Keimfreimachung von Gewürzen, Ernährungswirtschaft 5(1958) nr.1, 45-47.

Maxwell EJ, Chen DD (October 2008). "Twenty years of interface development for capillary electrophoresis-electrospray ionization-mass spectrometry". *Anal. Chim. Acta* 627 (1): 25–33.

McCarthy, G.J. "Walsh, Alan - Biographical entry". Encyclopedia of Australian Science. Retrieved 22 May 2012.

McIlvaine, T.C. (1921). "A buffer solution for colorimetric comparaison" (PDF). *J. Biol. Chem.* 49 (1): 183–186.

McLafferty, F. W.; Hertel, R. H.; Villwock, R. D. (1974). "Probability based matching of mass spectra. Rapid identification of specific compounds in mixtures". *Organic Mass Spectrometry* 9 (7): 690.

Mendham, J.; Denny, R.C.; Barnes, J.D.; Thomas, M (2000). *Vogel's textbook of quantitative chemical analysis* (5th. Ed.). Harlow: Pearson Education. ISBN 0-582-22628-7. Mendham, J.; Denny, R.C.; Barnes, J.D.; Thomas, M (2000). *Vogel's textbook of quantitative chemical analysis* (5th. Ed.). Harlow: Pearson Education. ISBN 0-582-22628-7.

Mikhail Tswett (1906) "Physikalisch-Chemische Studien über das Chlorophyll. Die Adsorption." (Physical-chemical studies of chlorophyll. Adsorption.) *Berichte der Deutschen botanischen Gesellschaft*, vol. 24, pp. 316–326. On page 322, Tsvet coins the term "chromatography": Original: " Wie die Lichtstrahlen im Spektrum, so it is werden in der Calciumkarbonatsäule die verschiedenen Komponenten eines Farbstoffgemisches gesetzmässig auseindergelegt, und lassen sich darin qualitativ und auch quantitativ bestimmen. Ein solches Präparat nenne ich ein Chromatogramm und die entsprechende Methode, die chromatographische Methode." Translation: Like light rays in a spectrum, so the different components of a mixture of pigments are dispersed in the calcium carbonate column following a set pattern, and [they] can be determined in there qualitatively as well as quantitatively. I call such a preparation a "chromatogram" and the corresponding method, the "chromatographic method".

Minck, F. (1896). Zur Frage über die Einwirkung der Röntgen'schen Strahlen auf Bacterien und ihre eventuelle therapeutische Verwendbarkeit. Münchener Medicinische Wochenschrift 43 (5), 101-102.

Mingjie Xu (2006). "Biomimetic silicification of 3D polyamine-rich scaffolds assembled by direct ink writing". *Soft Matter* 2 (3): 205–209.

Minton AP (2001). "The influence of macromolecular crowding and macromolecular confinement on biochemical reactions in physiological media". *J. Biol. Chem.* 276 (14): 10577–80.

Mistrik, R. (2004). A New Concept for the Interpretation of Mass Spectra Based on a Combination of a Fragmentation Mechanism Database and a Computer Expert System.in Ashcroft, A.E., Brenton, G., Monaghan,J.J. (Eds.), *Advances in Mass Spectrometry*, Elsevier, Amsterdam, vol. 16, pp. 821.

Mohr, Peter J.; Taylor, Barry N. (2005). CODATA recommended values of the fundamental physical constants: 2002. *Rev. Mod. Phys.* 77 (1): 1–107.

Mohr, Peter J.; Taylor, Barry N.; Newell, David B. (2008). CODATA Recommended Values of the Fundamental Physical Constants: 2006. *Rev. Mod. Phys.* 80 (2): 633–730.

Morlock, G., Oellig, C. (2009), CAMAG Bibliography Service 103, 5.

Morlock, Gertrud E.; Claudia Oellig, Louis W. Bezuidenhout, Michael J. Brett & Wolfgang Schwack (2010). "Miniaturized planar chromatography using office peripherals". *Analytical Chemistry* 82 (7): 2940–2946.

Newton, Isaac (1705). Oticks: Or, A Treatise of the Reflections, Refractions, Inflections and Colours of Light. London: Royal Society. pp. 13–19.

Niemann, H. B.; Atreya, S. K.; Bauer, S. J.; Carignan, G. R.; Demick, J. E.; Frost, R. L.; Gautier, D.; Haberman, J. A.; Harpold, D. N.; Hunten, D. M.; Israel, G.; Lunine, J. I.; Kasprzak, W. T.; Owen, T. C.; Paulkovich, M.; Raulin, F.; Raaen, E.; Way, S. H. (2005). "The abundances of constituents of Titan's atmosphere from the GCMS instrument on the Huygens probe". *Nature* 438 (7069): 779.

Nomenclature Committee of the International Union of Biochemistry (NC-IUB) (1979). "Units of Enzyme Activity". *Eur. J. Biochem.* 97 (2): 319–20.

Nurok, David (1989). "Strategies for optimizing the mobile phase in planar chromatography". *Chemical* Reviews 89 (2): 363–375.

O'Keefe MA, Allard LF. "Sub-Ångstrom Electron Microscopy for Sub-Ångstrom Nano-Metrology" (PDF). Information Bridge: DOE Scientific and Technical Information – Sponsored by OSTI. Retrieved 2010-01-31.

Optimizing the Analysis of Volatile Organic Compounds – Technical Guide" Restek Corporation, Lit. Cat. 59887A.

Oseen, C.W. (1926). *Presentation Speech for the 1926 Nobel Prize in Physics.*

Oura, K.; V. G. Lifshits; A. A. Saranin; A. V. Zotov; M. Katayama (2003).*Surface Science: An Introduction*. Berlin: Springer. ISBN 3-540-00545-5.

Park, Melvin A.; Callahan, John H.; Vertes, Akos (1994). "An inductive detector for time-of-flight mass spectrometry". *Rapid Communications in Mass Spectrometry* 8 (4): 317–322.

Parkins, William E. (2005). "The uranium bomb, the calutron, and the space-charge problem". *Physics Today* 58 (5): 45–51.

Passonneau, J.V., Lowry, O.H. (1993). *Enzymatic Analysis. A Practical Guide.* Totowa NJ: Humana Press. pp. 85–110.

Patterson, G. E.; Guymon, A. J.; Riter, L. S.; Everly, M.; Griep-Raming, J.; Laughlin, B. C.; Ouyang, Z.; Cooks, R. G. (2002). "Miniature Cylindrical Ion Trap Mass Spectrometer". *Analytical Chemistry* 74 (24): 6145.

Paul, W.; Steinwedel, H. (1953). "Ein neues Massenspektrometer ohne Magnetfeld". *Zeitschrift für Naturforschung A* 8 (7): 448–450.

Pawsey, Joseph; Payne-Scott, Ruby; McCready, Lindsay (1946). "Radio-Frequency Energy from the Sun". *Nature* 157 (3980): 158–159. Bibcode: 1946 Natur. 157. 158P.

Perrin, Jean (1909). Mouvement brownien et réalité moléculaire. *Annales de Chimie et de Physique.* 8e Série 18: 1–114. Extract in English, translation by Frederick Soddy.

Petrie, S. and Bohme, D. K. (2007). "Ions in space". *Mass Spectrometry Reviews* 26 (2): 258–280.

Physical Principles of Food Preservation: Von Marcus Karel, Daryl B. Lund, CRC Press, 2003 ISBN 0-8247-4063-7, S. 462 ff.

Pierre Bouguer, (1729). *Essai d'optique sur la gradation de la lumière* (Paris, France: Claude Jombert, 1729) pp. 16–22.

Po, Henry N.; Senozan, N. M. (2001). "Henderson–Hasselbalch Equation: Its History and Limitations". *J. Chem. Educ.* 78 (11): 1499–1503.

Pople, J.A.; Bernstein, H. J.; and Schneider, W. G. (1957). "The Analysis of Nuclear Magnetic Resonanace Spectra". *Can J. Chem* 35: 65–81.

Prescott, S. C. (1904). The effect of radium rays on the colon bacillus, the diphtheria bacillus and yeast. *Science* XX no.503, 246-248

Price, Phil (1991). "Standard definitions of terms relating to mass spectrometry. A report from the Committee on Measurements and Standards of the American Society for Mass Spectrometry". *Journal of the American Society for Mass Spectrometry* 2 (4): 336–348

Radiation. *The free dictionary by Farlex*. Farlex, Inc. Retrieved 2014-01-11.

Rendina, George. 1976. Experimental methods in modern biochemistry. Philadelphia, PA: Saunders, 46-55.

Riker JB, Haberman B (1976). "Expired gas monitoring by mass spectrometry in a respiratory intensive care unit". *Crit. Care Med.* 4 (5): 223–9.

Robert Bunsen and Gustav Kirchhoff. *Chemical Heritage Foundation*. Retrieved 2014-07-29.

Robert E. Finnigan. *Chemical Heritage Foundation*. Retrieved 23 January 2015.

Rudenberg, H Gunther and Rudenberg, Paul G (2010). "Chapter 6 – Origin and Background of the Invention of the Electron Microscope: Commentary and Expanded Notes on Memoir of Reinhold Rüdenberg". *Advances in Imaging and Electron Physics* 160. Elsevier.

Ruska, Ernst (1986). "Ernst Ruska Autobiography". Nobel Foundation. Retrieved2010-01-31.

Sabanay, I.; Arad, T.; Weiner, S.; Geiger, B. (1991). "Study of vitrified, unstained frozen tissue sections by cryoimmunoelectron microscopy". *Journal of Cell Science* 100 (1): 227–236.

Schnell, S., Chappell, M.J., Evans, N.D. Roussel, M.R. (2006). "The mechanism distinguishability problem in biochemical kinetics: The single-enzyme, single-substrate reaction as a case study". *Comptes Rendus Biologies* 329 (1): 51–61.

Schwartz, B. Effect of X-rays on Trichinae. Journal of Agricultural Research 20 (1921) 845-854

Schwartz, Jae C.; Senko, Michael W. and Syka, John E. P. (2002). "A two-dimensional quadrupole ion trap mass spectrometer". *Journal of the American Society for Mass Spectrometry* 13 (6): 659–669.

Scorpio, R. (2000). Fundamentals of Acids, Bases, Buffers & Their Application to Biochemical Systems. ISBN 0-7872-7374-0.

Shah, N; Sattar, A; Benanti, M; Hollander, S; and Cheuck, L (2006). "Magnetic resonance spectroscopy as an imaging tool for cancer: a review of the literature.". *The Journal of the American Osteopathic Association* 106 (1): 23–27. PMID 16428685.

Sheldon, Michelle T.; Mistrik, Robert; Croley, Timothy R. (2009). "Determination of ion structures in structurally related compounds using precursor ion fingerprinting". *Journal of the American Society for Mass Spectrometry* 20 (3): 370–376.

Siri, William (1947). "Mass spectroscope for analysis in the low-mass range". *Review of Scientific Instruments* 18 (8): 540–545.

Sloan, K. M.; Mustacich, R. V.; Eckenrode, B. A. (2001). "Development and evaluation of a low thermal mass gas chromatograph for rapid forensic GC-MS analyses". *Field Analytical Chemistry & Technology* 5 (6): 288.

Smith, P. A.; Lepage, C. J.; Lukacs, M.; Martin, N.; Shufutinsky, A.; Savage, P. B. (2010). "Field-portable gas chromatography with transmission quadrupole and cylindrical ion trap mass spectrometric detection: Chromatographic retention index data and ion/molecule interactions for chemical warfare agent identification". *International Journal of Mass Spectrometry* 295 (3): 113.

Soohwan Jang (2007). "Comparison of E-beam and Sputter-Deposited ITO Films for 1.55 μm Metal–Semiconductor–Metal Photodetector Applications". *Journal of the Electrochemical Society* 154 (5): H336–H339.

Sowell, Renã A.; Koeniger, Stormy L.; Valentine, Stephen J.; Moon, Myeong Hee; Clemmer, David E. (2004). "Nanoflow LC/IMS-MS and LC/IMS-CID/MS of Protein Mixtures". *Journal of the American Society for Mass Spectrometry* 15 (9): 1341–1353.

Sparkman, O. David (2000). *Mass spectrometry desk reference.* Pittsburgh: Global View Pub.

SPLEEM. National Center for Electron Microscopy (NCEM). Retrieved 2010-01-31.

Squires, Gordon (1998). "Francis Aston and the mass spectrograph". *Dalton Transactions* (23): 3893–3900.

Stein, SE; Scott DR (1994). "Optimization and testing of mass spectral library search algorithms for compound identification". *J Am Soc Mass Spectrom* 5 (9): 859–866.

Still, W. C.; Kahn, M.; Mitra, A. (1978). "Rapid chromatographic technique for preparative separations with moderate resolution". *J. Org. Chem.* 43 (14): 2923–2925.

Stryer, Lubert. *Biochemistry (Third Edition).* New York, NY: W.H. Freeman and Company, 1988. pp. 187-191.

Suzuki, M. and M. Tonouchi (2005). "Fe-implanted InGaAs terahertz emitters for 1.56μm wavelength excitation". *Applied Physics Letters* 86 (5).

Tanaka, K.; Waki, H.; Ido, Y.; Akita, S.; Yoshida, Y.; Yoshida, T. (1988). "Protein and Polymer Analyses up to m/z 100 000 by Laser Ionization Time-of flight Mass Spectrometry". *Rapid Commun Mass Spectrom* 2 (20): 151–3.

The Nobel Prize in Chemistry 2002: Information for the Public. The Nobel Foundation. 9 October 2002. Retrieved 2007-08-29.

The Scale of Things. Office of Basic Energy Sciences, U.S. Department of Energy. 2006-05-26. Retrieved 2010-01-31.

The word "chromatogram" first appeared in print in 1906:

Thermo Instrument Systems Inc. History". *International Directory of Company Histories* (Volume 11 ed.). St. James Press. 1995. pp. 513–514.

This account is based on the review in Mohr, Peter J.; Taylor, Barry N. (1999). CODATA recommended values of the fundamental physical constants: 1998. *J. Phys. Chem. Ref. Data* 28 (6): 1713–1852.

Thomas A., Carlson (1975). *Photoelectron and Auger Spectroscopy.* New York: Plenum Press. ISBN 0-306-33901-3.

Thompson, Michael; M. D. Baker; A. Christie; J. F. Tyson (1985). *Auger Electron Spectroscopy.* Chichester: John Wiley & Sons. ISBN 0-471-04377-X.

Thomson, J.J. (1913). Rays Of Positive Electricity and Their Application to Chemical Analysis. London: Longman's Green and Company.

TLC / HPTLC, DBS, Alox - Made in Switzerland. CAMAG. Retrieved 2014-08-16.

Todd MJ, Gomez J (2001). "Enzyme kinetics determined using calorimetry: a general assay for enzyme activity?". *Anal. Biochem.* 296 (2): 179–87.

Tsivou, M.; Kioukia-Fougia, N.; Lyris, E.; Aggelis, Y.; Fragkaki, A.; Kiousi, X.; Simitsek, P.; Dimopoulou, H.; Leontiou, I. -P.; Stamou, M.; Spyridaki, M. -H.; Georgakopoulos, C. (2006). "An overview of the doping control analysis during the Olympic Games of 2004 in Athens, Greece". *Analytica Chimica Acta* 555: 1.

Tswett, M. S. (1905). "О новой категории адсорбционных явлений и о применении их к биохимическому анализу" (O novoy kategorii adsorbtsionnykh yavleny i o primenenii ikh k biokkhimicheskomu analizu" (On a new category of adsorption phenomena and on its application to biochemical analysis)), *Труды Варшавского общества естествоиспытателей, отделении биологии* (Trudy Varshavskago Obshchestva Estestvoispytatelei, Otdelenie Biologii (Proceedings of the Warsaw Society of Naturalists [i.e., natural scientists], Biology Section)), vol. 14, no. 6, pp. 20–39.

Tswett, Mikhail (1906). "Adsorptionanalyse und chromatographische Methode. Anwendung auf die Chemie des Chlorophylls" [Adsorption analysis and chromatographic method. Application to the chemistry of chlorophyll]. *Berichte der Deutschen botanischen Gesellschaft* 24: 384–393.

Tureček, František; McLafferty, Fred W. (1993). Interpretation of mass spectra. Sausalito: University Science Books. ISBN 0-935702-25-3.

Verbeck G, Hoffmann W, Walton B (2012). "Soft-landing preparative mass spectrometry".*Analyst* 137 (19): 4393–4407.

Verbeck, GF and Ruotolo, BT and Sawyer, HA and Gillig, KJ and Russell, DH, G; Ruotolo, B; Sawyer, H; Gillig, K; Russell, D (2002). "A fundamental introduction to ion mobility mass spectrometry applied to the analysis of biomolecules". *J Biomol Tech* 13(2): 56-61.

Virgo, S.E. (1933). Loschmidt's Number. *Science Progress* 27: 634–49.

von Ardenne, M and Beischer, D (1940). "Untersuchung von metalloxyd-rauchen mit dem universal-elektronenmikroskop". *Zeitschrift Electrochemie* (in German) 46: 270–277.

Weisstein, Eric W. "Radiation". Eric Weisstein's World of Physics. Wolfram Research. Retrieved 2014-01-11.

Wemmer, David (2000). "Chapter 5: Structure and Dynamics by NMR". In Bloomfield, Victor A.; Crothers, Donald M.; Tinoco, Ignacio. *Nucleic acids: Structures, Properties, and Functions*. Sausalito, California: University Science Books. ISBN 0-935702-49-0.

Went, M. R.; M. Vos; A. S. Kheifets (2006). "Satellite structure in Auger and (*e*, 2*e*) spectra of germanium". *Radiation Physics and Chemistry* 75 (11): 1698–1703.

What is TLC/HPTLC. CAMAG. Retrieved 2014-08-16.

Widmaier, Eric P.; Hershel Raff; Kevin T. Strang (2008). *Vander's Human Physiology, 11th Ed.* McGraw-Hill. pp. 108–12. ISBN 978-0-07-304962-5.

Wienken, C. J. (2010). "Protein-binding assays in biological liquids using microscale thermophoresis". *Nature Communications* 1 (7): 100.

Williams, E. R. (2007). Toward the SI System Based on Fundamental Constants: Weighing the Electron. *IEEE Trans. Instrum. Meas.* 56 (2): 646–50.

Wüst, O. (1930). Procédé pour la conservation d'aliments en tous genres, Brevet d'invention no.701302.

Yu, Ling; Deling Jin (2001). "AES and SAM microanalysis of structure ceramics by thinning and coating the backside". *Surface and Interface Analysis* 31 (4): 338–342.

www.ingramcontent.com/pod-product-compliance
Ingram Content Group UK Ltd.
Pitfield, Milton Keynes, MK11 3LW, UK
UKHW021530300726
14060UKWH00011B/195